Rehabilitation of the Hand and Upper Limb

For Butterworth Heinemann:

Senior Commissioning Editor: Heidi Allen
Development Editor: Robert Edwards
Project Manager: Derek Robertson
Design Direction: George Ajayi

Rehabilitation of the Hand and Upper Limb

Edited by

Rosemary Prosser MSc BApSc CHT

Director, Sydney Hand Therapy and Rehabilitation Centre;
Consultant Hand Therapist, St Luke's Hospital Hand Unit,
Sydney, Australia

W. Bruce Conolly AM FRCS FRACS FACS

Associate Professor of Hand Surgery, University of New South Wales;
Clinical Associate Professor, Department of Surgery, University of Sydney;
Staff Surgeon, Sydney Hospital Hand Unit;
Director; Overseas Hand Surgery & Rehabilitation Projects,
St Luke's and Sydney Hospital Hand Units,
Sydney, Australia

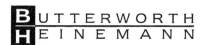

EDINBURGH LONDON NEW YORK OXFORD PHILADELPHIA ST LOUIS SYDNEY TORONTO

BUTTERWORTH-HEINEMANN
An imprint of Elsevier Limited

First edition 2003
  Reprinted 2005

ISBN 0 7506 2263 6

British Library Cataloguing in Publication Data
A catalogue record for this book is available from the British Library

Library of Congress Cataloguing in Publication Data
A catalogue record for this book is available from the Library of Congress

Note
Medical knowledge is constantly changing. As new information becomes available, changes in treatment, procedures, equipment and the use of drugs become necessary. The editors, contributor and the publishers have taken care to ensure that the information given in this text is accurate and up to date. However, readers are strongly advised to confirm that the information, especially with regard to drug usage, complies with the latest legislation and standards of practice.

The Publisher

your source for books, journals and multimedia in the health sciences
www.elsevierhealth.com

Working together to grow
libraries in developing countries

www.elsevier.com | www.bookaid.org | www.sabre.org

ELSEVIER   BOOK AID International   Sabre Foundation

Transferred to digital printing 2006

Printed and bound by CPI Antony Rowe, Eastbourne

Contents

Contributors

Editors

Rosemary Prosser
CHT MSc(Hand & Upper Limb) PGDSportSc&Ex BAppSc(Phty)
Director,
Sydney Hand Therapy & Rehabilitation Centre;
Consultant Hand Therapist,
St Luke's Hospital Hand Unit,
Sydney, Australia

W Bruce Conolly AM FRCS FRACS FACS
Associate Professor of Hand Surgery,
University of New South Wales;
Clinical Associate Professor,
Department of Surgery,
University of Sydney;
Staff Surgeon, Sydney Hospital Hand Unit;
Director,
Overseas Hand Surgery & Rehabilitation Projects,
St Luke's and Sydney Hospital Hand Units,
Sydney, Australia

Contributors

Jill Allen Grad Dip(Phty)
Physiotherapist, Principal, Private Practice
(Specialising in the Shoulder 1991–2001),
Chatswood, Sydney, Australia

Craig Allingham BAppSc(Phty) GDSportSc
CertMens' Health
Sports Physiotherapist; Director, Physiocare;
Adjunct Senior Lecturer,
School of Physiotherapy and Exercise Science,
Griffith University,
Queensland, Australia

Judith Davidson BAppSc(OT) MAppSc(Ergon)
Occupational Therapist,
Prince of Wales Hospital,
Randwick, Sydney, Australia

Victoria Frampton MCSP SRP
Hand Therapist, Private Practitioner, Canterbury;
Hand Therapy Advisor to East Kent Hospitals
Trust, Kent, UK

Karen Ginn PhD BSc GradDip(Manips)
Senior Lecturer,
School of Biomedical Sciences (Anatomy),
University of Sydney,
Lidcombe, Sydney, Australia

Claudia R Gschwind MD FRACS FMH(Switzerland)
Hand & Microsurgery Unit,
Royal North Shore Private Hospital,
Sydney, Australia

Timothy J Herbert FRCS FRACS
Emeritus Consultant,
Sydney and St Luke's Hospital Hand Units,
Sydney, Australia

Jeffery Hughes MBBS FRACS(Ortho) FAOrthA
Orthopaedic Surgeon, Private Practice,
Chatswood, Sydney, Australia

Elaine Juzl GDPhys MCSP
Clinical Specialist in Hand Therapy,
Wellington Hospital;
Partner,
NES Hand Therapy Training;
London, UK

Sandra Kay MClinSc(Hand & Upper Limb) BAppSc(Phty)
Hand Physiotherapist,
Physiotherapy Department,
Royal Adelaide Hospital,
Australia

Paul LaStayo PhD PT CHT
Assistant Professor,
Department of Physical Therapy,
Northern Arizona University,
Flagstaff, AZ, USA

Annette Leveridge DipCOT SROT
Private Practitioner,
Occupational Therapy Specialist,
Hand Therapy and Burns;
previously Head of Occupational Therapy Service,
Mount Vernon Hospital, UK

Amelia Lucas MHlthSc(Ortho Manips)
Practice Principal, Cabramatta, Sydney;
previously Senior Academic Associate,
CSU/AAOMT post-graduate Masters Degree,
Charles Sturt University,
Wagga Wagga, Australia

Jenny McConnell MBiomedEng GradDip(Manips)
BAppSc(Phty)
Physiotherapist, Private Practice,
Mosman, Sydney, Australia

Deirdre McGhee BAppSc(Phty) DipTCM(China) MATMS
Physiotherapist, Private Practice;
Lecturer,
University of Wollongong,
Wollongong, Australia

James A Masson MBBS(Hons) FRACS
Director,
Sydney Hospital Hand Unit,
Sydney, Australia

Bryce M Meads BHB MBChB FRACS(Orth)
Consultant Hand Surgeon,
Sydney and St Luke's Hospital Hand Units,
Sydney, Australia

Lisa Newell BAppSc(Phty)
Private Practitioner,
North Shore Private Hospital,
St Leonards, Sydney, Australia

Mark M J Perko MBBS FRACS
Orthopaedic Surgeon,
North Sydney Orthopaedic &
Sports Medicine Centre,
Sydney, Australia

Michael J Sandow BMBS FRACS
Head of Service, Hand and Upper Limb Service,
Department of Orthopaedic Surgery and Trauma,
Royal Adelaide Hospital,
Australia

Peter Scougall MBBS FRACS(Ortho) FAOrthA
Consultant Hand & Wrist Surgeon,
Sydney and St Luke's Hospital Hand Units,
Sydney, Australia

David H Sonnabend MD BSc(Med) FRACS
Professor of Orthopaedic and Traumatic Surgery,
University of Sydney and
Royal North Shore Hospital,
Sydney, Australia

Anne Wajon CHT MAppSc(Phty) BAppSc(Phty)
Director, Hand Therapy at Hornsby,
Hornsby, Australia

Douglass Wheen MBBS FRACS
Director, St Luke's Hospital Hand Unit;
Consultant Hand Surgeon,
Sydney Hospital Hand Unit,
Sydney, Australia

Maureen Williams AUA BA
Physiotherapist, North Shore Private Suites,
St Leonards, Sydney, Australia

Judith Wilton MS PGDHlthSc BAppSc(OT)
Director, Hand Rehabilitation Specialists,
West Perth, Western Australia, Australia

Preface

The outcome for any patient with a disorder of the hand or upper extremity depends on the mutual understanding and cooperation of the three main parties concerned: the patient, the surgeon and the therapist.

The surgeon must know the indications and rationale for, and results of surgery, as well as both the physiotherapy and occupational therapy aspects of hand therapy. The therapist, likewise, must know the indications and rationale for, and results of hand therapy, as well as those of surgical treatments. The patient must have an understanding of his or her pathology and his or her role in its management, along with the roles of the surgeon and therapist.

Although there have been great advances in surgery, e.g. tissue transplantation based on microsurgery techniques, and great improvements in many hand therapy techniques, the basic principles of hand surgery and hand therapy remain: thorough assessment/examination, accurate diagnosis and appropriate treatment of each individual patient and their problem.

Many years ago, the editors were invited to produce a text on the rehabilitation of the hand and upper limb that would be applicable in the clinical situation. This resulting book is for surgeons and therapists at all levels of experience and training who might be treating patients with a disorder of their hand or upper limb.

RP, WBC, 2003

Acknowledgements

We would like to express our thanks to: Dr Barbara Grunseit, Director of Clinical Services, St Luke's Hospital Complex and the Board of that hospital for making available the Hand Unit office staff; Pam Morris, St Luke's Hospital Hand Unit secretary for her assistance in the preparation of the manuscript, handling of correspondence and proof reading; and Mr David Robinson, St Luke's Hospital Hand Unit Medical Photographer, for producing many of the photographs and coordinating the illustrations. Appreciation for their support over many years goes to all members of St Luke's and Sydney Hospital Hand Units and Sydney Hand Therapy and Rehabilitation Centre.

We would like to convey our appreciation to our contributing authors, all of whom are recognised by their colleagues as experts in their particular field.

Finally, we thank Caroline Makepeace, who initiated the project, and Zoe Youd, Heidi Allen, David Burin and Derek Robertson who have helped bring this book to fruition.

RP, WBC, 2003

1

Introduction

A.   WOUND AND TISSUE HEALING

James A Masson

WOUND HEALING

Wound healing is a complex continuum of physiological, biochemical, cellular, molecular and immunological responses to tissue injury, regulated by growth factors and cytokines released from the wound itself (Fig. 1.1). The aim of wound healing is to restore structural and functional integrity to the damaged tissues. Traditionally, wound healing has been divided into three phases – the inflammatory phase, the proliferative phase and the remodelling phase[1] (Fig. 1.2).

Inflammatory phase

The inflammatory phase commences upon injury and lasts for approximately 72 hours. The first event in tissue injury is disruption of blood vessels, followed by a brief period of vasoconstriction and platelet degranulation. This initiates the clotting cascade, ending in the production of a fibrin clot. Activated platelets also initiate the plasminogen, complement and kinin cascades, resulting in vasodilatation and increased small vessel permeability, giving rise to tissue oedema. The activated platelet produces many growth factors which are chemotactic and mitogenic for inflammatory cells, such as neutrophils and monocytes, the latter transforming into macrophages.[2,3] The increased vessel permeability allows these

1

neutrophils and monocytes to pass out between the endothelial cells by a process of diapedesis.

In the initial stages of healing, the inflammatory cells eliminate bacteria and debris by phagocytosis. Neutrophils arrive in the wound within the first 6 hours and reach a peak at 24–48 hours. Wound healing can still progress normally in the absence of neutrophils. Macrophages first appear 48 hours after injury and remain in the wound until healing is complete. The macrophages are also responsible for recruiting the mesenchymal cells, which signal the transition to the proliferative phase. They are the most important cells in amplifying and sustaining the wound healing process.[4] T lymphocytes appear around the fifth day and play a part in the regulation of macrophage activities. They also secrete lymphokines, which affect endothelial cell behaviour and fibroblast recruitment and proliferation.[5]

Proliferative (fibroblastic) phase

The next phase of wound healing, also known as the granulation phase, commences 3–4 days after the initial injury and lasts approximately 2–4 weeks. The macrophages, which appeared during the initial inflammatory phase, continue to move into the wound. They secrete cytokines and growth factors which attract fibroblasts and new blood vessels. The fibroblasts lay down a loose matrix of fibronectin, hyaluronic acid and collagen into which the blood vessels grow. This composite of

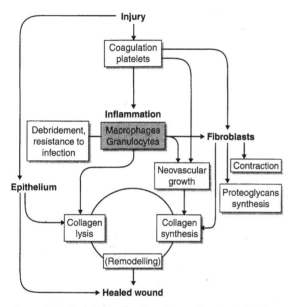

Figure 1.1 Overview of healing. (Reproduced with kind permission from Hunt TK: Basic principles of wound healing. J Trauma 30 (12 Suppl):S124, 1990.)

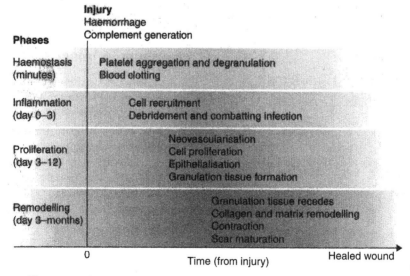

Figure 1.2 General time frame of the wound healing process. (Reproduced from Hom DB: The wound healing response to grafted tissue. Otolaryngol Clin North Am 27:14, 1994.)

fibroblasts, macrophages and new capillaries is known as 'granulation tissue'.

Within hours of injury, epithelial cells at the periphery of the wound and in residual dermal epithelial appendages restore epidermal continuity through the processes of mobilisation, migration, mitosis and cellular differentiation. During mobilisation, the cells immediately adjacent to the wound edge enlarge, flatten, detach from neighbouring cells and flow away from them. Migration continues until cells touch one another, producing contact inhibition. Epithelial mitosis actually begins within hours of injury, but intensifies during the proliferative phase. Fixed basal cells away from the wound edge multiply to replace the migrating cells, and the cells that have migrated also multiply. Once the wound has been bridged by a complete layer of epithelial cells, the cells differentiate from basal cells through the various stages of differentiated keratinocytes to produce a strátum corneum.

Remodelling (maturation) phase

During the final phase of wound healing, which begins about 3 weeks after the injury and lasts for several months, the extracellular matrix is reorganised. Both collagen synthesis and degradation are increased, so there is no net increase in collagen content. The type III collagen which was secreted initially is gradually replaced by mature type I collagen, which is highly cross-linked and reoriented in response to mechanical stress. There is an overall reduction in cell numbers (fibroblasts and macrophages) and a decrease in tissue vascularity.

Wound contraction is an active, essential part of the repair process which begins around the fifth day and lasts for 2 weeks. A specialised type of fibroblast within the wound, the myofibroblast, provides the contractile force.[6] The myofibroblast differs from the normal fibroblast in having some ultrastructural similarities to smooth muscle cells.

Myofibroblasts are present throughout the wound, not just at the periphery, so that the entire granulating surface of the wound acts as a contractile organ. There is a direct relationship between the rate of wound contraction and the

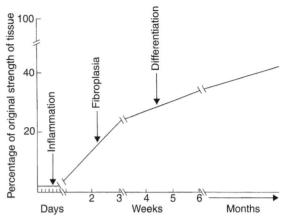

Figure 1.3 The three phases of wound healing, showing the phases of repair and the gain in tensile strength in each period. (Reproduced with permission from Boscheinen-Morrin J, Conolly WB: The hand: fundamentals of therapy. Oxford: Butterworth-Heinemann, 2000.)

number of myofibroblasts within the wound.[7] Wound contraction can be used to advantage by the surgeon and therapist, e.g. in fingertip wounds or the open palm technique in Dupuytren's contracture. The final result of the healing process is a mature scar, which may take up to 18 months from the time of the initial injury. The increase in wound tensile strength that takes place during the fibroblastic phase corresponds to the increasing levels of collagen within the wound.[8] The tensile strength of a wound never reaches the pre-injury state, and probably plateaus at about 80% of normal at approximately 60 days after injury[9] (Fig. 1.3).

FACTORS AFFECTING WOUND HEALING

There are many factors which can have an adverse affect on wound healing. Only those of clinical relevance to the hand surgeon and therapist will be discussed here.

Oxygen

Various steps in the wound healing process are particularly oxygen-sensitive: namely, collagen synthesis, angiogenesis and epithelialisation.[10] Therefore, the commonest reason that wounds fail to heal is an inadequate tissue oxygen tension. This may result from insufficient debridement of a traumatic wound, leaving necrotic tissue behind; unsatisfactory vascularity of tissues; tight suturing or postoperative swelling, producing wound tension; wound infection, which may compete for the available oxygen; or anaemia, with insufficient haemoglobin to transfer the available oxygen.

Infection

Infection decreases the oxygen level in the tissues and increases the breakdown of collagen. It also impairs angiogenesis and epithelialisation.[11]

Age

With increasing age, the phases of wound healing take longer, and the rate of cellular multiplication is slower. Tissues of elderly patients are also less resistant to ischaemia.

Smoking

Nicotine causes sympathetically induced vasoconstriction, producing localised tissue ischaemia, and decreased oxygen delivery. Smoke also contains carbon monoxide, which binds with haemoglobin to form carboxyhaemoglobin. The oxygen molecules then have to compete for free haemoglobin molecules for transport.

Steroids

Steroids arrest the inflammatory process. They inhibit wound macrophages and interfere with collagen formation, angiogenesis and wound contraction.[12]

Diabetes mellitus

Patients with diabetes mellitus have decreased oxygen delivery to the tissues due to stiff red blood cells and increased blood viscosity, making it more difficult for the corpuscles to negotiate the capillaries. Their haemoglobin also becomes glycosylated and competes with oxygen. In the initial inflammatory phase, the white cells of diabetics have a decreased ability to phagocytose and kill bacteria.[13]

ABNORMAL SCARS

When excessive accumulation of collagen occurs from increased collagen synthesis or decreased collagen breakdown during the proliferative and remodelling phases of wound healing, a hypertrophic scar or keloid may result.[14]

Hypertrophic scars are limited to the confines of the initial injury, whereas keloids extend beyond the original wound. Hypertrophic scars are much more common than keloids. In fact, the hand is quite a privileged site in terms of occurrence of true keloids. Hypertrophic scars are not infrequently seen in the palmar skin, whereas true keloids rarely are. The same cannot be said for the dorsum of the hand or the volar and dorsal forearm skin, especially in predisposed individuals, i.e. young dark-skinned or Asian individuals. Keloids seem to be hormone-sensitive, often worsening during pregnancy and resolving following menopause.

Management

Surgery is rarely indicated in the management of hypertrophic scars or keloids. Unless the abnormal scar followed a defined complication – e.g. wound infection, haematoma, dehiscence – further attempts at surgical correction will often only worsen the situation. Therefore, all non-surgical modalities should be exhausted before surgery is considered. Many modalities have been used experimentally and clinically. Once again, only those of clinical relevance in the hand patient will be discussed.

Pressure

It is thought that pressure decreases tissue metabolism and increases collagen breakdown by increasing the activity of collagenase.[15] The collagenase enzyme is heat-sensitive, with its activity increasing 1000-fold for every degree centigrade increase in temperature. Therefore, the local warming produced by a pressure garment may have its effect partially by this mechanism. However, as with all conservative measures, treatment should persist for at least 6 months and, in burns patients, often for up to 2 years.

Silicone gel

The exact mechanism of action of silicone gel is not known. It may be related to some effect of the silicone oil which bleeds from the gel, or perhaps the occlusive effect of the dressing.[16,17]

Intralesional steroids

Intralesional injection of steroids prevents excessive collagen deposition, and allows collagenase to correct the imbalance in collagen metabolism. Injection may be combined with excision. Important side effects are local hypopigmentation (which can be quite distressing in dark-skinned individuals), skin atrophy and telangiectasiae.

REFERENCES

1. Howes EL, Sooy JW, Harvey SC: Healing of wounds as determined by their tensile strength. JAMA 92:42, 1929.
2. Martin P, Hopkinson-Woolley J, McCluskey J: Growth factors and cutaneous wound repair. Prog Growth Factor Res 4:25, 1992.
3. Moulin V: Growth factors in skin wound healing. Europ J Cell Biol 68:1, 1995.
4. Clark RA et al: Role of macrophages in wound healing. Surg Forum 27:16, 1976.
5. Peterson JM et al: Significance of T lymphocytes in wound healing. Surgery 102:300, 1987.
6. Gabbiani G, Ryan GB, Majno G: Presence of modified fibroblasts in granulation tissue, and possible role in wound contraction. Experientia 27:549, 1970.
7. Rudolph R: Location of the force of wound contraction. Surg Gynecol Obstet 148:547, 1979.
8. Madden JW, Peacock EE: Studies on the biology of collagen during wound healing. III. Dynamic metabolism of scar collagen and remodeling of dermal wounds. Ann Surg 174:511, 1971.
9. Levenson SM et al: The healing of rat skin wounds. Ann Surg 161:293, 1965.
10. Hunt TK, Pai MP: The effect of variant ambient oxygen tensions on wound metabolism and collagen synthesis. Surg Gynecol Obstet 135:561, 1972.
11. Robson MC, Stenberg BD, Heggers JP: Wound healing alterations caused by infection. Clin Plast Surg 17(3): 485, 1990.
12. Stephens FO, Dunphy JE, Hunt TK: Effect of delayed administration of corticosteroids on wound contraction. Ann Surg 173:214, 1971.
13. Morain WD, Colen LB: Wound healing in diabetes mellitus. Clin Plast Surg 17(3):493, 1990.
14. Cohen IK et al: Collagen synthesis in human keloid and hypertrophic scar. Surg Forum 22:448, 1971.
15. Thomas DW et al: The pathogenesis of hypertrophic/keloid scarring. Int J Oral Maxillofac Surg 23:232, 1994.
16. Quinn KJ: Silicone gel in scar treatment. Burns 13:S33, 1987.
17. Sawada Y, Sone K: Hydration and occlusion treatment for hypertrophic scars and keloids. Br J Plast Surg 45:599, 1992.

B. THERAPY PRINCIPLES AND MODALITIES

Rosemary Prosser

Hand therapy, occupational therapy and physiotherapy require a knowledge of science and an appreciation of humanity. One needs a logical scientific basis in order to problem solve and set appropriate treatment goals. Developing treatment strategies requires a knowledge of various techniques, an understanding of the patient's ability and motivation to participate in the therapy programme, and having the appropriate therapy skills, materials and equipment available.

TREATMENT OF THE PATIENT

It is essential to understand the impact of upper limb dysfunction on each patient's ability to work, play sport, perform hobbies or general activities of daily living (ADL). As each patient is an individual, the response will be different and

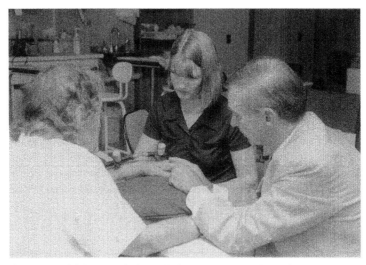

Figure 1.4 A joint consultation with the patient, therapist and surgeon assists in providing a cohesive postoperative plan with appropriate goals for the patient.

the treatment needs to be different. Therapy needs to be individually tailored after discussion with the doctor/surgeon and other medical professionals (Fig. 1.4). Postoperatively, it is important that the treating therapist receive relevant details of the surgery: such details may include the joint condition, tendon status, the amount of tension in repaired structures, degree of difficulty of surgery and any unusual findings (Fig. 1.5). This information will assist the therapist to tailor the therapy programme to the needs of the individual.

TREATMENT RATIONALE

Any hand therapy treatment should not cause pain for two reasons. First, over-vigorous treatment causes inflammation and may result in microtrauma to the tissues. The associated oedema infiltrates the tissues and causes fibrous tissue to be laid down with an increase in interstitial scarring.[1-4] Secondly, all therapy programmes require patient participation. Patient compliance will be much greater if the treatment is not painful.

Some type of gentle motion is needed within the first 2 weeks post-injury and postoperatively. Knowledge of the phases of healing, the structures

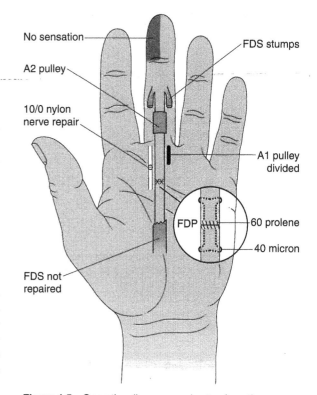

Figure 1.5 Operative diagrams and notes from the surgeon's operation report provide details which assist in the formulation of an appropriate individual therapy programme for the patient.

involved and the surgical techniques performed is essential for appropriate exercise prescription.

Body tissues respond to stress and strain factors.[1-4] For the stress to produce a change in length of tissues, it needs to be prolonged, gentle and pain free. This basic principle applies to splinting and has the potential to make a lasting change in the connective tissues.[2,5-7] These principles also apply in an exercise programme to mobilise stiff joints and soft tissues. The exercises should be done slowly and frequently during the day (4–6 × per day) and may take many months. The rehabilitation programme for the patient is a time-consuming undertaking. The patient's understanding and participation in this type of programme is necessary if the best result is to be achieved.

ASSESSMENT

Each section of this book will concentrate on assessment and treatment techniques, particular to the hand, wrist, elbow and shoulder. The aim of this chapter is to discuss some of the primary techniques that can be used for therapy in any part of the body.

Subjective/history

Assessment should involve, first, talking with the patient. We need to have a clear understanding of what the patient's problems and needs are. This requires good communication skills. When considering the impact of pain, a visual analogue scale (VAS) is helpful. Recording the area of pain and any associated physical findings on a body or arm chart gives clear information at a glance.

Objective: examination recording measurement

The second part of the assessment, the objective assessment, involves measurement of the patient's problem.

Evaluation of the problem and setting treatment goals is easier if the objective assessment is systematic. All tissues – including the skin, subcutaneous tissues, tendons, muscles, joints and bones – need to be assessed. The patient's coordination and dexterity also needs evaluation.

Observation of the hand/limb posture, skin creases, muscle bulk, fingertip pads and skin will give us information about the use and movement of the limb. Look at and feel the tissues before moving the muscles or joints.

Tissue assessment includes the following categories:

The skin

- work staining
- texture, smooth and/or shiny, calluses
- sweating
- hair growth
- nails
- wounds:
    closure
    granulation tissue
    sloughy or necrotic areas
- scars:
    colour
    thickness.

Soft tissues

- oedema – location and quality
- subcutaneous tissues – fingertip pulp bulk
- fascia – thickness, modules and tension
- tendons – position and alignment; integrity, intact or ruptured, decreased glide; size (thickness and swelling (chronic or inflamed)); and reflexes
- muscles – bulk; strength, which includes power grip, pinch grip and individual muscle strength and muscle charting; and tone.

Bones and joints

- bony alignment
- joint ligament integrity
- joint thickening or oedema
- joint range of movement: active and passive
- joint stiffness, torque range of movement
- accessory glide
- joint rhythm, e.g. scapulothoracic rhythm.

Limb function

How the limb functions also needs to be assessed, and is one of the most important parts of the assessment. The primary goal of all therapy programmes is to improve the functional use of the limb. Evaluation may include type of prehension, quality of motion, dexterity and coordination necessary for useful activity.

Useful measurement devices

These include the following:

- therapist's hands – feeling the soft tissues gives information on muscle activity, strength, apprehension, stiffness, flexibility and the general response of the tissues to movement
- goniometer to measure joint range
- force gauge for torque range of movement measures
- Jamar and pinch meter to record functional grip and pinch strength
- volumeter for oedema measurement
- monofilaments and a two-point discriminator for sensibility evaluation
- BTE, Valpar, Lido, West, Moberg Perdue or Crawford pegboard, Jebson Minnosota rate of manipulation and others to assess functional use.

When using measuring instruments we need to think about their validity and reliability. Is the instrument that you are using measuring what you need to know? Is it able to do repeated measures accurately?

Techniques and modalities of hand therapy

Massage

Indications. Scar tissue, tight muscles, trigger points, oedema.

Method. Massage should be done 3–5 min, distal to proximal 4–6 × per day if the full benefit is to be gained. The pressure should be firm but gentle.

Effects. Softens soft tissues and scars, relaxes muscle, decreases oedema and enhances proprioception.

Contraindications and precautions. Fragile skin, e.g. patients on steroids. A contact medium, e.g. lanolin or vitamin E cream, should be used. New skin grafts are often fragile and only tolerate the most gentle pressure.

Exercises

Indications. Stiffness in joints, tendons and neural structures, weak muscles, oedema and poor dexterity.

Method. Exercises may be active, passive or resisted. They may be used to improve range of motion, strength, coordination, dexterity, and nerve and tendon excursion. Frequency and duration of exercise depends on the patient's condition. An acutely inflamed joint may only tolerate exercise 2 × per day for 5 repetitions. A chronically stiff joint may need to be exercised hourly or second hourly, 2–3 sets of 10 repetitions.

Effects. Mobilises stiff joints and tendons, such as the tendon gliding exercises[8] (Fig. 1.6). Improves nerve excursion, such as the neural gliding techniques[9] (Fig. 1.7). Other exercise techniques such as hold/relax and contact/relax are useful in stretching out a tight tendon muscle unit. Exercises also strengthen muscles, decrease oedema and improve dexterity. Strengthening

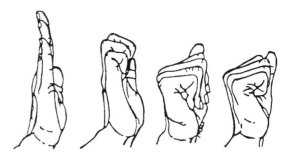

Figure 1.6 Tendon gliding exercises were first described by Whebe et al. These gliding exercises maximise differential glide of flexor digitorum superficialis (FDS) and flexor digitorum profundus (FDP). (Redrawn with permission from G van Strien: Postoperative management of flexor tendon injuries. In: Hunter J, Schneider L, Mackin E, Callahan A (eds), Rehabilitation of the hand. St Louis: Mosby, 1990:401.)

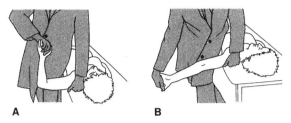

A   **B**

Figure 1.7 Upper limb tension test one (ULTT 1) first stage (A) and end stage (B). Neural tension testing and neural gliding exercises such as ULTT 1 are used in neural mobilisation when median nerve tethering is symptomatic.[9]

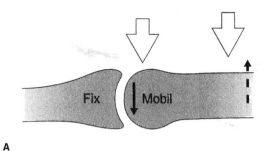

A

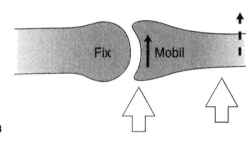

B

Figure 1.8 The convex concave rule states that the therapist should move a bone with a convex joint surface opposite to the direction of the restricted bone movement. A concave joint surface should be moved in the same direction of the restricted bone movement.[10] A: When the moving bone surface is convex and the restricted motion upwards (dotted arrow), the treatment direction is downwards (solid arrows). B: For a concave bone surface, the treatment direction is upwards (solid arrows), in the same direction as the restricted motion (dotted arrows).

may be localised to individual muscles or for particular muscle groups which work together functionally.

Contraindications and effects. Weak muscles should not be exercised when fatigued. Weak or frayed tendons may rupture if undue force is placed on them. If the tissues are already inflamed, exercise sessions need to be short and gentle so as not to aggravate the patient's condition.

Passive joint mobilisations (PJMs)

Indications. Stiff joints, decreased accessory glide.

Method. One joint surface is moved while the adjacent surface is stabilised. The gliding, sliding or rocking should be done in the plane of the movement occurring at the joint. Strict adherence to the convex concave rule is essential for physiological glide and avoidance of abnormal joint compression[10] (Fig. 1.8).

Effects. Movement of two joint surfaces on each other in a physiological manner increases accessory joint movement and thus motion.

Contraindications and precautions. Great care should be exercised with arthritic or acutely inflamed joints. An infected joint is a contraindication to PJMs.

Silicone gel pads, putty pads

Indications. Thick or raised scar.

Method. Silicone putty is mixed with a catalyst. The silicone mixture is then applied to the body part/scar and sets in approximately 3 min. Generally, silicone compression pads are worn

at night (Fig. 1.9). Gel sheets are commercially available. They can also be worn in the day as they do not inhibit motion in the same way as the thicker and more rigid pads.

Effects. Softens scar, decreases water content of scar and helps realignment of connective tissue matrix.[11]

Contraindications and precautions. Open areas, fragile skin, skin allergy.

Cold packs

Indications. Oedema, inflammation, pain.

Method. An ice pack or commercially available cold pack, e.g. Cryocuff, is applied to the swollen body part. Cold packs are most effective in the first 36–72 hours post-injury/surgery when oedema or inflammation is present.

Effects. Decreases oedema and inflammation and pain due to this.

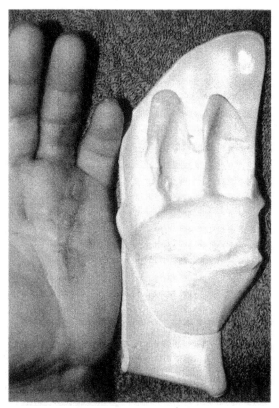

Figure 1.9 Silicone compression pad used to soften scar tissue is primarily worn at night, freeing the hand for activity and exercise in the day.

Contraindications and precautions. Nerve injury with cold intolerance, poor sensation, poor vascularity, e.g. following artery repair. Care when placing cold pack directly over a fresh wound.

Heat (hot packs)

Indications. Pain, tight soft tissues (tendons, muscles and joints).

Method. A skin test to determine the patient's sensibility to temperature is done first. The hot pack is usually wrapped in a towel or specifically made towelling cover to prevent overheating of the skin and then applied to the body part. The patient is instructed to notify the therapist if the hot pack is more than a comfortable warmth.

Effects. Increases pliability/flexibility of the soft tissues in preparation for exercise. This improves range and reduces the strain on the soft tissues. Increased circulation in the heated region may also lessen pain.

Contraindications and precautions. Infection, oedema. The patient should be skin tested for hot and cold sensation and given the appropriate warnings regarding burns from excessive heat.

Ultrasound

Indications. Sensitive scars, thick scar. Tight muscles, trigger points.

Method. Sound waves are administered to the patient through the sound head and a coupling medium, gel or water: 1 MHZ is used for treatment of deeper tissues (tissue penetration of approximately 65 mm); 3 MHZ is used for treatment of superficial tissues (tissue penetration of approximately 30 mm). Generally, low doses are used for acute problems (0.6 W) and higher doses (1.0 W) for chronic problems.

Effects. Improves circulation and decreases the tightness of soft tissues through micromassage effect. Vibration of nerve endings in muscle has a soothing effect. The micromassage also has a heating effect. Clinically, it appears to be helpful in decreasing the pain and sensitivity of hypersensitive scars.

Contraindications and precautions. The patient should be skin tested and given appropriate warnings about excessive heat. Poor sensation and infection are contraindications. Low doses should be used in areas where there may be superficial metal.[12] Plastics used in replacement surgery should be avoided.[12]

Interferential

Indications. Pain and/or oedema.

Method. The interferential pads are applied either side of the painful or oedematous area. They are applied to the body part for 15 min.

Effects. Decreases pain, muscle spasm and oedema, improves circulation. It is generally accepted that 70–150 Hz is used for pain control and acute problems and below 50 Hz is used for chronic conditions.

Contraindications and precautions. Poor sensation (detected by sharp/blunt skin test), metal in the area treated and infection.

Laser

Indications. Slow-healing wounds, pain (myofascial or from arthritis or joint trauma).

Method. Laser is applied to the skin. The skin should be cleaned with an alcohol wipe if necessary. If skin contact is not desired, as in wounds, the applicator is held just off the surface. The therapeutic window dosage is 0.5–$4.0\,J/cm^2$ for the skin. Higher doses (10–$32\,J/cm^2$) for subcutaneous tissues have been recommended. Painful areas are treated at the point of maximal pain, e.g. a trigger point. A scanning technique can be used for wounds. Five to six treatments is reported to be sufficient.[12]

Effects. Lasers of different wavelength have different penetration depths: 904 nm penetrates to subcutaneous tissues (2–4 nm) and red lasers 694.3 nm penetration is to skin only (1–2 nm). The laser light is absorbed by cytochromes in the mitochondria; this is believed to affect cell membrane permeability, including calcium transport.

Contraindications and precautions. Eye damage if the laser is focused directly on the eye. Protective goggles can be used. Neoplastic tissue, thrombosis and phlebitis are contraindications.

FES (functional electrical stimulation)

Indications. Poor muscle contraction, weak muscle, adherent tendon muscle unit.

Method. This electrical stimulation technique gives the muscle electrical impulses, causing contraction at a set number of repetitions. One electrode is placed over the motor point of the muscle and the other over the innovating peripheral nerve, proximal to the muscle. The patient is asked to voluntarily contract the muscle being stimulated in synchrony with the stimulated contraction. It is a faradic type of stimulation; therefore, the muscles need to be innovated.

Effects. Facilitates and enhances muscle contraction, tendon glide and strengthening. It is not a substitute for active voluntary contraction. It is a tool to enhance contraction.

Contraindications and precautions. Metal in the area, poor tolerance of the patient, poor sensation detected by sharp/blunt skin test, and infection are contraindications.

TENS (transcutaneous electrical nerve stimulation)

Indications. Pain, postoperative pain, nerve irritability, sensitive scar. For more details see Chapter 7E.

Method. The TENS electrodes can be applied over the peripheral nerve proximal to the painful area, over dematones, over nerve roots or sympathetic ganglion (Fig. 1.10). The frequency mode of the TENS will depend on the patient's condition.

Effects. Alters sensory input and decreases pain.

Contraindications and precautions. Sensitive skin, poor patient tolerance and poor sensation detected by sharp/blunt skin test.

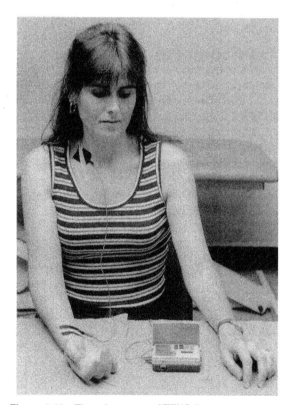

Figure 1.10 The primary use of TENS (transcutaneous electrical nerve stimulation) is for the relief of pain. Electrode placement is over the median nerve or stellate ganglion.

Compression pump

Indications. Oedema.

Method. Compression at approximately 30 mmHg is applied using a commercially available sleeve. Air is pumped into the sleeve in a cyclic rhythm, simulating a pumping action. It is usually applied for 20 min. Sequential pumps provide a better pumping action by sequentially inflating the distal to proximal compartments of the sleeve.

Effects. Decreases oedema – the pump increases the pressure gradient from interstitial tissues to capillaries, thus forcing excessive fluid back into the circulatory system centrally.

Contraindications and precautions. Infection, poor vascularity, care with lymphoedema (a sequential pump with low pressure only should be used, as high pressures collapse the lymph vessels; lymph drainage massage should be tried first).

Compression garments – wraps, gloves, and sleeves

Indications. Oedema, sensitive scars, hypersensitivity, immature or raised scar.

Method. Tubigrip or a Lycra material can be used. A custom-made sleeve or glove is made and fitted to the patient. Care should be taken so that the circulation to the limb is not restricted.

Effects. Decreases oedema, softens scar and helps connective tissue realignment.

Contraindications and precautions. Fragile skin, open wounds, care with unstable circulation, e.g. early post-replantation.

Splinting

Indications. *Static:* to support, rest or protect a body part; to enhance movement at a particular joint; and to improve hand function and prevent contractures. *Dynamic:* to elongate scar tissue, tendon muscle unit, joint capsular structures, skin and subcutaneous tissue and to facilitate use of the hand.

Method. Basic principles of splint construction are:

1. The larger the splint area, the lower the pressure on the tissues.
2. Bony prominences should be accommodated.
3. Avoid pressure on superficial nerves.
4. The angle of pull of a dynamic splint should be 90° to the longitudinal axis of the bone. The line of pull should be in the physiological line of movement.

Each splint needs to be custom-made for the patient. The effectiveness will depend on compliance, comfort, fit and the actual splint design and construction.[13]

Effects. The effects of the splint will depend on the indication, i.e. protection, enhancement of movement or function, to stretch a tight joint, tendon, skin or to prevent contractures.

Contraindications and precautions. Fragile skin, anaesthetic skin, care with infection, bony prominences and poor vascularity.

CPM (continuous passive motion)

Indications. Stiff joints, intra-articular fractures.

Method. The CPM (Fig. 1.11) should be worn for approximately 11 hours per day for at least 2 weeks.[14] CPM effectiveness can then be re-evaluated. CPM is part of the complete treatment. It is not treatment on its own.

Effects. Improves joint motion, assists in the healing of articular defects.

Contraindications and precautions. Infection, irritable joints and care with recent surgery.

Functional activity/activity programmes

Indications. To facilitate functional motion.

Method. A functional activity (Fig. 1.12) or strengthening programme is a very important aspect in return to work, sport, or simple domestic tasks. Strengthening often needs to be specific to the patient's requirements. Intense or stressed patients often do better with an appropriate activity programme rather than an exercise programme.

Effects. Improvement in functional use of the limb.

Contraindications and precautions. Do not exercise or do the activity into pain.

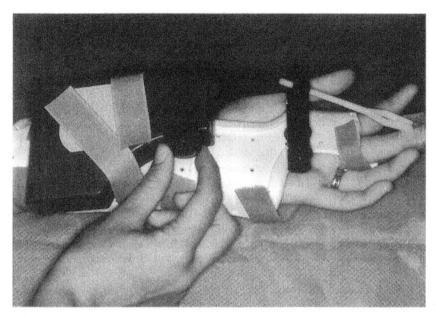

Figure 1.11 Continuous passive motion (CPM) applied to improve proximal interphalangeal (PIP) joint passive range.

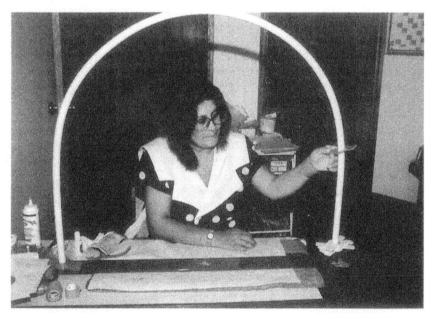

Figure 1.12 An activity programme is an important part of the patient's rehabilitation programme. It focuses the patient's attention on the activity and limb function rather than on a specific isolated motion. This particular activity requires shoulder flexion, extension, abduction and adduction; elbow flexion and extension; forearm rotation; wrist extension; a pinch grip; and coordination of all these movements.

REFERENCES

1. Bell-Krotoski J, Breger D, Breach R: Application of biomechanics for evaluation of the hand. In: Hunter J, Schneider L, Machin E, Callahan A (eds), Rehabilitation of the Hand. Philadelphia: Mosby, 1990:139–64.
2. Wilton J: Hand splinting. London: WB Saunders, 1997:9–13.
3. Brand P, Thompson D: Mechanical resistance. In: Brand P, Hallester A (eds), Clinical mechanics of the hand, 2nd edn. St Louis: Mosby, 1992:92–128.
4. Arem A, Madden J: Effects of stress on healing wounds intermittent noncyclical tension. J Surg Res 20:275–86, 1976.
5. Kottke F, Pauley D, Ptak R: The rationale for prolonged stretching for correction of shortening of connective tissue. Arch Phys Med Rehab 47:345–52, 1966.
6. Kolumban S: The role of static and dynamic splints, physiotherapy techniques and time in straightening contractures of the interphalangeal. Leprosy in India Oct:323–8, 1969.
7. Strickland J: Biologic basis for hand splinting. In: Fees E, Philips C (eds), Hand splinting, principles and methods. St Louis: Mosby, 1987:43–70.
8. Wehbe MA, Hunter JM: Flexor tendon gliding in the hand. Part I. Differential gliding. J Hand Surg 10A:575, 1985.
9. Butler D: Mobilisation of the nervous system. Melbourne: Churchill Livingstone, 1991:147–202.
10. Kaltenborn F: Mobilization of the extremity joints. Olaf Norlis Bokhander, Universitetsgaten, Oslo, 1980:26–8.
11. Ahn S, Monafo W, Mustoe T: Topical silicone gel sheeting for the prevention and treatment of hypertrophic scar. Arch Surg 126:499, 1991.
12. Low J, Reed A: Electrotherapy explained, 2nd edn. Oxford: Butterworth Heinmann, 1994.
13. Fess E, Phillips C: Hand splinting, 2nd edn. St Louis: Mosby, 1987.
14. Prosser R: The effectiveness of CPM for treatment of isolated joint stiffness following hand injury. Proceedings IFSHT 1st International Congress, Tel Aviv, Israel, 1987:31–4.

2

The hand

A. FUNCTIONAL ANATOMY AND ASSESSMENT

W Bruce Conolly and Rosemary Prosser

INTRODUCTION

The hand is really an extension of the brain. It serves three main functions: expression, sensation and prehension (combining precision pinch and gross grasp). The hand is a compact complex structure, consisting of five types of tissue:

1. skeleton (bone and joints)
2. muscle tendon units
3. nerves
4. vascular supply (blood and lymph)
5. skin and soft tissues.

THE SIGNIFICANCE OF APPLIED ANATOMY FOR THERAPISTS

The diagnosis and treatment of hand conditions by surgeons and therapists is dependent on a knowledge of the functional anatomy of the hand. Every surgical procedure involves the dissection of the delicate tissues of the hand. Therapy treatment requires an anatomical appreciation of the procedure undertaken.

THE SKELETON (BONES AND JOINTS) – Figure 2.1

The hand has 19 small long bones that form five rays radiating from the wrist, which comprises of eight carpal bones.

There is longitudinal arching of the rays and transverse arching across the metacarpals of the hand unit, giving it a three-dimensional configuration.

The wrist joint is the key joint of the hand. It is a complex joint, comprising the radiocarpal and intercarpal joints and the associated distal radio-ulnar joint (DRUJ). Wrist motion is complex and occurs at both the radiocarpal and midcarpal joints.

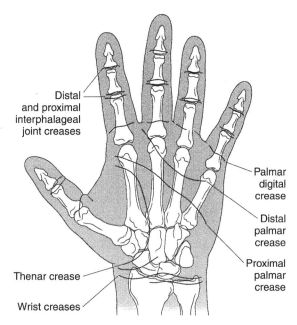

Figure 2.1 The skeleton of the hand and wrist, showing the bones and joints and creases.

THE CARPOMETACARPAL (CMC) JOINTS

The first CMC joint at the base of the thumb is a saddle joint that allows flexion and extension, abduction and adduction and some rotation. There is a strong ulnar oblique (beak) ligament attaching the ulnar side of the base of the first metacarpal to the trapezium. This is one of the primary stabilisers of this joint. The second and third carpometacarpal joints are the keystones of the transverse arch. These joints are relatively rigid. The fourth and fifth CMC joints are mobile, allowing cupping of the hand.

THE METACARPOPHALANGEAL (MCP) JOINTS – Figure 2.2A, C

These are condyloid joints that allow flexion and extension and abduction and adduction lateral movements on full extension.

The proper collateral ligaments (PCL) and accessory collateral ligaments (ACL) arise dorsal to the axis of rotation of the metacarpal heads. The PCL attaches to the base of the proximal

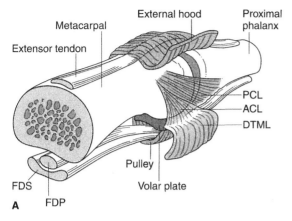

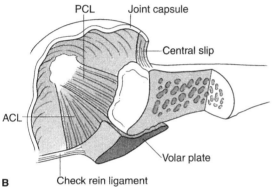

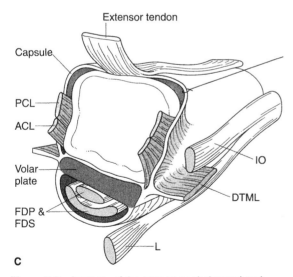

Figure 2.2   Anatomy of the metacarpophalangeal and proximal interphalangeal joints. A: The metacarpophalangeal joint from the outside. B: The proximal interphalangeal joint from the inside. (Adapted from Bowers with permission.) C: A cross-section of the metacarpophalangeal joint. (Adapted from Zancolli with permission.)

phalanx and the ACL to the volar plate. As a result of the cam effect of the head of the metacarpal and its volar flare, the PCL and ACL ligaments become tight on flexion and relaxed on extension. The MP joint is therefore stable in flexion and mobile in extension.

The ulnar PCL ligament of the thumb is the one most commonly injured and the ligament commonly involved in rheumatoid arthritis.

THE PROXIMAL INTERPHALANGEAL (PIP) JOINTS AND THE DISTAL INTERPHALANGEAL (DIP) JOINTS

These are bicondylar hinge joints with strong PCL and ACL ligaments to provide stability. They are equally tight in flexion and extension. There is a strong volar plate firmly attached to the base of the middle phalanx and loosely attached by means of a check rein ligament to the neck of the proximal phalanx (Fig. 2.2B). The volar plate is tight in extension.

MUSCLES AND TENDONS

There are 48 extrinsic muscles in the forearm and hand for control of hand function: 28 of these muscles are in the forearm, 14 in the extensor/ supinator and 14 in the flexor/pronator group. They arise from the humeral epicondyles, radius and ulna and become tendinous just proximal to the extensor and flexor retinacula. The excursion of the tendons varies from 18 to 85 mm. The median nerve innervates all the flexor pronator group except the flexor carpi ulnaris (FCU) and flexor digitorum profundus (FDP) to the ring and little fingers, which are innervated by the ulnar nerve. The radial nerve innervates all the extensor supinator group. The prime wrist movers are on the borders of the forearm. The long digit flexors and extensors occupy the intervening space. The long finger flexors are synergistic with the wrist extensors and vice versa.

In each digit the long flexor tendons and their synovial bursae run within a fibrous flexor sheath. Bow stringing of the tendons is resisted by the annular and cruciform pulley system (Fig. 2.3).

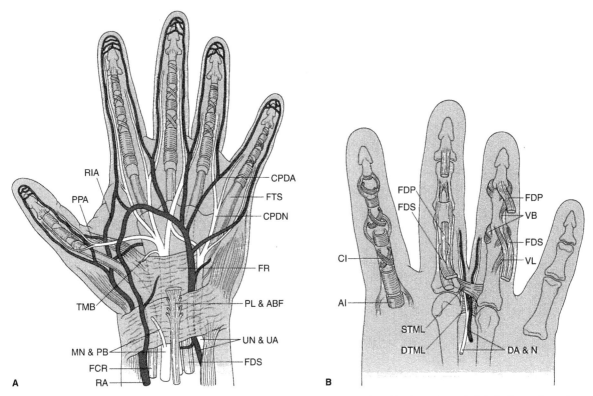

Figure 2.3 A: Deep volar anatomy, showing the structures at the carpal tunnel and in the palm and digit. B: Deep dissection of the digits and anatomy of the web space. Note the flexor tendon anatomy in the digit.

Independent finger flexion is provided by the flexor digitorum superficialis (FDS) acting on the PIP joints. Flexor pollicis longus (FPL) and FDP to the index are independent. FDP is otherwise a mass action muscle. The thumb, index and little fingers have independent extension. The extensor communi lack independence as they are tethered together over the body of the hand by variable oblique interconnections called juncturae (Fig. 2.4).

The extensors join the extensor hood and are maintained centrally over the metacarpal head by the radial and ulnar sagittal bands, which are anchored to the volar plate and intermetacarpal ligament (Fig. 2.5). In the digit there is an integrated extrinsic and intrinsic extensor mechanism supported by the retinacular ligaments.

Tendons are relatively avascular structures whose gliding is facilitated by a surrounding layer of tenosynovium. The tendon substance itself is surrounded by a thin fibrous and cellular layer called epitenon, which is adherent to the tendon surface.

THE INTRINSICS – See Figure 2.5

Twenty intrinsic muscles arise between the wrist and the metacarpophalangeal joints. They provide the balancing force between the extrinsic extensors and the extrinsic flexors. They may be divided into the central intrinsic muscles (the interossei and the lumbricals) and the peripheral intrinsic muscles (the thenar and hypothenar muscles).

There are five dorsal abducting interossei and three palmar interossei which adduct to the central middle finger digit. There are four hypothenar muscles: abductor digiti minimi (ADM), the opponens digiti minimi (ODM) and the flexor digiti minimi brevis (FDM), which act on the proximal phalanx of the little finger, and the

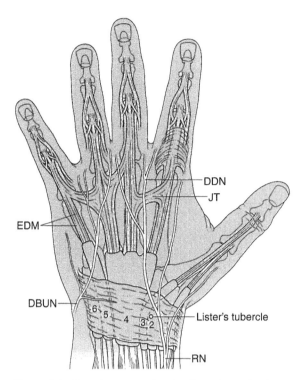

Figure 2.4 Dorsal anatomy showing the extensor tendons and extensor apparatus over the wrist and digits and the dorsal and superficial branches of the radial and ulnar nerves.

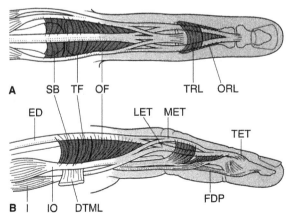

Figure 2.5 The intrinsic apparatus of the digit. A: Dorsal view. B: Lateral view. L, lumbrical; IO, interosseous; DTML, deep transverse metacarpal ligaments; SB, sagittal band; ST, transverse fibres; OF, oblique fibres; TRL, transverse retinacula ligament; ORL, oblique retinacula ligament; LET, lateral extensor tendon; MET, middle extensor tendon; TET, terminal extensor tendon.

palmaris brevis, which is a small subcutaneous muscle.

There are five thenar muscles, divided into the median nerve innervated muscles lying radial to FPL – opponens pollicis (OP), abductor pollicis brevis (APB) and part of flexor pollicis brevis (FPB) – and the ulnar nerve innervated muscles lying ulnar to FPL – FPB and adductor pollicis (ADP). The former group rotate the thumb, so its pad can oppose to the other digits at 180 degrees, i.e. opposition and pronation, and the latter group give the thumb its power of adduction.

The palmar interossei are inserted into the extensor expansion and the dorsal interossei insert between the base of the proximal phalanx and the extensor expansion.

There are four lumbrical muscles – the two radial ones arising from the radial side of the FDP of index and middle fingers and the ulnar two by two heads from the adjacent side of the FDP to the middle ring and little fingers. These muscles join the radial edge of the extensor apparatus expansion.

The extensor mechanism of the digit distal to the MCP joint is a combined intrinsic and extrinsic unit which extends the interphalangeal joints. The four lumbrical and seven interossei muscles contribute tendons called the lateral bands which lie volar to the MCP joint and dorsal to the IP joint axis, thus acting as MCP flexors and IP extensors.

The extrinsic extensor tendon continues down the centre of the proximal phalanx and inserts primarily at the base of the middle phalanx as a triangular ligament. At this level the lateral bands coalesce and continue to the distal phalangeal insertion. Intrinsic and extrinsic contributions to this coalescing mechanism are held together with ligamentous fibres which form a common unit. The excursion is small, the tendon thin and laceration may cause a critical change in the balance of the finger.

THE FASCIA AND RETINACULA –
Figure 2.6

Fascia varies from thin delicate strands and sheets to highly developed ligaments, pulleys and retinacular bands. The fascia forms sleeves in the forearm and hand and the complex system of

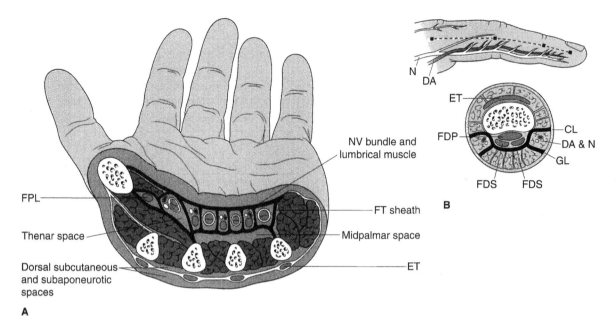

Figure 2.6   A: Cross-section anatomy at the mid palm level showing fascial spaces. B: Lateral view and cross-section of a digit.

fascial bands within each digit. It forms compartments for the passage of neurovascular structures, e.g. cubital tunnel and the musculotendinous units. At the wrist the deep fascia of the forearm condenses to form the extensor retinaculum and six compartments for the extensor tendons. In the digit, fascia forms the annular and cruciform pulley system. Such tunnels and compartments necessitate the coexistence of synovial bursae to facilitate tendon motion (see Fig. 2.3).

On the volar aspect, the deep fascia of the forearm merges with the palmar carpal ligament and this blends into the flexor retinaculum, one of the toughest ligaments of the body, being about 2.5 cm wide and 5–7 mm thick.

On the back of the hand the digital extensors lie between the superficial dorsal subcutaneous and the deeper subaponeurotic space formed by the dorsal fascia, which fuses with the palmar fascia laterally over the marginal metacarpals, especially at the MCP joints (see Fig. 2.4).

THE INNERVATION OF THE HAND –
Figure 2.7

The median, ulnar and radial nerves with a contribution from the lateral cutaneous nerves of

the forearm, supply the motor, sensory and autonomic requirements of the hand.

Cutaneous nerve supply

The common sensory innervation is shown in Figures 2.6 and 2.7. Variations are common. One should keep in mind the sensory innervation not only of the skin but also of the joints and muscles.

Radial nerve

The radial nerve (C5, 6, 7, 8, T1) arises from the posterior cord and spirals around the posterior aspect of the humerus in the spiral groove. It supplies the triceps and anconeus in the arm. Just above the elbow it gives branches to the brachioradialis (BR) and divides into its two terminal branches, the superficial and deep. The superficial branch gives branches to extensor carpi radialis longus (ECRL) and extensor carpi radialis brevis (ECRB). The deep branch, the posterior interosseous nerve, winds around the neck of the radius between the superficial and the deep layers of the supinator muscle and innervates all the supinator and extrinsic extensors of the wrist and digits – abductor pollicis longus (APL),

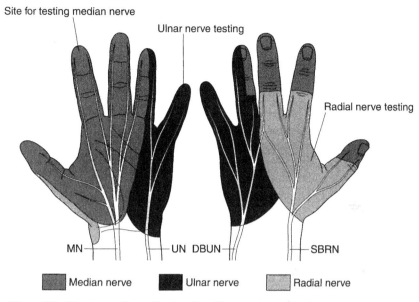

Figure 2.7 The innervation of the hand and forearm (cutaneous).

extensor pollicis brevis (EPB), extensor pollicis longus (EPL), EI (extensor indicus), EDM (extensor digiti minimi) and ECU (extensor carpi ulnaris).

Ulnar nerve

The ulnar nerve (C8, T1) arises from the medial cord of the brachial plexus. It pierces the medial intermuscular septum to pass from the flexor to the extensor aspect of the arm and then passes in the cubital tunnel posterior to the medial epicondyle and then into the forearm between the two heads of FCU. In the upper forearm it gives muscular branches to FCU and FDP to the ring and little fingers. In the distal third of the forearm it gives off its dorsal sensory branch and then passes with the ulnar artery through Guyon's space into the hand to give muscle branches to the hypothenar muscles as well as the deep motor branch which passes round the hook of the hamate to supply all intrinsic muscles of the hand except those supplied by the median nerve, terminating in the first dorsal interosseous muscle. The superficial sensory branch in the palm supplies the ulnar one and a half digits.

Median nerve

The median nerve (C5, 6, 7, 8 and T1) arises from the medial and lateral cords of the brachial plexus and passes down the arm with the brachial artery not giving any branches until it reaches the elbow. It enters the forearm beside the biceps and passes through or under pronator teres and then beneath the arch of the superficialis and shortly after gives off its anterior interosseous nerve, which supplies FPL, FDP to the index and middle fingers and pronator quadratus (PQ).

The median nerve itself supplies all the other flexors of the forearm, except those supplied by the ulnar nerve (FDP to the ring and little fingers and FCU). These branches may arise above the level of the elbow. In the distal forearm, after giving off the palmar cutaneous branch, the median nerve passes through the carpal tunnel and gives rise to its thenar motor branch and the sensory branches to the radial three and one half digits and the two radial lumbricals.

The median nerve then supplies 11 of the 14 of the extrinsic flexor pronator group and five of the 20 intrinsic muscles of the hand.

AUTONOMIC INNERVATION

The sympathetic nerves arise from the stellate ganglion lying behind the vertebral artery at the neck of the first rib. The postganglionic fibres are transmitted to the hand and upper limb mostly in the lower trunk of the brachial plexus. However, some fibres are transmitted by the blood vessels, the periarterial sympathetic plexus. The sympathetic nerves control all the autonomic functions of the hand and upper limb, including those identified with the parasympathetic system. There are no parasympathetic fibres as such in the upper limb. The sympathetic system plays a major role in the normal function and disorders of the hand and upper limb and, especially, as regards painful conditions, e.g. reflex sympathetic dystrophy.

THE VASCULAR SUPPLY OF THE HAND – See Figure 2.3

The radial and ulnar arteries form the superficial and deep palmar arches which, together with the interosseous arteries, supply the various structures of the hand.

Venous drainage is by way of the superficial and deep systems of veins. The superficial system begins with the dorsal venous arch. The arch receive blood from the palm not only around the borders of the hand but also by veins which perforate the interosseous spaces. Thus, the pressures on the palm on gripping fail to impede venous return.

Cephalic and basilic veins arise from the dorsal venous arches. These join the deep veins and the lymphatics. Deep veins in the hand and forearm accompany the arteries as venae comitantes.

There are two sets of lymphatic vessels: the superficial lymphatics run with the superficial veins and the deep lymphatics run with the arteries.

THE SKIN OF THE HAND

Various subcutaneous tissues are contained within the skin, which forms a glove over the hand and comprises about 5% of the body surface area. The dorsal skin is thin, mobile and elastic. It is thin (1–2 mm), soft and yielding and has a loose pliable subcutaneous layer to allow full flexion of the fingers and thumb. Apart from the dorsal aspect of the distal phalanges, this skin contains hair. The palmar, volar skin is 4 mm thick and tough to withstand wear. It covers a thick pad of fat traversed by fibrous septa and is richly supplied by nerve endings and sweat glands.

A system of creases adhering the skin to the deeper layers allows closure of the hand without the skin bunching up into folds. This skin has no pigment or hair. The volar skin is specialised for sensation and for precision and power gripping.

THE NAIL APPARATUS

This is a specialised epidermal appendage which supports and protects the fingertips and provides a mechanism for picking up and scratching. The nail grows about 0.1 mm a day.

VOLAR SURFACE ANATOMY – Figure 2.8

On the volar aspect, one can palpate the tubercle of the scaphoid and the ridge of the trapezium, the pisiform and the hook of the hamate at the wrist (Fig. 2.8). One can palpate the radial and ulnar arteries and the flexor carpi radialis (FCR), palmaris longus (PL) and flexor carpi ulnaris (FCU) tendon. Note the relation of the palmar creases to the underlying skeleton, as seen in Figure 2.1.

DORSAL SURFACE ANATOMY – See Figure 2.4

One can palpate the radial styloid, Lister's tubercle, the ulnar styloid and the base of the second metacarpal (styloid process).

ASSESSMENT OF THE HAND

The hand is a vital part of our body. It plays an important role in work, leisure activities, communication and personal relationships. Assessment of the hand is unique to each patient and involves assessment of an individual's needs.

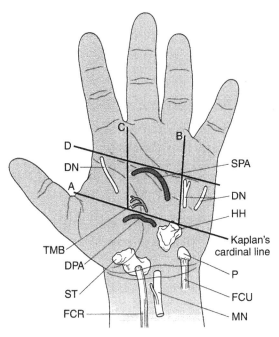

Figure 2.8 Volar surface anatomy.

Subjective assessment

In order to determine appropriate management of a patient's condition, an understanding and appreciation of the full nature of the problem is necessary.

The subjective assessment requires good communication skills and, often, some judicious inquiry. The location and nature of symptoms (pain, swelling, redness and stiffness) are plotted on a hand/arm chart (Fig. 2.9) with relevant details. Factors that provoke or relieve the symptoms are also recorded.

A thorough history of the mechanism of injury or aggravating activity is recorded. The mechanism of injury can provide information which helps to localise the injured tissues.

Objective assessment

Examination should follow the simple formula of look, palpate, move and measure.

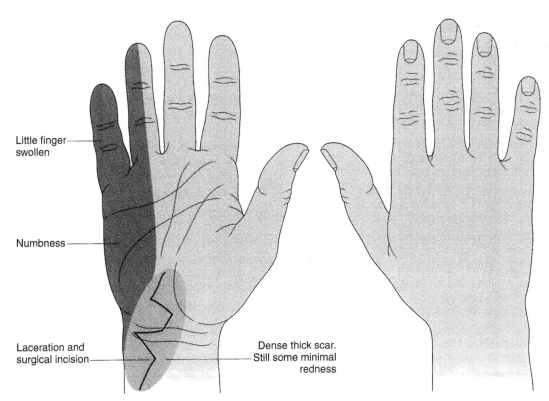

Figure 2.9 A hand chart provides information regarding symptoms such as pain, swelling, redness, pins and needles and numbness at a glance.

Observation

A great deal can be gathered from simple observation. The posture and use of the hand for simple activities gives information on pain, range of motion, dexterity and function. Particular areas and changes to note include:

- general colour of the hand
- the finger pads, for wasting and work staining
- intrinsic and extrinsic musculature for wasting
- the skin, for sweating, hair growth and texture (shininess and lack of creases)
- the nails, for length and texture
- wounds for redness, colour and degree of healing
- scars for redness, thickness and tenderness
- areas of oedema
- general bony alignment and tendon location.

Palpation

Palpation should be gentle, which allows the palpation of subtle changes in the tissues and helps gain the patient's confidence. Tissues examined should include:

- skin, for texture and sweating
- scar, for density and mobility (adhesions)
- swollen tissues for their quality of swelling (boggy or brawny)
- tendons for swelling, tension and crepitus
- muscles for tone and trigger points
- joints for swelling and tenderness
- any lumps or bumps for mobility or density
- joint accessory glide (the author prefers to do this component of the examination after range of movement measurement).

Measurement

Measurement can be done via instruments or using manual skills such as those required in manual muscle testing. When choosing a measuring instrument, consideration of validity, reliability and the need to compare the data with normal values is necessary. Measuring instruments with validity and reliability evaluation are the volumeter, the goniometer, monofilaments,

STI test and the Jamar grip dynameter.[1,2] Normal values have been published for the Jebson hand function test, Perdue pegboard and Minnesota rate of manipulation board.

Function and qualities of the tissues

Scar. A good measuring device has yet to be designed to quantify scar tissue. An experimental instrument to measure skin and scar density by applying a known force to the scar has been described in the literature[3,4] but is not used clinically.

Sensibility. There are a battery of tests used to measure sensibility. It is generally accepted that no one test gives a complete picture of the sensibility of the hand. Most therapists use a combination of tests. Sensibility tests can generally be categorised into density tests, threshold tests, functional tests and objective tests.

- Density tests include two-point discrimination and moving two-point discrimination.
- Threshold tests include pain, heat, cold and touch-pressure or monofilament tests (Fig. 2.10).
- Functional sensibility tests include the STI test, Moberg pick-up test, and the Dellon pick-up test. The STI, shape texture identification test, is the most standardised functional test. Active manipulation of objects is required in these tests. Sensibility is used in conjunction with cortical input, mobility, strength and coordination. This gives an indication of functional sensation.
- Objective tests include the Ninhydrin (triketohydrindene hydrate) sweat test, nerve conduction studies and the wrinkle test. These tests can be termed objective, as they do not require subjective interpretation of the stimulus by the patient. They can give useful information about nerve function in children and malingerers.

Oedema. Oedema measurements are often taken using a girth measurement technique. This can suffice for forearm or individual digit measurement but is inadequate for hand/palmar oedema measurement. The hand volumeter can

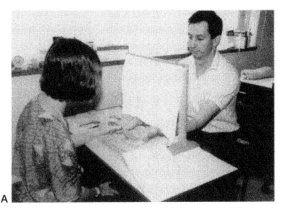
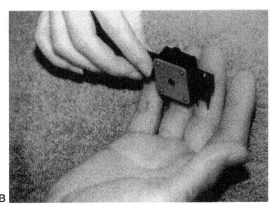

A

B

Figure 2.10 A: Light touch deep pressure testing is a threshold test using monofilaments. Each area of the hand and forearm can be tested. This gives the therapist a chart of sensibility which may range from normal to untestable or anaesthetic. It can be used to plot nerve recovery or as an indication of loss of nerve function. Testing should be done in a quiet room; the patient's hand is stabilised and vision occluded with a screen. B: Moving two-point discrimination is done in a similar manner. The two-point discriminator is moved from proximal to distal, longitudinally along the finger.

accurately measure oedema of the hand. Van Velze et al.[5] have shown that the dominant hand can be 10–15% larger than the non-dominant hand.

Joint range. Joint range of movement should be measured with an appropriate-size goniometer. Lateral placement compared with dorsal placement of the goniometer should be considered and may depend on the examiner's experience and the oedema and/or deformity present.[6–8] Generally, it is agreed that there is greater intra-tester reliability than intertester reliability so, where possible, sequential measurements should be made by the same therapist.

Active range of motion is the motion achieved at the joint by voluntary muscle contraction. Passive range of movement is the motion available at the joint when the muscle is relaxed. If the patient has full active range of motion, passive motion measures are not necessary.

Joint stiffness can be quantified by using a torque range of movement measuring method (Fig. 2.11) described by Brand and others.[4,8,9] Passive range of movement at predetermined forces is measured to give a stiffness curve, which gives an indication of the quality of stiffness.

Other aspects to be considered include the length of the muscle tendon unit where it crosses two or more joints. Insufficient resting length may interfere with range of movement measures,

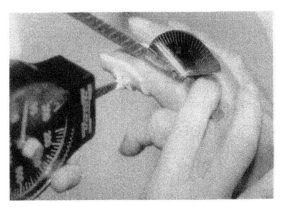

Figure 2.11 Torque range of movement (ROM) measurements provide an objective measure of the stiffness of a joint. ROM measures are taken at several different force levels, e.g. 100, 200, 300, 400, 600, 800 and 1000 g. The curve generated by plotting ROM against force applied is the torque curve or the stiffness curve for the joint. A steep curve indicates a hard end feel, a flatter curve a more springy end feel.

such as in the case of the tenodesis action at the wrist of the extrinsic hand muscles. When measuring the finger joints, the wrist should be positioned consistently in neutral.

Musculotendinous tightness in terms of limited excursion can be assessed manually. The muscle is placed in its maximal lengthened position and then gently stressed. Loss of joint range in the maximal lengthened position compared with better joint range with the muscle in the mid position is an indication of musculotendinous tightness.

Musculotendon units which are susceptible to shortening caused by oedema, trauma or immobilisation are the long flexors, long extensors, thumb web muscle and intrinsics. Testing for intrinsic tightness is shown in Figure 2.12.

Strength. The strength of each individual muscle can be measured manually. The completed muscle chart shows the strength of all muscles (graded 0–5) in the upper limb. A precise knowledge of the anatomy and function of the muscles is essential to be able to do this accurately. Where the muscle traverses more than one joint or has more than one action, special positioning may be required. Palpation of the muscle or tendon during testing is necessary if the muscle is weak.

A comprehensive description of muscle testing for the hand is described by Salter[10] and Tubiana et al.[11] Some of the more difficult muscles to test are FDS, extensor digitorum communis (EDC), lumbricals, palmar and dorsal interossei and opponens pollicis:

- FDS can be tested by flexion of the PIP joint, with the FDP excluded by trapping all other fingers in extension (Fig. 2.13).
- EDC action is isolated MP extension. If the IP joints are flexed while the patient extends the MP joints, then the action of the intrinsics is eliminated.
- The primary role of the lumbricals is initiation and flexion of the MP joints; however, they also act to extend the interphalangeal (IP) joints. The palmar interossei adduct the

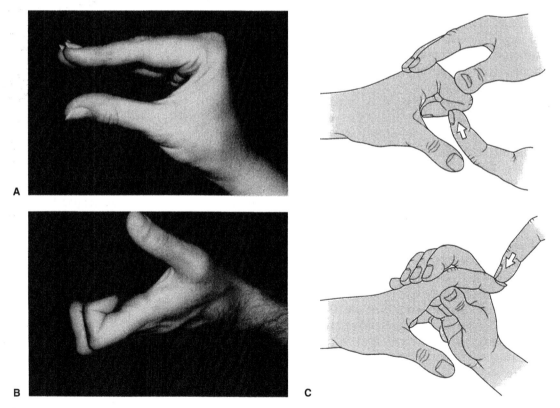

Figure 2.12 A: The intrinsic plus position – the intrinsics are contracting. B: The intrinsic minus position – the intrinsics are in their maximal stretch position, metacarpophalangeal (MP) extension and full interphalangeal (IP) flexion. C: Testing for intrinsic tightness. The intrinsics are tight if IP flexion is decreased with MP extension when the maximal stretch position is attempted. (From: The hand … Surgery of the hand. New York: Churchill Livingstone, 1983.)

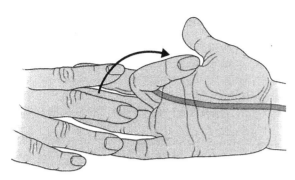

Figure 2.13 Testing flexor digitorum superficialis (FDS) muscle function. The flexor digitorum profundus (FDP) are eliminated by trapping the remaining fingers in extension.

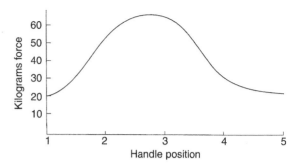

Figure 2.14 The typical bell curve that can be seen when testing grip strength. Maximal grip strength is achieved at the middle handle positions. Grip is lower with inner range (position 1) and outer range (position 5). As a result of the standard handle positions, the curve will peak sooner if the patient has a small hand.

fingers and the dorsal interossei abduct the fingers. Testing of the intrinsic muscles of the hand is performed simultaneously by resisting MP flexion and IP extension. Remember this action requires both lumbrical and interossei action. The dorsal and palmar interossei can be differentiated by testing finger abduction and adduction.

• Opponens pollicis is a deep thenar muscle which cannot be easily palpated. It rotates the thumb proximal phalanx into pronation and flexes the MP joint so that pulp-to-pulp apposition can be obtained. This is best tested by observing the amount of pronation achieved by the thumb and is evident in nail-to-nail opposition in the same plane. Resistance can then be applied in this position.

Functional grip strength can be measured with a Jamar dynamometer for cylindrical grip and with a B and L pinch gauge for 2 pt, 3 pt and lateral pinch grips. The Jamar dynamometer has high instrument reliability. It can measure a cylindrical grip at five adjustable spacings. There is a normal bell curve of grip strength (Fig. 2.14). Strength is greatest at the middle spacings and weakest at each end. A flat bell curve may indicate that maximal effort was not given.[12] However, Hamilton et al.[13] have shown that subjects with a weak grip will have a much flatter curve. Bechtol[14] reported a 5–10% difference between the dominant and non-dominant hand. A rapid exchange technique can be used to confirm grip measures. The Jamar dynamometer is exchanged at a 2–5 s interval and several measures

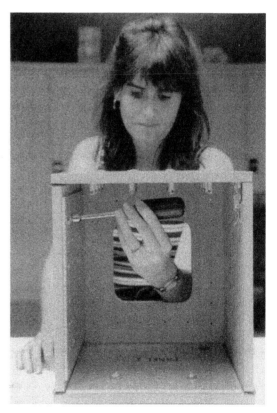

Figure 2.15 Valpar testing. This test assesses proficiency with various small hand tools.

are taken. This type of grip measurement can be more accurately recorded on a computerised evaluation system. Grip measures should fall close to the value recorded without the rapid exchange.

Inconsistent effort is indicated by inconsistent measures.

Several computerised measuring systems have become available. These systems are very expensive, but have the advantage that the range of movement and grip measures are recorded directly from the instrument. Sensibility and other measures need to be manually recorded. Multiple copies of the report/readings can be made easily. These instruments require the same sort of reliability and validity considerations as non-computerised instruments.

Functional testing

There is a huge range of functional testing apparatus available, including the Perdue, Crawford, Minnesota, West, Valpar (Fig. 2.15), Key and Isherhagen testing equipment. Basically, the most important factor for functional testing is that it should be functional and relevant for the patient being tested: an assembly worker in a computer factory will need different tests than a fitter and turner or a secretary. Job or task simulation or work site evaluation may provide the most relevant and accurate testing for the patient.

REFERENCES

1. Fess E: Reliability and validity in testing. Four hand assessment instruments [abstract]. J Hand Ther 5:236, 1992.
2. Bell-Krotoski J, Weinstein S, Weinstein C: Testing sensibility, including touch, pressure, two-part discrimination, point localisation and vibration. J Hand Ther 6:114–23, 1993.
3. Fess E: Documentation essential elements of an upper extremity assessment battery. In: Hunter J, Schneider L, Mackin E, Callahan A (eds), Rehabilitation of the hand. Philadelphia: Mosby, 1990:77–8.
4. Bell-Krotoski J, Breger D, Beach R: Application of biomechanics for evaluation of the hand. In: Hunter J, Schneider L, Mackin E, Callahan A (eds), Rehabilitation of the hand. Philadelphia: Mosby, 1990:139–64.
5. Van Velze C, Kluever I, Van der Merwe C, Comin D, Mennen U: The difference in volume of dominant and non dominant hands. J Hand Ther 4:6–9, 1991.
6. Hamilton GF, Lachenbruch PA: The reliability of goniometry in assessing finger joint angle. Phys Ther 49:465, 1969.
7. Cambridge C: Range-of-motion measurements of the hand. In: Hunter J, Schneider L, Mackin E, Callahan A (eds), Rehabilitation of the hand. Philadelphia: Mosby, 1990:82–92.
8. Flowers K, Pheasant S: The use of torque angle curves in the assessment of digital joint stiffness. J Hand Ther 1:69–75, 1988.
9. Breger-Lee D, Bell Krotoski J, Brandsma W: Torque angle of motion in the hand clinic. J Hand Ther 3:7–13, 1990.
10. Salter M: Hand injuries. Edinburgh: Churchill Livingstone, 1987:30–43.
11. Tubiana R, Thomine J-M, Mackin E: Examination of the hand and wrist. London: Martin Dunitz, 1996:205–24.
12. Aulicino P, Dupuy T: Clinical examination of the hand. In: Hunter J, Schneider L, Mackin E, Callahan A (eds), Rehabilitation of the hand. Philadelphia: Mosby, 1990: 43–4.
13. Hamilton A, Balnave R, Adams R: Grip strength testing reliability. J Hand Ther 7:163–70, 1994.
14. Bechtol C: Grip test. The use of a dynamometer with adjustable handle spacings. J Bone Joint Surg 36a:820–2, 1954.

B. METACARPAL AND PHALANGEAL FRACTURES

Peter Scougall and Rosemary Prosser

Metacarpal and phalangeal fractures are common injuries. Although they are sometimes regarded as trivial, they may result in significant stiffness and deformity, particularly if poorly treated. A force sufficient to cause a fracture will also cause soft tissue damage and predispose to stiffness. This may be aggravated by poor surgery and prolonged immobilisation.

Function can best be restored by anatomical reduction of the fracture in such a way that allows early comfortable mobilisation of the hand.

Consider the following factors when assessing a finger fracture:

1. Stability: a stable fracture will resist displacement when exposed to a

physiological load, an unstable fracture will not. Alignment must be maintained by treatment until healing restores stability. Instability may occur due to comminution, bone loss, loss of soft tissue support or unbalanced muscle action across the fracture. An undisplaced spiral fracture of the third metacarpal is well splinted by the intact bones and soft tissue on both sides. Displaced fractures of the border metacarpals and multiple metacarpal fractures are unstable.

2. Alignment, including angulation, shortening and malrotation. Malrotation is best assessed clinically, not on X-ray. Check nail alignment end-on in extension. Check digital scissoring in flexion. Compare with the opposite side.

3. Associated soft tissue injury: it is important to consider all the tissues which may have been injured, including skin, tendon, vessels and nerves.

4. Pre-existing disease: pre-existing osteoarthritis will predispose to stiffness. Pathological fractures may require more complicated treatment (tumour excision, bone grafting and fixation). Osteoporotic bone may be difficult to internally fix.

5. Patient factors: many factors will influence treatment and results, including age, general health, occupation, expectations, compliance and motivation.

Unfavourable prognostic factors after finger fractures include open injury, comminution, significant associated soft tissue injury and prolonged immobilisation. Three of these four factors are determined by the injury. Only one, the duration of immobilisation, is determined by the treatment. Early motion is beneficial.

After phalangeal fractures, Strickland et al.[1] noted that immobilisation for less than 4 weeks resulted in 80% normal motion. Immobilisation for greater than 4 weeks reduced finger motion to 66% of normal or less. Results are improved by early motion. Stable fractures can be moved early.

Unstable fractures should be stabilised to allow early motion.

THERAPY FOLLOWING CLOSED REDUCTION

It is most important for the hand therapist to know if the fracture is stable or not. A stable fracture can be treated by early gentle active motion. The goals of therapy are:

1. support the hand and fracture in the acute stage
2. control oedema
3. maintain or restore motion
4. restore joint and tendon glide
5. restore strength
6. restore functional use.

The hand is supported in a POSI splint (position of safe immobilisation) – wrist 20–30 degrees extension, MPs maximal (70 degrees) flexion and IPs extended (0 degree) (Fig. 2.16). Rest only those joints immediately adjacent to the fracture. The splint should allow motion of all other joints. Early oedema control will help prevent excessive scar formation and subsequent adhesions. Active and assisted active motion is started as soon as possible. Stretching techniques including passive joint mobilisations and splinting, static (Fig. 2.17) or dynamic, can be commenced once there is some clinical union (4–6 weeks).

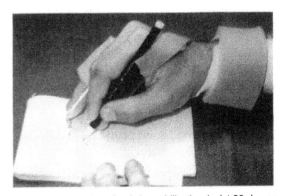

Figure 2.16 Position of safe immobilisation (wrist 30 degree extension, MPs in 70 degree flexion and IPs extended) for proximal phalangeal fracture of the little finger. Only the joints and digit adjacent to the fracture are splinted. This enables motion to prevent stiffness and function of the uninjured digits.

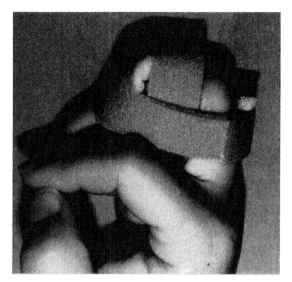

Figure 2.17 A flexion strap used to stretch the extensor apparatus and DIP joint into flexion.

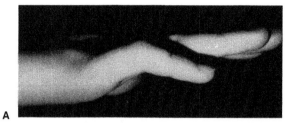

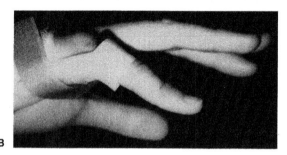

Figure 2.18 A: Hyperextension of the MP joint accompanied by PIP joint extensor lag following undisplaced fracture of the MC. B: A three-point blocking splint prevents MP hyperextension and facilitates PIP extension.

Important points

1. Isolated joint motion should always be included in the therapy programme.

2. Specific exercises to glide the tendons will prevent tendon adhesion to bone. For example:
   - EDC exercises for metacarpal fractures
   - FDS/FDP gliding individually and differentially for proximal and middle phalangeal, fractures.

3. Ensure that the fracture is not rotating: spiral and oblique fractures are more likely to do this. If the fracture unites in a malrotated position, digital scissoring will result. This interferes with functional grip. Buddy strapping helps maintain alignment in the early stages. If scissoring is apparent and cannot be controlled by buddy strapping, surgical fixation of the fracture is required.

4. The greater the soft tissue injury and swelling, the greater the scarring and adhesion formation. This may limit hand function more than the fracture itself in the long term. It is important to treat the soft tissues early in order to minimise the scarring. Massage, compression therapy, cold packs and gentle exercise are the primary modalities and techniques used.

5. Immobilisation for 4 weeks in a POSI splint may cause intrinsic muscle tightness. This should be monitored and intrinsic stretches instigated if required.

6. Poor active PIP joint extension with essentially normal passive extension may become apparent following fracture or joint injury. This may be due to altered biomechanics of the extensor mechanism, habitual posturing or a relative lengthening of the extensor tendon due to skeletal shortening at the fracture site. Intrinsic strengthening and controlled intrinsic PIP extension with the MP in neutral or slight flexion is required. A small hand-based three-point MP extension block splint will prevent the habitual posturing (Fig. 2.18).

SURGICAL MANAGEMENT

Many fractures are well treated non-operatively and, until recently, most were. Due to improved materials and techniques, particularly those developed by the Swiss AO/ASIF group,[2,3] operative treatment is now preferred for many injuries. Non-displaced and stable injuries are treated non-operatively. Immobilisation is often unnecessary

Table 2.1   Treatment of unstable fractures

Non-operative	Operative
Traction	Percutaneous K-wire
Splint	Open reduction and internal fixation wire (screws, plate)
Plaster	External fixateur

and may be harmful. A temporary splint in the 'safe' position may be used for 1 week (metacarpophalangeal joints flexed to 70 degrees or more; interphalangeal joints extended), followed by mobilisation according to soft tissue requirements.

A variety of techniques are available for the treatment of unstable fractures (Table 2.1).

The final choice will depend on the nature of the injury, the experience of the surgeon and various factors related to the patient.

Some displaced injuries can be realigned by closed reduction. Immobilisation for up to 3 weeks is required, followed by protected active mobilisation. Rotation is controlled by buddy taping.

With current techniques, most displaced and unstable fractures are better treated operatively. Early surgical treatment involving anatomical reduction and rigid internal fixation will enable early active mobilisation. The indications for open reduction and internal fixation are:

1. inability to achieve or maintain a satisfactory position closed
2. displaced intra-articular fracture
3. fractures associated with significant soft tissue injury, e.g. open fracture, nerve, vessel or tendon injury
4. pathological fractures and non-union.

Surgery must be well planned and carefully performed. Surgical dissection should be minimally traumatic, so as to preserve the blood supply to bone and soft tissue. Fixation should be strong enough to allow motion, without the need for additional external support. Bone defects should be grafted early. Inadequate internal fixation is worse than none at all, as the risks of surgery are combined with the disadvantages of immobilisation.

Many fixation techniques are available,[4] including:

1. K-wire: these wires are widely available and K-wire fixation is technically easy. Minimal dissection is required and the wires may be inserted percutaneously. Disadvantages include lack of rigid fixation and absence of compression. K-wires merely act as an internal splint. The benefit of internal fixation and early motion may be lost, as additional external support is often required. Protruding wires may cause skin irritation and pin tract infection. Pin protrusion and skewering of soft tissues may make hand therapy and splinting awkward.

2. Composite wiring: K-wires may be combined with a wire loop to provide additional stability and some compression. One example is tension band wiring, a technique used to fix displaced olecranon and patella fractures. Distraction forces due to the pull of the attached muscle are converted to compression forces at the fracture site. This technique is not often used in hand fractures. Composite wiring is contraindicated when there is bone loss or comminution.

3. Intramedullary fixation with a Steinman pin may be useful for some transverse fractures, but is not appropriate for oblique, spiral or comminuted injuries. The technique is relatively easy, and fixation is stable enough to allow early motion. Rotational malalignment and rod migration may be problems. If rod removal is ever required – e.g. infection – it may be difficult, as the pin is buried within the bone.

4. Screw fixation using techniques recommended by the Swiss AO/ASIF group provides rigid fixation with compression. This technique is ideally suited to fixation of long oblique and spiral fractures, whose length is at least twice the diameter of the bone. Screws are also appropriate for certain articular fractures – e.g. unicondylar fractures. Screw fixation is technically demanding and requires special equipment but will provide excellent fixation and allow early mobilisation.

5. Plate fixation: plates provide excellent fixation and may be used for a variety of complex and unstable injuries (Fig. 2.19). Many plate

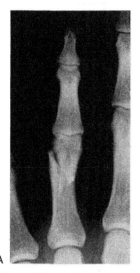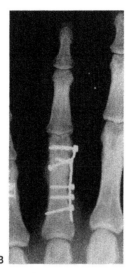

Figure 2.19 A: Comminuted, unstable fracture of the proximal phalanx. B: Open reduction and condylar plate fixation allows early mobilisation.

designs are available. The implant provides longitudinal stability and resists bending and torsion. Surgery is technically demanding but if properly performed, early mobilisation is possible. Supplemental lag screws may be used when the obliquity of the fracture permits. Bone defects should be stabilised early with bone graft. If a plate bridges a bone defect it may break due to cyclic bending stresses. Plates are bulky and may cause tendon irritation and adhesions. Removal is often required.

6. External fixation is indicated for certain complex injuries, including:

- Extremely comminuted fractures or fracture dislocations where internal fixation is technically impossible.
- Open injuries associated with extensive soft tissue trauma and contamination.

A variety of external fixateurs is available, including hinged and spring-loaded devices, which allow early motion while the fixateur is in place. These can be difficult to manage.

External fixateurs maintain length and stability and allow ready access for wound care. They must be carefully supervised, however, and may be associated with various problems, including pin tract infection, osteomyelitis, fracture through the pin holes and injury of important structures at the time of pin insertion.

There are many options available for the treatment of hand fractures. The final decision depends on the nature of the injury, the experience of the surgeon and the expectation and needs of the patient. It is usually best to aim for anatomical reduction and stabilisation of the fracture, followed by early mobilisation of the hand according to soft tissue requirements. Many simple injuries can be managed non-operatively. More complex fractures, particularly those associated with soft tissue injury, are usually better managed by operative techniques.

Details of treatment will vary and must be modified according to the needs of the individual patient. The following sections are summaries of treatment principles of phalangeal and metacarpal fractures.

FRACTURES OF THE DISTAL PHALANX

Distal phalangeal fractures may be classified as tuft, shaft or articular fractures. Tuft fractures are usually due to crush injuries. The fracture itself is less important than the associated soft tissue injury. Nail bed lacerations are common and there is a high risk of late nail deformity. This risk can be minimised by meticulous surgical repair of the nail bed. Drainage of subungual haematoma may relieve pain. Significantly displaced fractures of the distal phalanx may require internal fixation, e.g. K-wire or Herbert screw.

Therapy

The fracture is immobilised for 2–3 weeks for comfort. Fibrous union is common and rarely requires surgical treatment. Treatment of the soft tissue injury is the primary aim of therapy.

Specific tips

Digital nerve compression or contusion can be the most significant long-term problem. Hypersensitivity of the fingertip can be quite disabling. Desensitisation techniques (see Chapter 7A),

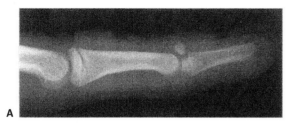

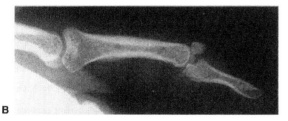

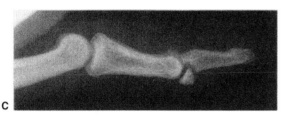

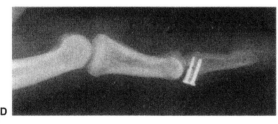

Figure 2.20 Mallet fractures: A: Small bone fragment, joint in good position. Treat in a splint. B: Large bone fragment, joint dislocated. Open reduction and internal fixation is indicated. C: Large bone fragment involving more than one-third of the joint surface. Open reduction is indicated. D: Open reduction and screw fixation of a large bone fragment.

TENS (transcutaneous electrical nerve stimulation) and an activity programme may be required.

Intra-articular fractures

Intra-articular fractures may be:

- Mallet injuries. The dorsal avulsion fracture is attached to the extensor tendon. Treatment depends on the size of the fragment and the position of the joint (Fig. 2.20). If the DIP joint is subluxed on a lateral X-ray and the fragment

is large (involving more than one-third of the articular surface),[5] surgical treatment is advised. Methods vary, but usually the fracture is internally fixed with K-wires or a screw. The repair may be protected by a transarticular K-wire for 4 weeks if required. A further 2–4 weeks of extension splintage is required if there is an extension lag.

If the joint is not subluxed, the injury can be managed the same as a closed mallet injury with no fracture: extension splintage of the DIP joint for 6–8 weeks and early PIP joint mobilisation (see Chapter 2E).

- A volar fracture may be associated with avulsion of the profundis tendon. If diagnosed early, primary tendon repair to bone is advised. Treatment options vary following late diagnosis. Choices include no treatment, two-stage flexor tendon reconstruction, tenodesis or DIP fusion.

- Epiphyseal injuries. In the younger child these are usually Salter–Harris[6] type I injuries. The nail plate is displaced and there is nearly always a transverse laceration of the nail matrix. Treatment involves irrigation and debridement, repair of the nail bed, fracture reduction and replacement of the nail plate beneath the proximal nail fold. An extension splint is applied for 3 weeks.

Salter–Harris type III injuries occur in adolescence. The treatment is similar to the adult mallet injury with a dorsal avulsion fracture.

FRACTURES OF THE MIDDLE AND PROXIMAL PHALANGES

These fractures may be extra- or intra-articular.

Extra-articular fractures

Therapy

Undisplaced and stable injuries are treated by protected early mobilisation. The hand may be splinted in the safe position for comfort for a brief period (7–10 days). Mobilisation exercises are then commenced with buddy taping for protection until the fracture is healed. Therapy includes isolated and composite flexion and extension

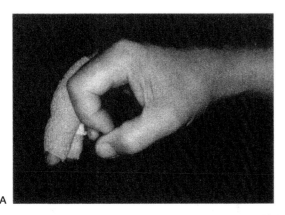
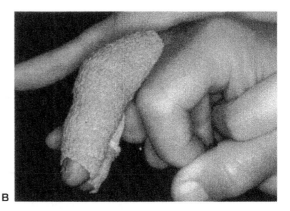

Figure 2.21 Fracture of the proximal phalanges of the middle and ring fingers. Both composite (A) and isolated (B) flexion and extension exercises are necessary. Often greater range of motion can be achieved with isolated joint exercise. The proximal phalanx is gently stabilised, enabling better PIP joint flexion to be achieved.

(Fig. 2.21) and tendon gliding exercises. Graded resisted exercise and activity is commenced at 4–6 weeks, depending on clinical union. Measures to address stiffness such as passive stretching and splinting can also be commenced at this time.

Specific tips

Specific attention to oblique retinacular ligament length and extrinsic/intrinsic balance may be necessary if full function is to be restored.

Judicious attention to PIP joint active and passive extension is essential. The PIP joint has a propensity to develop a flexion contracture due to oedema, stronger flexor muscles, volar plate anatomy and the joint resting position (see Chapter 2J). Prevention and early intervention will minimise this problem.

Displaced fractures

Displaced fractures require reduction. Unstable fractures require stabilisation (i.e. external splint or internal fixation), until healing provides stability.

If a satisfactory position is achieved after closed reduction, and the fracture is stable, the fracture is immobilised with the hand in the 'safe' position for 3–4 weeks. Protected mobilisation is then commenced. Therapy is similar to that for undisplaced fractures.

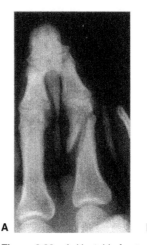
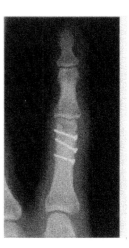

Figure 2.22 A: Unstable fracture of the proximal phalanx with malrotation clinically. B: Open reduction with screw fixation.

If irreducible or unstable after reduction, open reduction and internal fixation is required. Displaced spiral and comminuted fractures are likely to require internal fixation (see other indications for open reduction and internal fixation above). After anatomical reduction and rigid internal fixation (Fig. 2.22), early mobilisation (within a few days of surgery) may then be commenced, according to soft tissue requirements.

Intra-articular fractures

Intra-articular fractures require anatomical reduction in order to prevent joint incongruity and

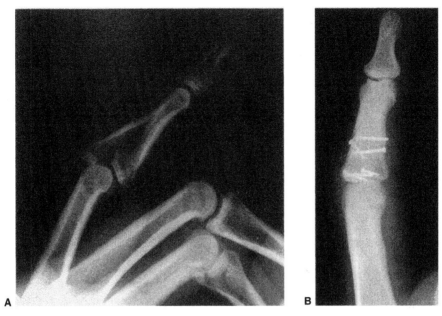

Figure 2.23   A: Displaced, intra-articular fracture dislocation of the PIP joint in a professional footballer. B: Open reduction, internal fixation allows for early mobilisation.

post-traumatic arthritis. Undisplaced fractures may be managed non-operatively. This usually involves a variable period of immobilisation in the 'safe' position (often 1–3 weeks). The splint is removed 4–6 times a day for gentle active exercises. Buddy taping can be used during exercise sessions to support the fracture.

Displaced intra-articular fractures require open reduction and internal fixation. Fixation with screws and plates is preferable but technically difficult (Fig. 2.23). Metaphyseal defects require early bone grafting. Internal fixation should be strong enough to allow early mobilisation in order to reduce the risk of post-traumatic stiffness.

Highly comminuted intra-articular fractures and fracture dislocations are very difficult to treat. Internal fixation of multiple small fragments may be technically impossible. Treatment with an external fixator or traction device is often indicated. Occasionally, primary arthrodesis or joint replacement is required.

Fractures of the condyles are common sporting injuries. Undisplaced fractures are potentially unstable but may be managed non-operatively,

by splinting and protected early motion. Careful follow-up (both clinical and X-ray) is essential to be certain that the fracture position does not change. It is important to avoid malunion, as this will result in articular incongruity leading to post-traumatic arthritis.

Displaced unicondylar fractures are best treated by open reduction and internal fixation. Lag screws provide better fixation but K-wires are also used. Bicondylar fractures are usually displaced. Open reduction and internal fixation (mini screws) is indicated but may be technically difficult. Protected motion is commenced within a few days of surgery. Even after ideal treatment, residual stiffness and extensor lag are not uncommon.

Avulsion fractures may be associated with significant soft tissue injuries. These are particularly important in the PIP joint. Dorsal avulsions from the base of the middle phalanx indicate detachment of the central slip of the extensor mechanism. Lateral avulsions indicate collateral ligament injuries. Large, displaced fragments require open reduction and internal fixation. Small fragments in an acceptable position may be treated non-operatively. The small fragment is ignored and

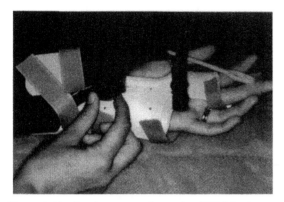

Figure 2.24 Continuous passive motion (CPM) for the PIP joint following proximal phalangeal fracture. A custom-made splint provides better fit, patient comfort and proximal phalanx stabilisation than the commercially available splint.

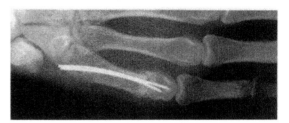

Figure 2.25 This clinically malrotated fracture of the neck of the fifth metacarpal (boxer's fracture) has been treated with closed reduction and fixation using the 'bouquet' technique.

the finger treated as if there were a ligament injury only.

Therapy

Salter et al.[7] and others have shown that continuous passive motion (CPM) enhances healing following articular fractures. Early active and passive motion for intra-articular fractures is recommended. A fracture must be stable to allow active motion and the application of the CPM device (Fig. 2.24). CPM is most effective if it is used for approximately 11 hours per day for at least 2 weeks following the injury.[8] CPM should be combined with massage, exercise and other appropriate therapy techniques for the best results. A POSI splint to rest the hand between CPM and exercise sessions is utilised for 4–6 weeks.

METACARPAL FRACTURES

Metacarpal fractures may involve the head, neck or shaft. Metacarpal head fractures are unusual. If possible, these intra-articular injuries should be reduced anatomically and internally fixed to allow early motion. In the presence of extensive comminution this may be impossible. Treatment alternatives then include external fixateur, joint replacement or non-operative treatment (brief

splinting followed by early mobilisation to mould the articular surface).

Metacarpal neck fractures are common. Often referred to as 'boxer's' fracture, they are in fact rare in professional boxers. The injury tends to occur in amateur fighters inspired by the will to defeat a stronger opponent such as a wall. The little and ring fingers are usually involved. Treatment is controversial.

Due to greater carpometacarpal motion in the ring and little fingers, angulation is better accepted in these digits. Just how much angulation is acceptable is controversial. The functional result is frequently good with no treatment. Even though reduction is easy, maintaining the reduction may be difficult with non-operative treatment. Many complications after this fracture are due to the treatment rather than the injury. Stiffness occurs due to prolonged immobilisation, digital nerves may be injured by percutaneous K-wires and infection and non-union may follow operative reduction. It is often difficult to improve the end result of this injury with surgery.

Indications for operative treatment of metacarpal neck fractures include malrotation, severe angular deformity and complete displacement of the head off the shaft. Various fixation techniques are used, including percutaneous K-wires or plate and screws. The 'bouquet' technique, as described by Foucher[9] is particularly useful (Fig. 2.25). Intramedullary fixation is achieved with several prebent K-wires inserted through the base of the metacarpal. The wires are arranged to be spread out in the metacarpal head like a bouquet of flowers, maintaining reduction by fixation in the subchondral bone. Early mobilisation is possible.

Metacarpal shaft fractures may be transverse, oblique, spiral or comminuted. Mild residual angulation is acceptable, particularly in the ring and little fingers, and is often more of a cosmetic rather than a functional problem. Malrotation is poorly tolerated, as it leads to digital scissoring and is more likely to occur after oblique or spiral fractures. Multiple fractures are unstable. Fractures of the border digits (index and little finger) are less stable than those involving middle and ring fingers. Most shaft fractures can be treated by closed reduction.

Open reduction and internal fixation is required for irreducible or unstable fractures and those associated with significant soft tissue injury (see above). Rigid fixation with plate and screws is preferred.

Fracture dislocation of the carpometacarpal joints more commonly involves the ring and little fingers. Not infrequently, this injury is missed. A true, lateral X-ray is required to make the diagnosis. Treatment involves closed reduction and percutaneous K-wire fixation. Postoperatively, a forearm-based ulnar gutter splint is applied and finger motion is commenced early.

If the dislocation presents late (over 4 weeks following injury), it is better to accept the position. Arthrodesis can be performed later if required.

Therapy

Following closed or open reduction the hand is immobilised in the safe position for 4–6 weeks. Active exercises are commenced within the first week following open reduction and by the second week following closed reduction. Passive motion is commenced at 3 weeks, along with light activity.

Specific tips

The extensor tendon has a great propensity to adhere to the healing fracture. Early active flexion and extension to prevent limiting adhesion formation is essential (Fig. 2.26).

Oedema control is also very important. Oedema tends to collect in the more mobile dorsal skin of the hand, further increasing the likelihood of adhesion of the extensor tendon.

THUMB FRACTURES

Residual deformity is better accepted in the thumb than in the fingers, due to the greater range of motion of the basal joint. Intra-articular fractures should be reduced anatomically to minimise the risk of stiffness and post-traumatic arthritis.

Treatment of most fractures is similar to that of the other digits. A few injuries require special mention.

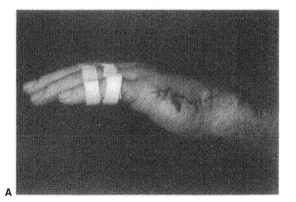
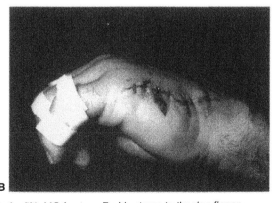

Figure 2.26 Active extension (A) and flexion (B) following ORIF of a fifth MC fracture. Buddy straps to the ring finger provide some support and encourage little finger motion. Care should be taken so that the buddy straps don't block flexion. Coban with coban buddy straps or a double Lycra stall are viable options which also address oedema.

Skier's thumb

Skier's thumb involves rupture of the ulnar collateral ligament of the metacarpophalangeal joint of the thumb. The ligament injury may be associated with an avulsion fracture from the base of the proximal phalanx. Large fragments should be reduced and internally fixed if significantly displaced. If the displaced fragment is small, it may be excised and the ligament repaired to bone.

Undisplaced fractures are treated non-operatively (see Chapter 2C).

Bennett's fracture

A Bennett's fracture is a fracture subluxation of the thumb carpometacarpal joint. The important anterior oblique ligament is attached to the volar fragment, which remains in the correct place. The remainder of the base of the metacarpal subluxes

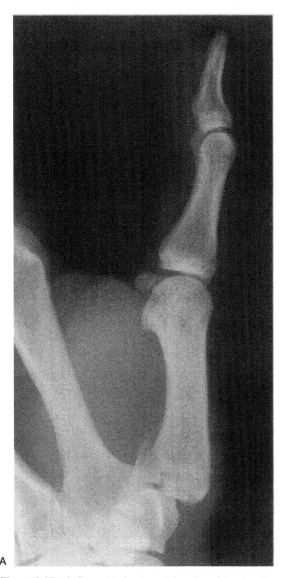

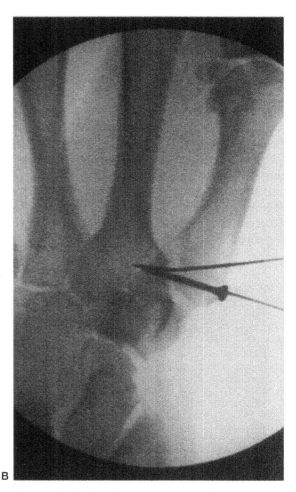

A   B

Figure 2.27   A: Bennett's fracture dislocation of the thumb carpometacarpal joint with a large bone fragment. B: Anatomical reduction and screw fixation enable early mobilisation.

due to the action of the attached abductor pollicis longus. This important intra-articular fracture deserves anatomical reduction.

If the volar fragment is large and the bone is strong, open reduction with lag screw fixation is preferred (Fig. 2.27), especially for young active patients. With this technique, anatomical reduction is possible and rigid fixation using the screw enables early mobilisation. Closed reduction and K-wire fixation is a reasonable alternative, particularly if the volar fragment is small.

Rolando fracture

A Rolando fracture is a comminuted Y- or T-shaped intra-articular fracture of the base of the thumb metacarpal. Open reduction and plate fixation is preferable but technically impossible if the comminution is excessive.

Therapy following thumb fractures

Distal phalangeal fractures in the thumb are treated in the same way as those in the fingers. Proximal phalangeal fractures are splinted with a hand-based splint, immobilising the MP joint only if the fracture is proximal. If the fracture involves the neck or head of the phalanx distally, the IP joint may be included. The splint is worn for approximately 3–4 weeks and for an additional 2 weeks for heavy activity or vulnerable circumstances such as sports or parties.

Metacarpal fractures are supported in a forearm-based splint including the MP joint with the thumb in palmar abduction. Oedema control measures are commenced early (within the first 48 hours after injury), along with early active exercises for each joint. Graded resistance is commenced at 4–5 weeks post fracture.

Specific tips

1. It is important to maintain the thumb abduction in order to avoid web contracture. Splint in comfortable maximal abduction. Maintain range of motion with early exercises.
2. Thumb stability is vital for hand function. Pinch grip and manipulation of objects depend upon it. If for various reasons internal fixation is not possible and the fracture remains unstable, splintage time may extend to 6 weeks.
3. IP joint stiffness following proximal phalanx or metacarpal fractures may be the result of tendon adhesions or secondary joint stiffness. Interphalangeal joint motion must be commenced early, within the first 2 weeks following the injury. Both active and passive interphalangeal joint exercises can be commenced within the first few days following splint application. A flexion strap may be necessary if IP joint flexion is not 50% of the uninjured side by 2 weeks post injury.

REFERENCES

1. Strickland JW, Steichan JB, Kleinmann WB, Hastings H, Flynn, M: Phalangeal fractures. Factors influencing digital performance. Orthop Rev II:39–50, 1982.
2. Muller MF, Algower M, Schneider R, Willenegger IT: Manual of internal fixation. Techniques recommended by the AO-ASIF group, 3rd edn. Berlin: Springer-Verlag, 1992.
3. Heim U, Pfeitter KM: Internal fixation of small fractures. Techniques recommended by the AO-ASIF group. Berlin: Springer-Verlag, 1988.
4. Green, DP: Operative hand surgery, 3rd edn. Edinburgh: Churchill Livingstone, 1993.
5. Lubahn JD: Mallet finger fractures: a comparison of open and closed technique. J Hand Surg 14A:394–6, 1989.
6. Salter RB, Harris WR: Injuries involving the epiphyseal plate. J Bone Joint Surg (Am) 45:587–622, 1963.
7. Salter RB, Clements MD, Ogilvie-Harris et al: The healing of articular tissues through continuous passive motion: essence of the first ten years of experimental investigation. J Bone Joint Surg 64B:640, 1982.
8. Prosser R: Continuous passive motion for isolated joint injuries. Proceeding from International Federation of Societies of Hand Therapist, First Congress, Tel Aviv, 1989:31–4.
9. Foucher MD: "Bouquet" osteosynthesis in metacarpal neck fractures: a series of 66 patients. J Hand Surg 20A:286–90, 1995.

C. DISLOCATIONS AND LIGAMENT INJURIES IN THE DIGITS

Peter Scougall and Rosemary Prosser

PROXIMAL INTERPHALANGEAL JOINT

Dislocations and subluxations of the PIP joint are common. The initial injury often seems trivial, although stiffness and swelling may take many months to settle, and sometimes never resolve completely. Rehabilitation is frequently prolonged.

PIP joints are stable bicondylar hinge joints. The inherent stability of the articular surfaces is supplemented by soft tissue attachments on all four sides. The paired collateral ligaments reinforce the lateral capsule and, together with the volar plate, attach to the volar third of the middle phalanx. Dorsally, the joint is stabilised by the extensor mechanism, in particular the central slip. At least two of these structures must be disrupted for instability to occur.

Dislocations may be dorsal, lateral, volar or rotary.

Dorsal dislocations

Dorsal dislocations are the most common. Closed reduction is usually possible and the joint is generally stable once reduced (Fig. 2.28). Usually, the volar plate and at least one collateral ligament are torn; injuries usually heal with non-operative treatment.

Therapy

Stable dislocation post-reduction. After reduction, protected mobilisation is commenced early. The protocol is modified according to the nature of the injury, soft tissue swelling and ligamentous laxity of the patient. If the joint is stable after reduction, and the patient does not have ligamentous laxity (i.e. adjacent PIP joints do not hyperextend), motion can be commenced early. The finger is buddy taped to an adjacent digit for 2–3 weeks. Taping should be continued for several

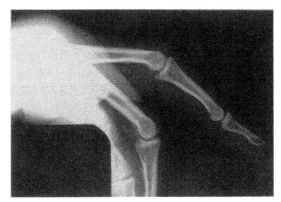

Figure 2.28 Reduced dorsal PIP joint dislocation. An avulsion fracture of the volar plate is evident. These injuries are usually stable after closed reduction. Stiffness is a greater risk than instability. Mobilise early.

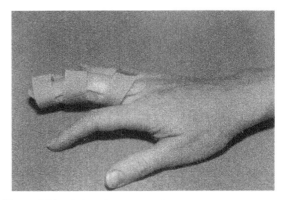

Figure 2.29 A dorsal blocking splint preventing PIP extension beyond 30 degrees is applied if the joint hyperextends after relocation or if there is generalised ligamentous laxity. Exercises can be done in the splint.

months during strenuous activities, including sport.

Dislocation with hyperextension tendency post-reduction. If there is extensive soft tissue swelling, or the patient has generalised ligamentous laxity, a dorsal extension block splint is applied with the PIP joint in slight flexion (30 degrees) for 10 days (Fig. 2.29).

Protected exercises are commenced as soon as the acute inflammation has settled (day 3–5). At 10–14 days, the joint is reassessed. If there is a continuing tendency for the joint to hyperextend, the dorsal blocking splint is reapplied for a

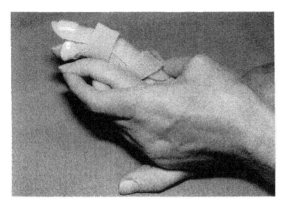

Figure 2.30 Early attention to DIP flexion range is necessary to prevent tightness and adhesion of the extensor mechanism and oblique retinacular ligament over the middle phalanx.

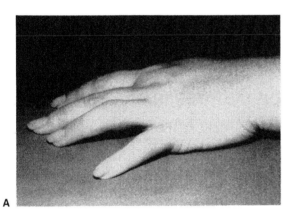

A

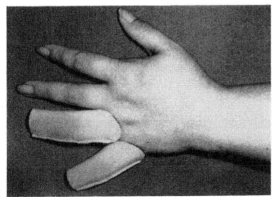

B

Figure 2.31 Four weeks following PIP joint dislocation. Neoprene sleeves for flexion contractures of the ring and little finger PIP joints were made and fitted. These were worn for 8 weeks by this patient with complete resolution of the flexion contractures.

further 2 weeks. If the joint is stable, exercises may be increased and the joint gradually extended. Resisted exercises are delayed until week 6.

Specific tips

Stiffness is common after this injury; instability is rare. DIP joint stiffness may occur due to adhesions of the extensor mechanism or oblique retinacular ligament (ORL). This can be a greater problem than PIP joint stiffness. Both active and passive DIP flexion should be commenced as soon as possible, usually by day 2 (Fig. 2.30).

PIP joint stiffness can be treated with stretches, passive joint mobilisations and splintage, generally from week 6 onwards.

An irritable PIP may remain inflamed and reactive for many months. These joints should be treated gently. A neoprene sleeve may be the only extension splintage they can tolerate (Fig. 2.31).

Dorsal fracture dislocation

A dorsal fracture dislocation involves an avulsion fracture from the volar aspect of the middle phalanx. If this fragment involves more than 40% of the joint surface, the joint will be unstable after reduction and surgical treatment is required. If reduction and fixation of the fragment is not possible, a volar plate arthroplasty is indicated. If unreduced, a fracture dislocation will lead to post-traumatic osteoarthritis and may eventually require joint replacement or arthrodesis.

Lateral dislocations

Lateral dislocations involve rupture of one collateral ligament and at least partial rupture of the volar plate. Closed reduction is usually possible and rehabilitation is similar to that for dorsal dislocations.

Volar dislocations

Volar dislocations are rarer but more complex than dorsal dislocations. They usually involve disruption of the extensor mechanism, in particular the central slip, with the consequent risk of button hole deformity (boutonnière) of the finger. Surgical treatment is more frequently required for volar dislocation, because the injury is more commonly either irreducible or unstable after reduction.

If closed reduction is successful, careful follow-up (both clinical and X-ray) is essential, as recurrent volar subluxation can occur.

If the joint is either irreducible, or unstable after reduction, open reduction and repair of the extensor tendon is indicated. The repair can be protected by a transarticular K-wire for 2–3 weeks. PIP splinting in extension is continued for a further 4 weeks.

Therapy

Volar dislocations with central slip disruptions. Whether open or closed, volar dislocations with central slip disruption should be treated in a PIP extension splint for 6–8 weeks. A static splint is applied for the first 2–3 weeks and may then be exchanged for a Capener. The Capener splint will maintain extension while allowing a few degrees of motion. Ensure oedema is well controlled. Coban or a lycra stall may be applied beneath the splint.

DIP motion is commenced early, within the first week to prevent lateral band and ORL adhesion. At 4–6 weeks, PIP motion is added to the programme. The timing of PIP motion will depend on the strength and density of the healing tendon and joint structures. Initially, short arc motion (0–60 degrees) only is allowed. At 6 weeks postoperative, unrestricted PIP motion is commenced. Other therapy programmes are discussed in Chapter 2E.

Rotary subluxation

Rotary subluxation is a rare variant of volar dislocation, which is usually irreducible closed. One lateral band usually separates from the central slip and is displaced volarly. Closed reduction is not possible, because the joint becomes trapped between the displaced lateral band and the central slip. Clinically, the diagnosis is suggested by incomplete PIP extension after attempted closed

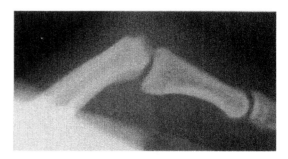

Figure 2.32 Rotary dislocation of the PIP joint is rare but important to recognise. The PIP joint buttonholes between the lateral band and the central slip and becomes locked in this position. Malrotation of the PIP joint can be seen on the lateral X-ray. One phalanx is lateral and one oblique.

reduction. Lateral X-rays demonstrate malrotation of the joint (Fig. 2.32). One phalanx appears lateral and one oblique. The joint is stable after open reduction and stabilisation of the displaced lateral band. Active mobilisation can be commenced at 2 weeks postoperatively.

DISTAL INTERPHALANGEAL JOINT

The anatomy of the DIP joint is similar to that of the PIP joint. Dislocations of the DIP joint are rare, and are usually dorsal or lateral when they occur. Closed reduction is usually possible. Instability is rare, and joint mobilisation can be commenced after about 2 weeks of protective splinting.

Occasionally, closed reduction is prevented by soft tissue interposition (volar plate, flexor tendon) or a bone fragment. Open reduction is then required. Open dislocation should be treated by thorough wound irrigation and debridement in the operating room.

METACARPOPHALANGEAL JOINT

The MP joints are condyloid in shape and stabilised by specialised structures on all sides. The volar plate is continuous with the transverse metacarpal ligament and allows some hyperextension of the joint. The collateral ligaments are tighter in flexion than extension. This stabilises the joint laterally in full flexion and allows some finger abduction and adduction in extension.

The thin dorsal capsule is reinforced by the extensor mechanism.

Dorsal dislocations

Dorsal dislocations of the MP joint may be simple or complex.

Simple dorsal dislocations

Simple dislocations are reducible closed. The joint is stable after reduction.

Therapy

Early motion is commenced in a dorsal extension block splint in 30–40 degrees of flexion within the first week following reduction. The splint may be required for 3–4 weeks. Therapy follows the same basic programme as described for PIP joint dislocations. Gentle passive stretches can be started at week 3 if the joint is stiff. Resisted exercises are not commenced till week 6.

Complex dorsal dislocations

In complex dislocations, closed reduction is prevented by the flexor tendons and intrinsic muscles, which form a noose around the narrow metacarpal neck. Attempted closed reduction only tightens this noose, preventing the tendons passing over the wider metacarpal head and thereby blocking reduction. Open reduction is required. Surgical release of the A1 pulley reduces the tension in the muscle–tendon noose and allows reduction of the joint.

Therapy

Postoperatively, the joint is immobilised in slight flexion (30–40 degrees) for 4–6 weeks. Interphalangeal (IP) joint flexion and extension is commenced within the first week. MP joint motion within the protective dorsal extension splint is commenced at 2 weeks. Gentle passive flexion stretches can be instituted at 3 weeks if the joint is stiff. Resisted activity is delayed until 6 weeks post-reduction.

Specific tips

Clinical experience treating MP joint dislocations indicates that some of these joints take many months to settle. Joint irritability may be troublesome for up to 6 months. Extension range should be monitored closely. If a lag is present at 4 weeks post-reduction, intermittent extension splintage and emphasis on extension exercises may be necessary.

Volar dislocations

Volar MP dislocations are extremely rare. Open reduction is indicated if the injury is irreducible closed.

THUMB

MP joint of the thumb – ulnar collateral ligament injury

Disruption of the ulnar collateral ligament of the MP joint of the thumb is a common injury, occurring due to forced radial deviation (abduction). This injury is often referred to as 'skier's thumb', although the term 'gamekeeper's thumb' is also used.

If the ligament is completely torn, it usually ruptures at its distal insertion and is then displaced to lie superficial to the adductor aponeurosis (Stener lesion).[1] It cannot heal in this displaced position and will lead to chronic joint instability if not repaired to bone. For this reason, complete ruptures of the ulnar collateral ligament should be treated by open surgical repair. Clinically, this diagnosis is suggested by joint laxity of greater than 30 degrees and the absence of a firm end point on examination. Joint mobility varies from person to person. Compare the clinical laxity of the injured thumb with the opposite side. Surgery usually confirms the presence of a Stener lesion and may also reveal an associated rupture of the dorsal capsule and volar plate. The joint may be subluxed. The ulnar collateral ligament is usually avulsed off the middle phalanx and should be repaired to its correct position on the bone. There are various ways to achieve this.

Intraosseous sutures or a Mitec suture anchor are both effective. Postoperatively, a plaster or splint is applied for 4 weeks with the MP joint in slight flexion.

Partial ruptures (less than 30 degrees laxity, firm end point on examination) can be treated in a hand-based thumb splint, immobilising the MP joint for 4 weeks. X-rays may demonstrate an associated avulsion fracture (Fig. 2.33). The location of the bone fragment will suggest the position of the injured ligament. Undisplaced fractures can be treated in a splint or cast. Small displaced fragments can be removed at the time of ligament repair. Large displaced fragments can be internally fixed with mini screws or K-wires.

Therapy

The MP joint is immobilised in a hand-based splint for 4 weeks (Fig. 2.34). Early IP joint motion is commenced within the first week. The patient is permitted to do light activity within pain limits, while wearing the splint.

At 4 weeks, MP joint motion is commenced. The splint is worn for 2 more weeks for moderate to heavy use of the hand. At 6 weeks, a graded resisted exercise programme is started.

Specific tips

Thumb stability is essential for strong functional pinch. MP joint instability due to chronic laxity or lengthening of the ulnar collateral ligament will significantly reduce pinch strength and will predispose to secondary osteoarthritis in the joint. In cases of severe ligament damage, it is acceptable to sacrifice some MP joint motion as long as stability is restored.

Limited IP joint flexion caused by extensor pollicis longus (EPL) and extensor apparatus tightness and adhesions is evident early and should be dealt with early. Clinically, if the IP joint flexion is not approximately 50% of the uninjured thumb at 2 weeks, further intervention is required. A flexion cuff is easily fitted. It is worn intermittently for between 2 and 6 hours per day, depending on the joint stiffness (Fig. 2.35).

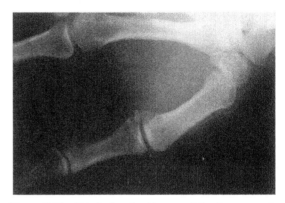

Figure 2.33 Skier's thumb with an avulsion fracture at the base of the middle phalanx.

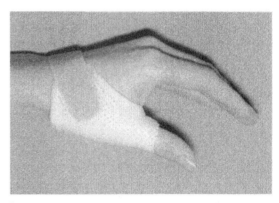

Figure 2.34 MP ulnar collateral ligament injuries are immobilised in a hand-based splint for 4–6 weeks. The interphalangeal (IP) joint is left free. Early IP active flexion is essential to prevent extensor pollicis longus tightness and adhesion.

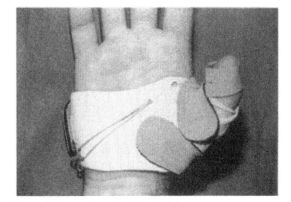

Figure 2.35 At 2 weeks if the IP joint range of motion is not 50% of the uninjured thumb, a dynamic flexion assist cuff is fitted to the splint. This is used between 2 and 6 hours per day, depending on the joint stiffness and patient tolerance.

Carpometacarpal joint

Most CMC joint injuries are fracture dislocations, already discussed in the section on metacarpal fractures.

CMC dislocations are usually dorsal, and may be missed if a proper lateral X-ray is not performed. Closed reduction and percutaneous K-wire fixation is indicated for fresh dislocations. Late injuries can sometimes be treated by open reduction, but may require arthrodesis if symptoms warrant.

CMC joint of the thumb

This is a saddle-shaped joint with a large range of motion. The small amount of inherent joint stability provided by the concave articular surfaces is augmented significantly by soft tissue attachments. The volar ligament is probably the most important stabiliser of the joint, particularly for pinch. It passes from the trapezium to the volar beak of the metacarpal.

Acute thumb dislocations are usually reducible closed. Cast immobilisation for 4 weeks may be adequate but careful follow-up and repeat X-ray is essential, as the injury is quite unstable and joint subluxation can occur in the plaster. It may be safer to maintain anatomical reduction with percutaneous K-wire fixation of the joint for the duration of cast immobilisation (4 weeks).

If an anatomical position cannot be achieved closed, open reduction is indicated. The important volar ligament can be reconstructed with a strip of flexor carpi radialis (FCR) tendon passed through a drill hole in the base of the metacarpal.

Therapy

CMC joint immobilisation can be achieved with a forearm-based spica cast. This may be changed at 2–3 weeks to a hand-based splint which immobilises the MP joint as well as the CMC.

If open reduction has been required, the sutures are removed at 2 weeks and wound/scar care commenced. IP joint exercises are started within the first week. MP joint exercises are commenced weeks 3–4. Between weeks 4 and 6 the splint may be worn intermittently for support during moderate to heavy use. Alternatively a neoprene support may be adequate at this stage. At 4 weeks, CMC joint exercises are commenced. At 6 weeks, a graded resisted programme can be started.

Maintenance of thumb web span by ensuring the thumb is in palmar abduction in the splint has been discussed in the previous chapter on thumb fractures.

Dynamic and serial static splinting, passive joint mobilisations (PJMs) and stretches can be started at 2 weeks for the IP joint, 4 weeks for the MP joint and 4–6 weeks for the CMC joint.

REFERENCE

1. Stener G: Displacement of the ruptured ulnar collateral ligament of the metacarpophalangeal joint of the thumb. A clinical and anatomical study. J Bone Joint Surg 44B:869–79, 1962.

FURTHER READING

Green DP: Operative hand surgery, 3rd edn. Edinburgh: Churchill Livingstone, 1993.

Rockwood LA, Green DP, Bucholz RW: Fractures in adults, 3rd edn. Philadelphia: Lippincott, 1991.

D. FLEXOR TENDON INJURIES

Michael Sandow and Sandra Kay

INTRODUCTION

Flexor tendon lacerations remain a challenge for the hand surgeon and therapist with the ultimate aim to restore maximum function with expediency and safety in a range of clinical situations. To achieve this goal, suture techniques and their specific postoperative therapy protocols have evolved over the years from programmes of complete immobilisation, through early controlled motion, to the current interest in early active motion.

Specific biomechanical factors during the rehabilitation period must be considered, as successful flexor tenorrhaphy relies on the suture material and its grasp on the tendon for at least the first 3 weeks, irrespective of the type of repair.[1] The benefits of an active mobilisation protocol following repair have been well recognised.[2] However, risk of rupture increases the technical demands placed on the surgeon initially and the therapist postoperatively; the myriad of different repair techniques available suggest that no single approach has been universally successful.

Although the flexor tendon has important biological properties in terms of nutrition and tissue interaction, it is a critical component of the force couple that produces flexion and extension of the interphalangeal joints. A satisfactory repair technique should be biomechanically sound, biologically inert and uncomplicated. There must be a consistent treatment concept which incorporates a specific repair and a specific postoperative therapy protocol so that the tenorrhaphy has sufficient integrity to resist postoperative rehabilitation forces. A flexor tenorrhaphy that has sufficient strength for a passive mobilisation protocol, e.g. Kleinert's technique,[3] may be inappropriate for an active protocol where stresses across the repair may be substantially greater, producing an unacceptable rupture rate. The results using the Savage and Risitano[4] multi-strand repair and subsequent studies by Silfverskiöld and May[5] highlight the importance of stronger repairs for an active flexor tendon mobilisation protocol. Elliot et al.[6] identified a high rupture rate in patients undergoing active mobilisation with a two-strand repair, suggesting that multi-strand repairs are more appropriate. However, passive mobilisation protocols remain an important alternative following flexor tenorrhaphy, despite increasing interest and reported advantages of an active motion regimen.

Tenorrhaphy techniques

To achieve a satisfactory repair, the severed tendon ends must be joined with sufficient strength, minimal tendency to gap and with as little interference to tendon glide and nutrition as possible. There are a large number of repair alternatives and these, plus important biomechanical aspects of the repair, are well summarised by Evans and Thompson[7] Ex-vivo porcine tenorrhaphy work in our laboratory[8] showed that the modified Kessler technique (Fig. 2.36A), even with an epitendinous repair, had inadequate tensile strength and high inherent gapping potential (Fig. 2.36B), making it less suitable for active mobilisation when compared with a modification of the Savage multistrand repair. As a result of this work we now use a *four*-strand single-cross grasp repair (Fig. 2.36C) with 4–0 or 3–0 braided polyester suture for most flexor tendon repairs. This has been demonstrated to have sufficient tensile strength (median tensile strength 4–0 = 45 N, 3–0 = 80 N) to allow safe *active* mobilisation (Fig. 2.37).

Postoperative management

Postoperative immobilisation

Early work by Mason and Allen[9] and later by Potenza[10] suggested there was a loss of tendon tensile strength immediately following repair, which led to a reluctance to stress repaired tendons early. A 3-week period of immobilisation was thought necessary to ensure sufficient extrinsic adhesion formation and tendon strength to prevent rupture when active motion began. However, this postoperative immobilisation resulted in adhesion formation, joint stiffness, loss of tendon glide and frequent poor outcomes.[2] More recent work by Wagner et al.[1] and Aoki et al.[11] has shown that there is minimal loss of tenorrhaphy

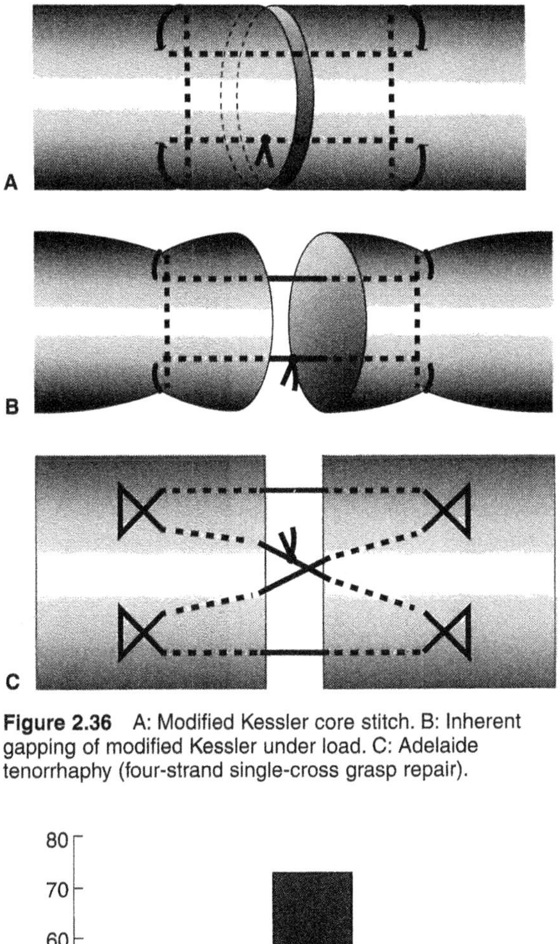

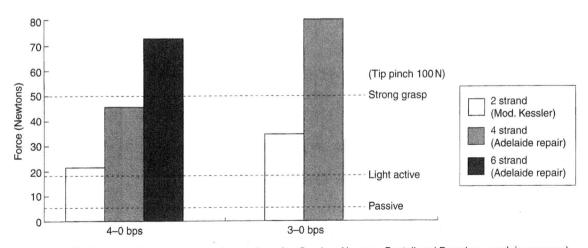

Figure 2.36 A: Modified Kessler core stitch. B: Inherent gapping of modified Kessler under load. C: Adelaide tenorrhaphy (four-strand single-cross grasp repair).

strength if the repair is carefully stressed, thus providing little support for delayed mobilisation.

Early controlled motion

Kleinert[3] in the 1950s developed a technique of dynamic splinting where a dorsal blocking splint maintained the wrist in almost full flexion, the metacarpophalangeal (MCP) joints in moderate flexion and the interphalangeal (IP) joints straight. Flexion of the digit was achieved passively by rubber band traction followed by active extension. Thus, the repaired tendon was theoretically protected from the stresses of active contraction. The improved outcomes with this technique were viewed with scepticism initially but were crucial in showing that early mobilisation could improve results.

Subsequently, Duran and Houser[12] reported a technique of controlled passive motion also using a dorsal blocking splint and rubber band traction, but incorporating a series of passive interphalangeal joint exercises which promoted differential motion of the flexor tendons to maintain independent excursion and prevent adhesions.

There have been progressive modifications to these original protocols. The position of the wrist was relaxed to mid-flexion with greater flexion of the MCP joints[13] and Slattery and McGrouther[14]

Figure 2.37 Median strength of repairs (porcine ex-vivo: after Sandow, Nawana, Bentall and Downing – work in progress) and strength required for various hand activities (after Schuind et al.[18]). Repairs were performed with single knot per tenorrhaphy.

added a palmar pulley to the splint to facilitate gliding between the separate flexor tendons. The Washington regimen[15,16] modified and combined both the Kleinert and Duran protocols.

Early active motion

Early active motion following tendon repair is not a new concept;[17] however, the increased risk of rupture and claims that no available suture technique could withstand the force of active motion[18,19] have deterred widespread use. Stronger and more complex repair techniques have been developed in an effort to address this increased tensile requirement.[7] Small et al.[20] were the first to publish a large series of patient results using a two-strand core repair. Although they achieved 80% good or excellent outcomes, this was accompanied by a 6% rupture rate in a series with only a 75% follow-up, suggesting the true rupture rate may have been much higher. In a previous series from our hospital,[8] with a complete qualify follow-up (100%), it was noted that there was disproportionately poorer recovery of motion in those patients who failed to return for scheduled review and who were difficult to locate for their final assessment.

Joint contracture prevention

Proximal interphalangeal (PIP) joint contractures have been a frequently reported complication of postoperative management, so digital straps or splints (Fig. 2.38) to reduce the risk of PIP joint contracture have been added to a number of regimens without appearing to increase rupture rate.[5,8,21]

Wrist position

The position of the wrist in postoperative splinting remains controversial. Traditionally, some measure of wrist flexion was adopted to reduce stress on the repaired tendon.[3] Gratton[22] reported that wrist flexion would diminish ease of finger flexion, thereby reducing the tendency for accidental hand usage, whereas Small et al.[20] suggested that placing the hand in a position of function may increase its normal use and thus increase the risk

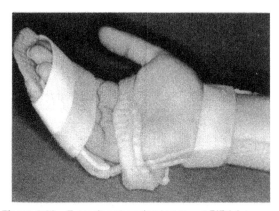

Figure 2.38 Extension strapping to prevent PIP joint contractures.

of rupture. More normal tendon excursion was achieved by Strickland[23] using a dynamic splint to allow combined wrist flexion/finger extension and wrist extension/finger flexion. Savage[24] identified that the major restraint to active finger flexion was passive extensor tension and that this decreased with wrist extension. He recommended that wrist extension of 45 degrees was the optimum position for postoperative active mobilisation, as it maximally relaxed the finger extensors, thereby reducing the minimum force required for active interphalangeal joint flexion (see Fig. 2.40). However, a position of 30 degree flexion remains the most commonly recommended position,[5,23] although Sandow and McMahon[8] adopted a position of neutral to 20 degree extension. Evans and Thompson[7] showed that modest wrist extension did not significantly increase the flexor tendon tension or work of flexion but did decrease passive extensor muscle tension.

ADELAIDE FLEXOR TENORRHAPHY PROTOCOL

The aim of treatment is to restore maximum function to the injured digit. As treatment depends on associated injuries, this protocol provides guidelines for the management of the flexor tendon only and will be considered under the following headings:

- skin incision
- tenorrhaphy technique

- protection of tendon during tendon healing
- restoration of joint range of motion and strength
- oedema control
- scar management
- prevention of interphalangeal joint contracture.

Skin incision

To retain palmar veins and thus minimise post-operative swelling, transverse incisions should be avoided, and thus extension of a partial transverse laceration is not necessarily appropriate. Where possible, a modified mid-lateral incision is used[25] to facilitate digital flexion and reduce oedema.

Tenorrhaphy technique

The repair technique used must have sufficient strength to resist the forces of active motion. A four-strand single-cross grasp repair with 3–0 braided polyester suture (see Fig. 2.36C) should have sufficient tensile strength for safe post-operative active mobilisation. As it is generally not possible to adjust the tension of each strand at the end of the repair, it is critical that the tendon ends remain accurately approximated throughout the repair. This is typically achieved with the standard technique of transfixing hypodermic needles. However, this method of tendon stabilisation does not easily permit adjustment of tendon coaptation during the repair and precludes movement of the tendon within the flexor sheath until the needles are removed. A coaptation device (Pactan®, Wright Medical Technology) (Fig. 2.39) maintains approximation of the tendon ends and allows adjustment during repair. As the needles do not transfix the tendon and sheath, the tendon can be advanced or retracted for better access.

For smaller tendons, a 4–0 braided polyester suture is sufficient. A 5–0 nylon epitendinous repair is generally performed, but typically only on the palmar aspect of the tendon. The epitendinous suture is used to prevent catching due to irregularity or gapping of the tendon edge and

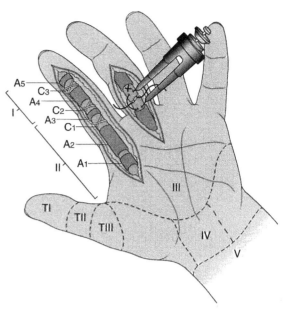

Figure 2.39   Anatomy of flexor pulleys (index finger) and partial insertion of Adelaide repair facilitated by tendon coaptation using the Pactan® repair device (Wright Medical Technology) (middle finger). Zones of flexor tendon injury are included (I–V).

does not contribute significantly to the overall strength of the repair.

Protection of tendon during tendon healing

Splinting

0–6 weeks. Postoperative dressings are carefully applied to avoid restricting finger flexion and circumferential bandages are not used around the fingers. A dorsal blocking thermoplastic splint is custom-made within 5 days of tendon repair to replace the plaster splint applied by the surgeon in the operating theatre, to continue to maintain a position of wrist extension 20–30 degrees, MCP flexion 80–90 degrees and full IP joint extension (Fig. 2.40). A moulded palmar bar proximal to the distal palmar crease keeps the hand firmly within the splint. A Velcro® elastic strap maintains finger extension at night and between exercise sessions (see Fig. 2.38).

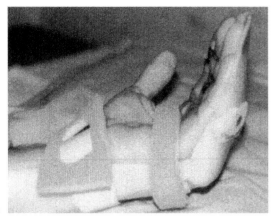
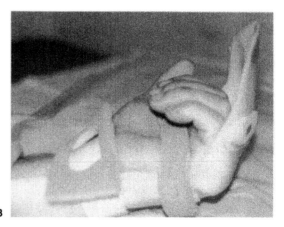

A   B

Figure 2.40 Postoperative splint (wrist 30 degree extension, MCP 80–90 degrees flexion, DIP, PIP straight) with range of motion at 1 week.

6–8 weeks. The dorsal blocking splint is removed but may be retained at night or in 'at risk' situations during the day. Buddy tapes provide additional protection for the injured digit for a further 2 weeks once the protective splint is removed and functional activity begins.

Patient education and advice

Education is paramount to ensure patient compliance. Time must be taken to explain the postoperative protocol, the time frame for recovery and essential precautions. Patients must be instructed not to remove the splint or use the hand for the first 6 weeks and to keep the hand elevated to avoid swelling. Patients need to understand that the hand should be protected from strenuous activity for 12 weeks and that any loss of active finger flexion must be reported to the surgeon or therapist as soon as possible.

Restoration of joint range of motion and strength

Exercise programme

0–6 weeks. The exercise programme is frequently commenced under the guidance of the surgeon in the recovery room, if the patient is

sufficiently cooperative. Long-acting local anaesthetic is injected adjacent to the finger wound to facilitate postoperative pain control. The use of major regional anaesthesia will delay the return of motor function to the arm and, although providing good postoperative analgesia, precludes immediate active motion. The exercise programme generally comprises 10 passive full finger flexion movements, and then 5 active finger extensions to the limit of the splint, alternating with 5 active assisted flexion contractions which can include 'place and hold' techniques if active flexion is poor. Initially, the patient must remain in the splint at all times. The exercises should be carried out every hour while awake and performed slowly, *gently* and without force. Written instructions provide a useful reminder of the home programme. Full active digital flexion should be possible by the postoperative day 7 (Fig. 2.40).

At 4 weeks the splint may be removed to use the tenodesis wrist action to facilitate active digital flexion as the wrist moves into active extension, and then active digital extension as the wrist moves into flexion. However, this additional exercise requires close supervision by the therapist when introduced.

6–12 weeks. Following splint removal at 6 weeks, light activities of daily living should be

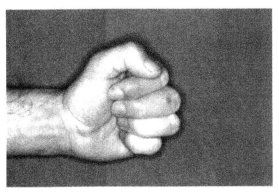

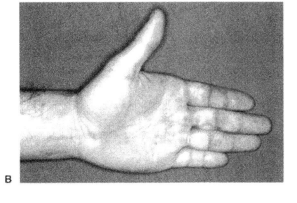

A   **B**

Figure 2.41   Flexion (A) and extension (B) at final review.

encouraged, as should combined wrist and finger flexion and extension movements and tendon gliding exercises.

From 8 weeks, light resistive exercises can be included and activities of daily living increased. Work-hardening programmes can begin from 10 weeks and a return to full duties by 12 weeks is encouraged (Fig. 2.41).

Oedema control

0–12 weeks. In the initial postoperative phase it is essential to control swelling using moderate elevation and gentle active exercises. Initially, compression wraps and finger stalls should be avoided as they will add to the work of flexion and thus may stress the repair during active mobilisation. However, light Coban® wrapping from 4 weeks may be helpful, and residual swelling addressed vigorously from 6 weeks with Coban® wrap, finger stalls and elastic gloves.

Scar management

0–6 weeks. Initially, scars can be dressed with an adhesive semiporous polyester dressing such as Hypafix®. Once wounds have healed, gentle scar massage may commence and the patient should be instructed to do this once or twice daily at home.

6–12 weeks. Thickened woody scars can be treated with more intensive massage and the application of silicone and other contact media.

Prevention of interphalangeal joint contracture

0–6 weeks. While in the splint, ensure that the MCPs are fully flexed to 80–90 degrees (remould the dorsal blocking splint if necessary) and that the hand is held firmly within the splint by the palmar bar, wrist strap and digital extension strap. Foam wedge extension blocks can also be inserted between the proximal phalanx and the splint to encourage full active PIP joint extension. When performing extension exercises, a finger placed on the dorsum of the proximal phalanx to block the MCP into flexion will also assist in maximising digital PIP extension.

6–12 weeks. From 6 weeks, static gutter splints can be moulded over the volar surface of the finger at the limit of *active* digital extension, and dynamic extension splints can be incorporated into the programme from 8 weeks postoperatively.

CONCLUSION

Flexor tendon repairs remain a challenge for the hand surgeon and therapist. However, recent work suggests that an active mobilisation protocol with a strong tenorrhaphy will afford the most predictable restoration of function. Based on biomechanical data, a four-strand single-cross grasp repair employed as part of the Adelaide tenorrhaphy technique has been shown to be successful in providing a reliable repair which will withstand the forces of active mobilisation. There would seem little reason to delay commencing active mobilisation when the adhesions that form will only become more resilient with time. An early active motion protocol appears to offer a less complicated regimen and delivers more normal physiological forces to the hand. There is evidence that a tendon which is appropriately stressed will avoid the critical postoperative weakening previously reported in immobilised tendon repairs.

However, it is crucial that any decision on the appropriate technique for flexor tenorrhaphy must take into account the specific biomechanical requirements of the rehabilitation phase. Best outcomes will be achieved when both the tenorrhaphy technique and postoperative programme are selected to suit available rehabilitation facilities, with input from both hand therapist and surgeon.

REFERENCES

1. Wagner WF Jr, Carroll C IV, Strickland JW, Heck DA, Toombs JP: A biomechanical comparison of techniques of flexor tendon repair. J Hand Surg (Am) 19A:979–83, 1994.
2. Gelberman RH, Woo SL-Y: The physiological basis for application of controlled stress in the rehabilitation of flexor tendon injuries. J Hand Therapy 2:66–70, 1989.
3. Lister GD, Kleinert HE, Kutz JE, Atasoy E: Primary flexor tendon repair followed by immediate controlled mobilisation. J Hand Surg (Am) 2A:441–51, 1977.
4. Savage R, Risitano G: Flexor tendon repair using a "six strand" method of repair and early active mobilisation. J Hand Surg (Br) 14B:396–9, 1989.
5. Silfverskiöld KL, May EJ: Flexor tendon repair in zone II with a new suture technique and an early mobilization program combining passive and active flexion. J Hand Surg (Am) 19A:53–60, 1994.
6. Elliot D, Moiemen NS, Flemming AFS, Harris SB, Foster AJ: The rupture rate of acute flexor tendon repairs mobilised by the controlled active motion regimen. J Hand Surg (Br) 19B:507–12, 1994.
7. Evans RB, Thompson DE: The application of force to the healing tendon. J Hand Ther 6:266–84, 1993.
8. Sandow MJ, McMahon M: Single-cross grasp six-strand repair for acute flexor tenorrhaphy. Atlas Hand Clin 1:41–64, 1996.
9. Mason ML, Allen HS: The rate of healing of tendons. An experimental study of tensile strength. Ann Surg 113:424–56, 1941.
10. Potenza AD: Philosophy of flexor tendon surgery. Orthop Clin N Am 17:349–52, 1986.
11. Aoki M, Kubota H, Pruitt DL, Manske PR: Biomechanical and histologic characteristics of canine flexor tendon repair using early postoperative mobilization. J Hand Surg (Am) 22:107–14, 1997.
12. Duran RJ, Houser RG: Controlled passive motion following flexor tendon repair in zones 2 and 3. In: Symposium on Tendon Surgery in the Hand (AAOS). St Louis: Mosby, 1995.
13. Strickland JW: Management of acute flexor tendon injuries. Orthop Clin N Am 14:827–49, 1983.
14. Slattery PG, McGrouther DA: A modified Kleinert controlled mobilisation splint following flexor tendon repair. J Hand Surg (Br) 9B:217–18, 1984.
15. Chow JA, Thomes LJ, Dovelle S, Milnor WH, Seyfer AE, Smith AC: A combined regimen of controlled motion following flexor tendon repair in "no man's land." J Plast Recon Surg 79:447–53, 1987.
16. Chow JA, Thomes LJ, Dovelle S, Monsivais J, Milnor WH, Jackson JP: Controlled motion rehabilitation after flexor tendon repair and grafting. A multi-centre study. J Bone Joint Surg 70B:591–5, 1988.
17. Harmer TW: Tendon suture. Boston Med Surg J 808–10, 1917.
18. Schuind F, Garcia-Elias M, Cooney WP III et al: Flexor tendon forces: in vivo measurements. J Hand Surg (Am) 19A:291–8, 1992.
19. Strickland JW: Biologic rationale, clinical application, and results of early motion following flexor tendon repair. J Hand Ther 2:71–83, 1989.
20. Small JO, Brennan MD, Colville J: Early active mobilisation following flexor tendon repair in zone 2. J Hand Surg (Br) 14B:383–91, 1989.
21. Lee H: Double loop locking suture: a technique of tendon repair for early active mobilization. Part II: clinical experience. J Hand Surg (Am) 15A:953–8, 1990.
22. Gratton P: Early active mobilisation after flexor tendon repairs. J Hand Ther 6:285–9, 1993.
23. Strickland JW: The Indiana Method of flexor tendon repair. Atlas Hand Clin 1:77–103, 1996.
24. Savage R: The influence of wrist position on the minimum force required for active movement of the interphalangeal joints. J Hand Surg (Br) 13B:262–8, 1988.
25. Hall RF Jr, Vliegenthart DF: A modified mid-lateral incision for volar approach to the digit. J Hand Surg (Br) 11B:195–7, 1986.

E. EXTENSOR TENDON INJURY, REPAIR AND THERAPY

Rosemary Prosser and W Bruce Conolly

INTRODUCTION AND PATHOLOGICAL ANATOMY

Extensor tendons on the back of the hand are thin and flat with longitudinal fibres. Horizontal mattress sutures are needed for their repair. Extensor tendons have a shorter excursion and a less powerful lever action than flexor tendons.

The extensor system has its own intricacy and complexity. A tiny cut to divide the central slip if unrecognised and untreated may lead to an irreversible flexion contracture of the PIP joint and a hyperextension contracture of the distal interphalangeal (DIP) joint.

The extensor tendons are covered by thin untethered dorsal skin and lie close to the underlying skeleton. Injuries involving the skeleton then often involve the extensor apparatus.

SURGICAL TOPOGRAPHY

The location of a tendon injury in relation to the underlying skeleton will influence the deformity, function and impairment and the nature of treatment. Figure 2.42 shows the eight zones of extensor tendon injury of the fingers, thumb, hand and wrist.

INDICATIONS AND CONTRAINDICATIONS

Closed injuries are best treated by splintage for 6–8 weeks.

In open injuries there may be only a small degree of tendon retraction because of the abundance of interconnecting components, e.g. the retinacular fibre system over the joints and the intertendinous vincula between the tendons and the back of the hand. One exception is the EPL tendon which, if divided proximal to the MP joint, will retract strongly into the distal forearm because of the lack of interconnecting structures.

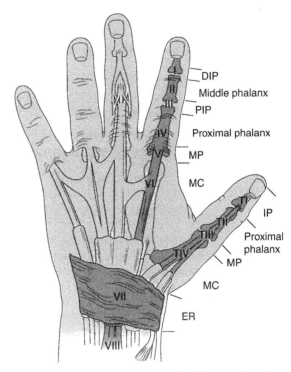

Figure 2.42 Zones of extensor tendon injury and repair. Note that there are eight zones for the finger, hand and wrist and four for the thumb. Zones I–VIII are shown. DIP = distal interphalangeal joint, PIP = proximal interphalangeal joint, MP = metacarpophalangeal joint, MC = metacarpal, IP = interphalangeal, ER = extensor retinaculum.

ZONE 1: MALLET INJURIES

The DIP joint is extended by two mechanisms, the thin terminal extensor tendon and the oblique retinacular ligament (ORL), both of which insert into the epiphysis at the base of the distal phalanx, blending with the dorsal joint capsule. Open injuries may involve the extensor apparatus, skin, bone and joint.

Closed injuries are best treated by extension splintage of the terminal joint for 6–8 weeks. Surgery to repair a ruptured extensor tendon in this area is difficult and often produces disappointing results.

If a piece of bone that is avulsed is sufficiently large as to allow the main fragment of the terminal phalanx to sublux volarward, then reduction of the subluxation by temporary fixation with a Kirschner wire is necessary. The avulsed fragment can be wired back into place if it is of sufficient size, i.e. greater than 30% of the joint surface.

Where there is open tendon injury, a few small sutures are used to oppose the tendon ends, but the prime treatment is extension splintage.

Post-injury and surgery management

The primary stay of treatment is splintage (Fig. 2.43A,B). Constant splinting 24 hours per day, with a 10-min skin airing interval for 6–8 weeks is necessary. The joint should be immobilised in neutral or slight hyperextension if possible. When the splint is removed for skin care, the DIP joint must be continually supported in hyperextension. The PIP joint is exercised to prevent stiffness at this level (Fig. 2.44).

After 6–8 weeks, the splint is discontinued in the day; gentle gross extension and flexion and daily activities are encouraged. The splint is continued at night for a further 2 weeks.

At week 8–12, depending on when the splint was removed, isolated DIP flexion is commenced.

Over the next 4 weeks a graduated resisted exercise and activity programme is carried out.

Attrition ruptures can be identified by the history. An attrition rupture usually occurs with a trivial incident which was not painful, such as tucking in the sheets while bedmaking. Attrition ruptures take longer to heal – up to 10 weeks of splinting may be required.

Specific tips

- This is not a demanding post-injury or surgery programme. Many patients just need individual guidance on the timing of the appropriate exercise and splint-wearing schedule.
- If the PIP joint is hypermobile and there is a tendency for the PIP to hyperextend, the PIP joint may need to be splinted in slight flexion while the DIP is being splinted in extension, if this tendency is not corrected with DIP extension splinting alone.

ZONE 2

Zone 2 lacerations are less common than zone 1 and 3 injuries and are often part of a complicated injury with skin loss and/or underlying fractures. The same principles apply as for surgery in zone 1.

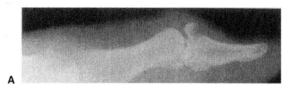

A

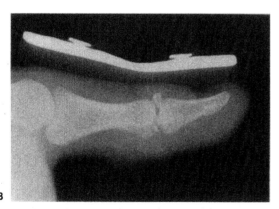

B

Figure 2.43 A: X-ray of a mallet injury in which a fragment of distal phalanx was avulsed. B: Reduction of the fragment and also extensor lag by splinting in slight hyperextension, as seen on X-ray.

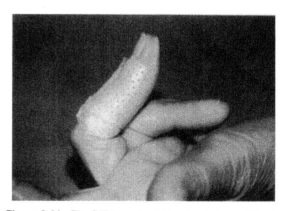

Figure 2.44 The PIP joint should be able to be mobilised to approximately 80–90 degrees while the DIP joint extension splintage is maintained.

ZONE 3: CENTRAL SLIP RUPTURES

Suspected closed ruptures can be tested by resisting PIP extension with the MP held in flexion. If there is excessive tone at the DIP joint, then central slip rupture should be suspected.

Closed or open injuries of the extensor apparatus over the PIP joint can produce a buttonhole deformity, which if untreated becomes a fixed flexion contracture of the PIP joint and a fixed DIP hyperextension contracture of the DIP joint.

Closed injuries are treated conservatively with a PIP extension splint.

In open injuries, surgical exploration and repair are mandatory. Most surgeons favour splinting the PIP joint in extension with a Kirschner wire for 2–3 weeks (Fig. 2.45), then carrying on further external splintage for a further 4–6 weeks, while maintaining DIP motion.

Post-injury and surgery management

Therapy post-injury and surgery are similar. The PIP joint is splinted constantly in extension for 2 weeks in a static digit splint or PIP digit cast.

DIP joint flexion is commenced within a few days of surgery or after the splint/cast application. This helps prevent oblique retinacular ligament tightness; it also pulls the extensor mechanism distally, reducing tension at the repair/injury site.

From weeks 2–6, a Capener splint is worn constantly (Fig. 2.46). PIP joint flexion and extension is usually commenced between 2 and 3 weeks. The patient is instructed not to flex beyond

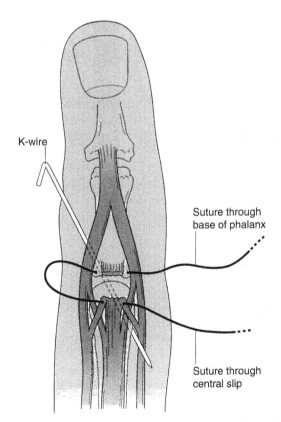

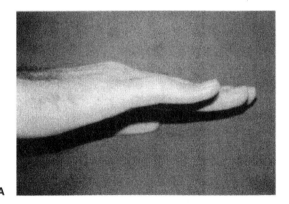

A

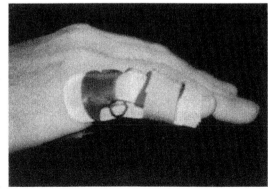

B

Figure 2.45 Repair of open central slip (buttonhole) zone 3 injury. The central slip is sutured to the base of the middle phalanx either to any remaining stump of tendon or through a drill hole through the bone. The lateral bands should lie in their normal dorsal position. A transarticular K-wire was passed across the PIP joint, avoiding the lateral bands for temporary splintage to enable early DIP joint exercises.

K-wire

Suture through base of phalanx

Suture through central slip

Figure 2.46 A Capener splint is worn from 2–6 weeks post-injury/surgery following central slip rupture. A Lycra sleeve is fitted under the Capener to control oedema.

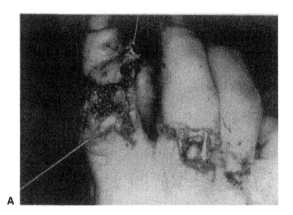

A

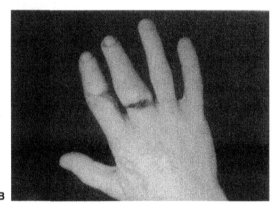

B

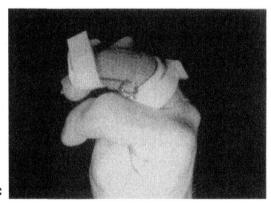

C

Figure 2.47 A: Gun shot injury showing significant soft tissue injury to the index and middle finger. The middle finger had loss of extensor tendon substance; the index finger extensor tendon was repaired. B: Healing at 4 weeks. C: Range of flexion at 8 weeks. Both digits were treated with static extension splintage from 2 weeks, then dynamic Capener splints for 6 weeks (plus 2 weeks at night only) for the index finger and 8 weeks (plus 2 weeks at night only) for the middle finger. Both digits gained flexion to the distal palmar crease and within 10 degrees of complete extension.

30 degrees until week 5 or 6. In cases of severe trauma where dense adhesion formation is likely to occur, free active flexion is encouraged from week 2 (Fig. 2.47). Maximal range of flexion is encouraged within the Capener splint. The splint is worn at all times.

At week 6 the patient is weaned from the Capener splint in the day. It is still worn at night for a further 2–4 weeks. Full gross flexion is allowed and light resisted activity is commenced. Full resisted activity should be aimed to be achieved by 12 weeks post-repair or initial splinting.

Early short arc (30 degree) active motion has been described in the literature:[1] a dorsal and volar blocking splint may be used to achieve this. In this programme, early active flexion and extension to 30 degrees is commenced as soon as the splint is applied, i.e. within the first week. DIP flexion is commenced immediately to stretch the ORL and improve DIP flexion. Full gross flexion and light resistance are commenced at week 6 and splinting is discontinued.

An early controlled motion programme in which the digit is splinted in an outrigger splint with a 30 degree flexion stop has also been described.[2] Active flexion to 30 degrees is allowed in the splint; the rubber band traction provides the passive extension force. The splint is worn for 4 weeks; at this time active PIP joint extension is initiated.

Specific tips

- A compression digit sleeve or wrap should always be worn under a Capener splint to prevent oedema at the PIP joint.
- Good patient compliance is vital for an early active motion programme to be considered.
- If an extensor lag is evident after removal of the splint, a further 2 weeks of splinting may be necessary. During this time, gross flexion exercises may need to be discontinued.

ZONE 4

Zone 4 lacerations are usually simple transverse lacerations proximal to the insertion of the intrinsic tendon.

Post-injury and surgery management

The MP and PIP joints are splinted in extension for 4–6 weeks. Night-time protective splintage is continued for 2 more weeks. DIP joint motion is commenced immediately. At 4 weeks gentle active exercises for the MPs and PIPs in isolation – i.e. MP motion with the PIP held in extension and vice versa. The exercise programme is graduated over the next 4 weeks.

ZONES 5 AND 6: MP AND MC LEVEL

Zone 5

Laceration of the extensor tendon over the MCP joint often involves laceration through into the joint. If this occurs as part of a punch penetrating injury, primary wound toilet and irrigation of the joint and antibiotics should be carried out as soon as possible and tendon repair delayed until there is no sign of wound infection.

Zone 6

Here, where the tendons are thin and flat, the suture technique must grasp the tendon ends securely to prevent rupture and neatly to minimise adhesions (Fig. 2.48).

It is essential for these patients to regain flexion and a fist. Failure of full flexion may be a bigger problem than failure of full extension.

Postoperative management of zones 5 & 6

Following repair, the MP joints should be splinted in extension for 4–6 weeks constantly and for a further 2–4 weeks at night and for at-risk situations, e.g. travel and social functions. The PIP joints may also need to be splinted in extension if the disruption to the tendon is in the distal region, i.e. over the MP.

A static or dynamic splint can be used. The type of splint used must be assessed by the therapist and surgeon. A dynamic splint allows early movement and is reported to give less stiffness. It is, however, much more expensive to fabricate and more cumbersome to wear. A static splint is easier to fabricate and more economical but does increase postoperative stiffness if a conservative programme is followed.

The conservative static splint programme does not permit small-range MP joint flexion and extension until 3 weeks post-repair. The splint rests the wrist in approximately 30 degrees of extension, the MPs in 30 degrees flexion and the IPs in full extension (0 degrees) (Fig. 2.49).

Active DIP exercises can be commenced immediately. PIP joint exercises can be commenced immediately if the repair is proximal: if it is distal, PIP exercise may not be commenced until week 3. At 2 weeks, the sutures are removed and wound care is commenced. At 3 weeks, active MP exercises are commenced. Both extensor digitorum

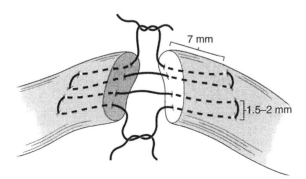

Figure 2.48 Technique for extension tendon repair. Note the double horizontal mattress suture.

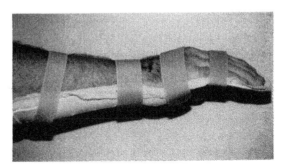

Figure 2.49 Static splinting for extensor tendon repair zones 5 and 6 is simple and inexpensive. The wrist is in 30 degrees extension, MPs in 30 degrees flexion and IPs, if included, in full extension (0 degrees).

communis (EDC) and composite extension are practised: first in inner range, then progressing to greater ranges over the next 2–3 weeks.

Light resisted activity is started at 6 weeks; full resisted activity is not permitted until 12 weeks post-repair.

The early controlled motion programme requires a dynamic splint with a 30 degree flexion block for 6 weeks.[3] In the first 6 weeks active IP exercises and active MP flexion to 30 degrees is carried out. The splint provides a passive extension force from 30 degrees to neutral. The splint is removed at 6 weeks and full gross flexion and light resisted activity is permitted.

The Norwich active extensor tendon programme,[4] reported in the literature, utilises a resting static splint that holds the MPs in some flexion and the IPs in full extension and the wrist in extension. The patient practises gross extension and EDC action of the digits while still in the splint: i.e. active extension with the wrist held in extension to protect the repair as soon as the splint is applied. The splint is worn for 6 weeks.

Howell[5] also reports on an immediate controlled active motion programme. The wrist is splinted in extension (20 degrees). Flexion of the involved digit(s) is limited by splintage in 15 degrees more extension than the other digits in a digit-based splint. The splint is worn for 4–6 weeks. Active motion of the IPs and MPs is permitted with the splints on as soon as the splints are applied.

Specific tips

- Extensor tendon adhesion over the metacarpals is a common problem. Early oedema control, including compression wraps or garments, diligent massage plus early controlled motion are the main techniques that will reduce this problem. Patients who scar densely or those who also have a bony injury may need special attention to minimise this. If dense scar and tendon adhesion are obvious by week 4, then splints should be discarded and therapy concentrated on regaining motion.

- Buddy strapping may help encourage extension once the splint is removed.

ZONES 7 AND 8: THE WRIST LEVEL

Zone 7

In this zone, extensor tendons in the six compartments are really in a synovial-lined fibro-osseous tunnel similar to the flexor apparatus in the digit. Divided extensor tendons tend to retract and become tethered. The same technique is used as for flexor tendons with a meticulous junction which will glide in this fibro-osseous tunnel. At least part of the extensor retinaculum should be preserved to prevent bow stringing.

Zone 8

Extensor tendon injuries proximal to the extensor retinaculum should be sutured the same as for flexor tendons severed above the wrist. The wrist is splinted in extension for 6 weeks due to the poor vascularity of the distal end of the wrist extensor tendons.

Post-surgical management of zones 7 and 8

The wrist is splinted in 30–40 degrees of extension for 6 weeks. Wound and scar care follow the usual guidelines. Active wrist extension is commenced in week 4. Light resisted activity is started in week 6 and upgraded gradually over the next 6 weeks.

THE THUMB

Tendon injuries in zones 1 and 2 – i.e. over the terminal joint and the proximal phalanx – are treated in the same way as zones 1 and 2 in the fingers. At the metacarpophalangeal joint there is no central slip, and injuries in this area and in zone 4, over the metacarpal, are treated as in zone 6 on the back of the hand.

Postoperative care

The thumb is splinted in extension and radial abduction for approximately 4–6 weeks and a further 2 weeks for sleep. Radial abduction prevents thumb web contracture. Active exercises are commenced at approximately 3 weeks post-repair. Resistance is commenced at 6 weeks.

Specific tip

If the patient has IP hyperextension, the thumb should be splinted in hyperextension: if it is not, then the normal hyperextension used for pinch will be lost.

RESULTS AND COMPLICATIONS

As with all tendon repairs, the main complications are adhesions and joint stiffness, or rupture of the repair. In the case of extensor tendon repair, the results are affected by the presence of associated injury (fracture, joint injury, skin loss).

EXTENSOR TENDON RECONSTRUCTION

Extensor tendons over the dorsum of the hand and digit can lose function from loss of substance or adhesions from injury, infection or disease, e.g. rheumatoid arthritis.

Extensor tendon function can be restored directly by delayed tendon repair, tendon transfer, tendon graft (Fig. 2.50) or tenolysis in the case of adhesions, or indirectly by joint arthrodesis.

In particular, extensor tendon grafting is indicated where there is multiple loss of extensor tendon at the back of the hand. These grafts will have a proximal junction in the distal forearm proximal to the extensor retinaculum and distally to the extensor hood over the MCP joints. Occasionally, two-stage extensor grafting is carried out using a preliminary silicone spacer.

It is wise to splint such grafted areas for 6 weeks; active extension can be delayed until 4 weeks postoperatively. The post-surgical therapy programme is similar to that following zones 5 and 6 extensor tendon repair.

Occasionally, smaller grafts are needed to replace the lost mechanism over the PIP joint and

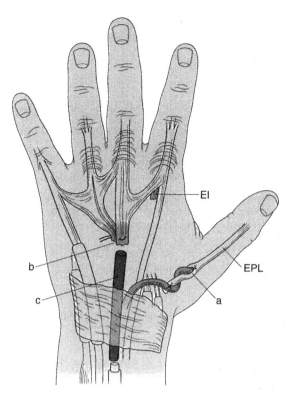

Figure 2.50   Some types of extensor tendon reconstruction: (a) EI to EPL; (b) EDC of ring finger sutured to EDC of middle finger; (c) interposition graft for EDC of middle finger with proximal junction at the distal forearm.

the same principles of prolonged splintage and delayed active exercise are followed.

Postoperative management following two-stage grafting

After the first stage, the hand is rested in a static volar splint, which holds the wrist in 30 degrees extension, MPs in 30 degrees of flexion and IPs in full extension. The splint is worn for approximately 4 weeks.

The surgery and incision is extensive; the silicone spacer rod is also a foreign body. For these reasons, the patient often needs 3–7 days of rest in the splint before commencing exercises. During this period, oedema and wound management is essential. This takes the form of elevation, cold packs and gentle compression wraps if appropriate.

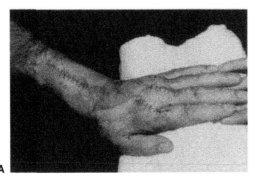 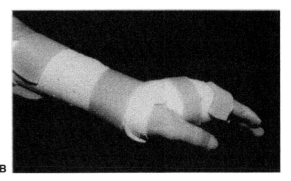

A   B

Figure 2.51 A: Extensor tendon reconstruction grafting 1 week postoperative. B: Splinting maintains the wrist in 30 degrees extension, MPs in 30 degrees flexion, and IPs are permitted to flex to approximately 60 degrees.

Exercises commence 3–7 days postoperative, with both active and passive movements. The MPs can only be extended passively.

The silastic rod(s) needs to be in place for at least 3 months so that a tunnel for the new tendon is formed. During this time strong vigorous activity is discouraged, as this may cause the rods to dislodge.

Postoperative management after the second stage – extensor tendon grafting

Therapy following this stage is similar to the post-extensor tendon repair programme for zones 5–8. Splinting following extensor tendon grafting second stage can be seen in Figure 2.51.

REFERENCES

1. Evans R, Thompson D: An analysis of factors that support early active short arc motion of the repaired central slip. J Hand Ther 5:187–201, 1992.
2. Walsh M, Rinehimer W, Muntzer E, Patel J, Sitler M: Early controlled motion with dynamic splinting versus static splinting for Zones III and IV extensor tendon lacerations: a preliminary report. J Hand Ther 7:232–6, 1994.
3. Evans I: Therapeutic management of extensor tendon injuries. In: Hunter J, Schneider L, Mackin E,

Callahan A (eds), Rehabilitation of the hand, 4th edn. Philadelphia: Mosby, 19:492–511, 1994.
4. Sylaidis P, Youatt M, Logan A: Early mobilization for extensor tendon injuries. J of Hand Surg (Br & Eur) 22B (5):594–6, 1997.
5. Howell J: Management of extensor tendon injuries of the fingers. The Upper Limb Symposium Course Proceedings, 4–6 July 1997.

F. TENDINITIS, TENOSYNOVITIS AND TENDON ENTRAPMENT

Rosemary Prosser and W Bruce Conolly

INTRODUCTION

Tendinitis and tenosynovitis are both conditions which involve inflammation and swelling of the tendon, the tendon synovium or the tendon sheath. This limits glide and thus the ability for the muscle tendon unit to contract, stretch and perform its function.

PATHOLOGICAL ANATOMY

The flexor tendon excursion varies from 18 mm to 85 mm.[1] In each digit the long flexor tendons and their synovial bursae run within a fibrous flexor sheath. Bow stringing of the tendons is resisted by the annular and cruciform pulley system.

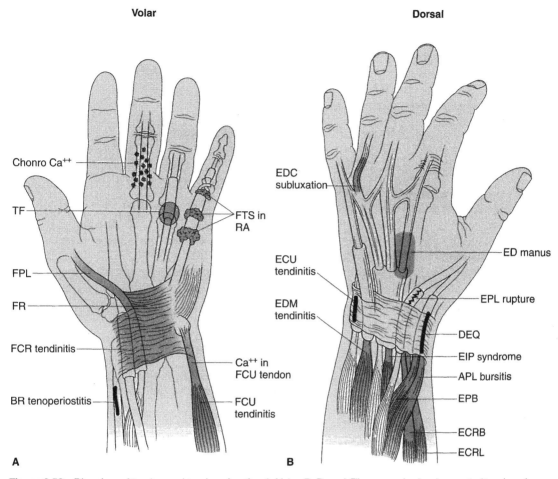

Volar

Chonro Ca^{++}

TF

FTS in RA

FPL

FR

FCR tendinitis

Ca^{++} in FCU tendon

BR tenoperiostitis

FCU tendinitis

A

Dorsal

EDC subluxation

ED manus

ECU tendinitis

EPL rupture

EDM tendinitis

DEQ

EIP syndrome

APL bursitis

EPB

ECRB

ECRL

B

Figure 2.52   Disorders of tendon and tendon sheaths. A: Volar. B: Dorsal. There may be involvement of tendons in any of the six extensor compartments. (Reproduced with permission from Conolly WB: Atlas of hand surgery. New York: Churchill Livingstone, 1997.)

Tendons are relatively avascular structures whose gliding is facilitated by a surrounding layer of tenosynovium. The tendon substance itself is surrounded by a thin fibrous and cellular layer called epitenon which is adherent to the tendon surface. The tendons and their associated structures of synovium, tendon sheath and retinaculum (Fig. 2.52) may be affected by:

- local anatomical anomalies
- occupational factors (forced repetitive activity in musicians and athletes and certain occupations)
- trauma, either a single episode or repeated
- irregularity after fracture

- metabolic factors, including diabetes, rheumatoid arthritis, etc.
- inflammation and infections.

CLINICAL FEATURES AND DIAGNOSIS

- The patient may present with an acute, subacute or chronic disorder.
- The symptoms include pain over the site of the tendon disorder aggravated by movement with blocking, catching or triggering. There may be pain referred to a distal joint in a

trigger condition or proximally up the muscle tendon unit.

- The physical signs include local swelling and tenderness with decreased movement.
- Crepitus and sometimes an associated neuritis of the overlying cutaneous nerves.
- There may be a palpable ganglion or swelling of the tendon sheath.

INVESTIGATIONS

1. Plain X-rays may be indicated to check the underlying skeleton and to exclude calcification.
2. Ultrasound imaging can show enlargement of the tendon and the presence of synovitis, tendon rupture or associated ganglion.
3. Relevant blood and pathology tests for rheumatoid arthritis, diabetes, gout and tuberculosis may be indicated.

CONSERVATIVE MANAGEMENT OF TENDON AND TENDON SHEATH DISORDERS

- A precise and comprehensive assessment is necessary to determine which structures are affected. Specific tests for the tendon are essential. Finkelstein's test, which involves wrist ulnar deviation (UD) and thumb adduction with MP flexion, is a good indicator for de Quervain's tenosynovitis. Trigger finger triggering or crepitus can be assessed by palpation over the A1 pulley. Good anatomical knowledge of the tendon path, the pulleys it passes through and its specific action is essential for accurate assessment.
- Where there is severe inflammation in association with constriction of the tendon a rigid low-temperature thermoplastic splint (Fig. 2.53) is used until the pain has settled. This may take from 2 to 6 weeks; during this time, joint motion should be monitored. After this period, a flexible neoprene support (Fig. 2.54) may be necessary to give support while motion and strength are being gained.
- Electrophysical agents such as ultrasound or ice may assist in decreasing acute pain and inflammation. Once inflammation has settled,

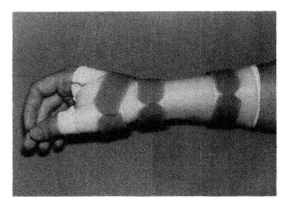

Figure 2.53 A low-temperature thermoplastic splint used in the conservative management of De Quervain's tenosynovitis. This is a radial thumb post splint in palmar abduction made from 1.6 mm splinting material.

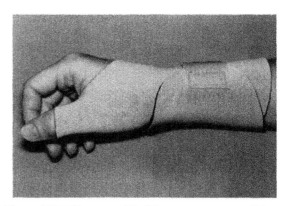

Figure 2.54 Wraparound flexible neoprene support. This type of support gives some support to the thumb and wrist without immobilising the area. It may facilitate weaning from a rigid splint and act as a reminder not to over-stress the thumb EPB and abductor pollicis longus (AbdPL).

heat may be more effective in terms of pain relief and increasing soft tissue mobility.

- After 1 or 2 weeks of splinting a gentle progressive exercise programme is begun to prevent joint stiffness and tendon adhesions. The exercise programme is progressed slowly and monitored closely. Initially, only gentle stretches are used. If pain and irritability are controlled, active exercise is commenced. Several weeks later, resisted exercise and activity are added. The ultimate goal is to improve the entire muscle–tendon unit function in terms of endurance, range and strength.
- Long-term activity modification may be necessary for recovery and prevention of recurrences.

SPECIFIC TIPS

1. De Quervain's tenosynovitis – this condition is common in new mothers and renovators. It is usually aggravated by radial and ulnar deviation activity: lifting and holding a growing baby or using a paint brush or paint scraper. It is important to cease aggravating activity; activity modification can be very effective. In the mother's case, alternate lifting and breast-feeding holding positions need to be adopted. The breast-feeding mother is more susceptible to aggravation of the condition due to the hormonal effect on the soft tissues.

2. Trigger finger – a night MP and IP extension splint may be necessary to completely rest the tendon. A day-time extension splint (Fig. 2.55) described by Evans et al.[2] has limited impact on function and rests the tendon where it passes through the A1 pulley. Conservative treatment should be trialled for 4–6 weeks.

CORTICOSTEROID INJECTIONS FOR DISORDERS OF TENDON AND TENDON SHEATHS

Most of the inflammatory conditions of the tendon and its associated structures respond, at least temporarily, to steroid injections. It is preferable to use a soluble steroid preparation. The various risks and benefits of steroid injection should be discussed with the patient prior to the injection. In particular, patients should be warned of possible fat atrophy and skin depigmentation. This is particularly important in dark-skinned races. When performing the injection, care needs to be taken to avoid intraneural or intratendinous

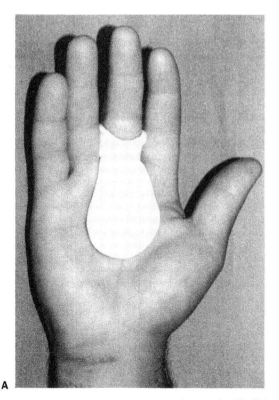
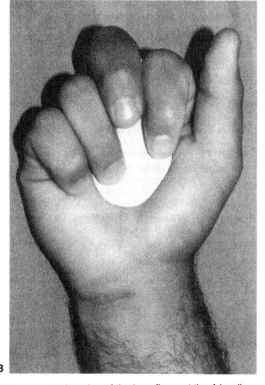

Figure 2.55 Small digit-based trigger finger splint (A). This splint prevents triggering of the long flexor at the A1 pulley by limiting MP flexion. There is good patient compliance, as it allows enough flexion to make a reasonably functional grip, enabling most patients to work with the splint on (B). It is usually worn for 6 weeks if the trigger is being managed conservatively.

injection. Infection in the area is a contraindication to corticosteroid injection.

A steroid injection is only part of an overall treatment plan that involves initial rest, analgesia and splintage followed by progressive increase in activity as appropriate.

- The technique for corticosteroid injection involves the injection of 2–3 ml of triamcinolone mixed with an equal volume of 1% Xylocaine (lignocaine) given into the tenosynovial space proximal and distal to the relevant pulley sheaths. Injection can be performed up to three times every 3–6 weeks. A 2 ml syringe and a 25-gauge needle is used for injection proximal and/or distal to the A1 pulley.[3]

OPERATIVE TREATMENT

Operative treatment may include surgical decompression of the fibrous tendon sheath, resection of inflamed synovia and resection of an associated ganglion. Rarely is there an indication for excision of calcium deposits or repair or reconstruction of the tendon system.

INDICATIONS FOR SURGERY

In general, all these disorders of the tendon and tendon sheaths should be managed conservatively for 6–8 weeks. If there is not marked improvement by then, surgery is indicated.

NONSPECIFIC INFLAMMATORY CONDITIONS
FCR tendinitis

FCR tendinitis may be secondary to arthritis of the first carpometacarpal (CMC) or scaphotrapezial trapezoid (STT) joint. The tight FCR tendon sheath is incised through a volar Z-shaped incision. Care should be taken to avoid damage to the palmar cutaneous branch of the median nerve, the lateral cutaneous nerve of the forearm and the superficial branch of the radial nerve.

Postoperative management

The wrist is splinted for approximately 2 weeks. During this time the splint is removed for gentle limited-range wrist motion within pain limits. A soft support may be beneficial for several weeks after this. If there is CMC or STT involvement, the thumb may need to be included in the splint.

At 2 weeks a very gentle stretching and graded exercise programme is commenced. Ice and ultrasound can be helpful in reducing early inflammation. In the authors' experience, a graded resisted activity programme is often more effective than a formal resisted exercise programme.

Underlying arthritis should be treated if it is symptomatic (see Chapter 4).

CONSTRICTIVE STATES: STENOSING TENOVAGINITIS

This condition gives rise to a disproportion between the tendon, which may be thick from hypertrophy or injury, and the tunnel, which may be narrowed from degenerative thickening or post-traumatic fibrosis.

De Quervain's disease

The APL, which often has several slips, and EPB can be in a combined or in separate tunnels in the first dorsal compartment. The retinacular roof may be very thick and even have an associated ganglion. There may also be an associated radial neuritis. The compartment is released by either an oblique, longitudinal or transverse incision (Fig. 2.56).

There should be a 95% success rate.[4] Complications which may occur include radial neuritis or neuroma, an unsightly scar, an unreleased EPB or volar subluxation of APL.

Postoperative management

Rigid splintage of the thumb and wrist for 1–2 days after surgery may be necessary. Subsequently, a neoprene support (see Fig. 2.54) is used for a further 3–4 weeks until the tendon has gained sufficient extensibility and strength. Exercises in

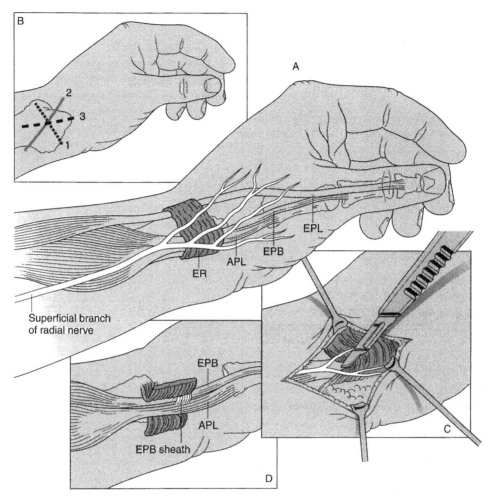

Figure 2.56 Release of De Quervain's condition: A: The anatomy of the first extensor compartment and the superficial branch of the radial nerve. B: A transverse incision leaves the best cosmetic scar but exposure may be compromised and there is probably more risk of injury to the superficial branch of the radial nerve. For this reason an oblique incision in the line of the radial nerve is probably safest. C and D: Incise and expose the tendons of APL and EPB. There may be two separate compartments. There may be multiple divisions of APL. Apply traction each to APL and then to EPB to demonstrate there is unrestricted glide and action of each tendon individually on the CMC joint and the MP joint, respectively.

terms of short arc wrist flexion/extension, radial and ulnar deviation and very gentle abductor pollicis longus (AbdPL) and EPB gliding within pain limits are commenced within the first post-operative week. A graded programme moving from active to resisted exercise is used. If radial neuritis is present, desensitisation techniques, TENS (transcutaneous electrical nerve stimulation) and other therapy techniques such as interferential and neural gliding may be needed.

The programme should be monitored closely and not progressed too quickly. Progression should be assessed on an individual basis.

Trigger finger and trigger thumb

Triggering is invariably at the A1 pulley. The A1 pulley is released through a transverse oblique or longitudinal approach. A full glide of the released tendon, FDP, FDS and FPL should be noted.

Postoperative management

Full passive extension of the digit at operation should be maintained by passive and active exercises, which are started within the first week postoperation. Emphasis should be on IP extension and flexion, with the MPs in extension. Splintage may be necessary after operation for early return to work or if progress is slow. A small MP volar extension splint (see Fig. 2.55) is adequate during the day. A hand-based digit extension splint may be necessary at night. There may be a slow recovery in diabetics and patients with associated Dupuytren's disease or osteoarthritis.

Intersection syndrome: oarsman's wrist

This condition is reported in the literature as being particularly associated with rowers,[5] due to repetitive wrist motion with the thumb in abduction. The APL becomes irritated as it crosses the radial wrist extensors, ECRL and ECRB proximal to Lister's tubercle. Surgical release is only occasionally indicated.

Conservative management involves primarily soft tissue massage, ECRL and ECRB stretches, electrotherapy, eccentric strengthening and, occasionally, splinting in the acute stage. Activity modification, especially in rowers, in terms of training intensity and technique may be required.

EPL tendinitis

This condition can occur after distal radial fractures and may be complicated by tendon rupture. Conservative treatment follows the general guidelines outlined above. In cases of failed conservative treatment, the EPL tendon is re-routed from its third compartment or Lister's tubercle removed. Tendon rupture is treated by EPL transfer using EIP.

REFERENCES

1. Simmons BP, De La Caffiniere JY: Physiology of flexion of the finger. In: Tubiana R (ed.), The hand. Philadelphia: WB Saunders, 1981:384.
2. Evans RB, Hunter JM, Borkhatter WE: Conservative management of the trigger finger: a new approach. J Hand Ther 1:59–68, 1988.
3. Harvey F: De Quervain's disease: surgical or nonsurgical treatment. J Hand Surg 15A:83, 1990.
4. Lamphier TA, Pepi JF, Brush CH, Ostrogen J: De Quervain's disease. J Int Coll Surg 31:192, 1959.
5. Grundberg AB, Reagan DS: Pathologic anatomy of the forearm: intersection syndrome. J Hand Surg 10A:299, 1985.

G. BURNS

Elaine Juzl and Annette Leveridge

INTRODUCTION

A major burn with severely burnt hands is one of the biggest challenges a hand therapist will encounter. Involvement of the skin and underlying structures can result in the development of contractures and functional limitations. It is vital that the team approach is used.

PATHOPHYSIOLOGY

The initial reaction of the body to a burn is to try to dissipate heat by dilating blood vessels, making the skin more erythematous.

Continuing heat increases the permeability of the walls of the blood vessels, leading to leakage into surrounding tissues. This causes the local circulation to become sluggish, and the heat forces cells to die.

Fluid loss starts immediately, mainly into the damaged tissues and surrounding areas, resulting in gross oedema.

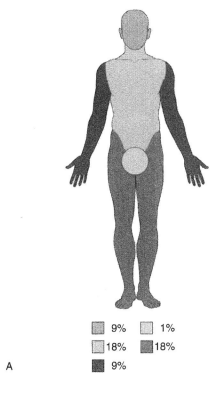

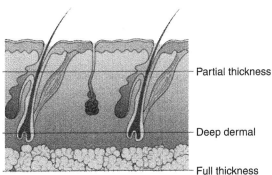

B

Figure 2.57 Surface areas of the body (A) and classification of burns (B).

The depth of skin damage affects the surgical management and subsequent rehabilitation of burn injury (Fig. 2.57).

Partial-thickness burn (superficial dermal). This type of burn heals spontaneously in 10–21 days. Tissue destruction involves the epidermis and superficial layers of the dermis. Protein-rich tissue fluid exudes from the wound. A crust (eschar) forms and separates some days later, revealing healed skin underneath.

Deep dermal burn. The epidermis and a significant amount of the dermis is destroyed; blistering occurs. Spontaneous healing may take 3–4 weeks. The burn is best skin grafted within 3–5 days before dead tissue is colonised by bacteria. Graft take is usually excellent with minimal scarring, allowing early and rapid rehabilitation.

Full-thickness skin loss. Accessory structures – e.g. nerve endings, hair follicles, sweat and sebaceous glands – have been destroyed in the burn. The wound is charred or watery in appearance with no blistering and is insensitive to pin prick. Large areas will only heal by application of a skin graft.

Classification of burn injury

Thermal burns

Thermal burns include:

- scalds, usually partial skin loss
- flame and contact burns, usually full-thickness loss with some partial-thickness area
- flash burns, generally partial thickness.

Chemical burns

Chemical burns are usually full-thickness burns. The chemical penetrates into deeper tissue if not catalysed; therefore, the chemical formula of the substance must be known.

Electrical burns

Electrical burns are generally full-thickness burns. There will be an entrance and exit burn, with damage between the two.

The severity of shock relates to the surface area of the skin damage rather than the depth of burn. The area of burn injury can be approximately estimated by using the 'rule of nines' (Fig. 2.57).

The temperature and duration of the burn will determine the amount of tissue destruction.

ASSESSMENT

As soon as the patient is admitted, a full assessment is carried out to ascertain the cause, severity and depth of the burn. Burns of the hands often accompany large degree burns. Life-threatening factors such as fluid resuscitation and inhalation injuries will therefore be dealt with first.

The depth of the burn. This is the most important factor in predicting the healing and outcome of the burn. Assessment must be made before the application of any preparations.

Burns to the dorsum of the hands. The hands are often used in a reflex action to protect the face, so that burns to the dorsal surface are more common than the palmar surface. There is often associated extensor tendon damage because the skin is thinner and the tendons closer to the surface.

The circulation to the digits. This needs to be assessed and monitored. A surgical release or escharotomy may need to be performed as a matter of urgency, particularly in the case of circumferential burns.

Other hand conditions and injuries. Conditions such as rheumatoid arthritis and fractures need to be assessed. Assessment of range of movement, muscle power, dexterity and function will be carried out at regular intervals as a record of progress, a means of 'highlighting' areas of concern and for liaison between professionals.

REHABILITATION – KEY ELEMENTS

The purpose of rehabilitation is to maintain mobility, prevent the development of contractures and promote hand and limb function. The key elements affecting the treatment of burns include:

Pain. Superficial and deep dermal burns of the hands can be particularly painful, because the dense nerve network is still intact. This can make rehabilitation a very challenging experience, as uncontrolled pain will contribute to postural deformities and affect patient compliance. Regular analgesia such as intravenous morphine will be necessary. Supplementary Entonox (nitrous oxide + oxygen mixture) may be required for treatment. Pain will reduce once skin cover has been achieved.

Oedema. After burn injury there is a massive inflammatory reaction with consequent swelling

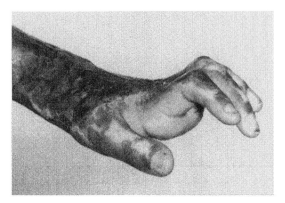

Figure 2.58   Hand burn – intrinsic minus deformity position. (Reproduced with permission of Nelson Thornes Ltd from Therapy for the Burn Patient, Leveridge, 1991.)

of the whole hand. An oedematous hand adopts the 'position of deformity' (Fig. 2.58).

Periods of immobility. After skin grafting there will be a period of immobilisation, which may be prolonged if further grafts are required. The hand is splinted in the position of safe immobilisation.

Reduced cooperation. Prolonged periods of bed rest and length of stay in hospital as well as pain are factors which may make it difficult for the patient to cooperate with treatment. Other contributory factors are the patient's age, i.e. the young and the elderly, and mental and social status prior to burn injury.

Contractile properties of scar tissue. The normal healing process of the skin results in the formation of a scar that has contractile properties. Prolonged inflammation followed by simultaneous epithelialisation from wound edges, wound closure by myofibroblasts and a rapid increase in the formation of collagen by fibroblasts produces contractile scar tissue.

HAND THERAPY

Early rehabilitation

From the moment the general condition of the patient is stable, rehabilitation commences and is directed towards functional independence.

Positioning

Elevation. Positioning is vital. The upper limb needs to be elevated using a Bradford sling to

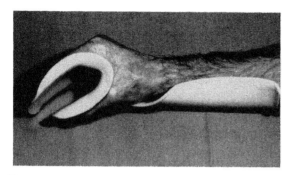

Figure 2.59 Hand in Pansplint anti-deformity position. (Reproduced with permission of Nelson Thornes Ltd from Therapy for the Burn Patient, Leveridge, 1991.)

prevent and/or reduce swelling and so lessen the likelihood of contractures. It will be necessary to take the arm out of the sling at regular intervals for exercises: e.g. full elbow extension for burns of the flexor aspect of the elbow. If the patient is ventilated and sedated, it may be possible to rest the arm on a raised table to achieve elevation while keeping the elbow extended.

Splints. The anti-deformity positions can be maintained by using pillows or rolled towels, or splints may be needed (Fig. 2.59). Superficial burns with a full range of movement should not need splinting but any patient finding it difficult to maintain range, or with a burn of greater depth, will need splinting.

Splinting

In acute burns, splints may be needed to:

1. maintain joints in the safe position
2. to help overcome the effects of oedema
3. to protect an exposed tendon.

The safe or anti-deformity position (rather than the functional position) is indicated for burns to the dorsum of the hand, circumferential burns and volar wrist burns:

- wrist: 30–40 degrees
- MCP joints: 60–70 degrees flexion (70 degrees flexion maintains the collateral ligaments at their maximum length)
- IP joints: full extension
- thumb: full abduction and slight extension to preserve the first web space.

Splinting regime for palmar burns:

- wrist: neutral position
- palm: dorsal or volar 'pan splints' holding hand in extension to prevent palmar contractures
- MP and IP extension, finger abduction and thumb abduction and extension.

In the case of ventilated or uncooperative patients, splinting should be continuous and splints only removed for exercise and dressing change. The therapist must be particularly vigilant about pressure areas and alter splints as necessary.

Wrist

When there is a tendency for the wrist to be held in flexion, a volar wrist extension splint in neutral to 10 degrees of extension can be worn.

Shoulder/elbow

If there is a burn on the flexor aspect of the elbow, there may be a need for a static extension splint. A burn under and around the axilla needs an 'aeroplane' splint to abduct the shoulder to 90 degrees.

Exercise

Hands will be dressed in plastic hand bags to keep burns protected from infection and moist while allowing unlimited exercise and function. An antibacterial agent such as silver sulphadiazine (Flamazine) can be used in the bag.

Active exercise will be the treatment of first choice, although assistance may need to be given by the therapist to achieve maximal range of movement. Active exercise helps reduce swelling by pumping the fluid proximally, maintains normal tendon glide and reduces the formation of adhesions.

All joints need to be put through their full range in isolation and as a mass movement. Full distal interphalangeal joint (DIP) flexion needs to be encouraged when making a fist, as this is often lacking. It is important to remember web and lumbrical stretches in order to prevent any stiffness. Rigorous attention to full range, good positioning and elevation in the early stages can prevent oedema and further complications of joint stiffness later.

Exposed tendons

If involvement of the extensor mechanism is suspected, certain precautions need to be considered:

- The hand should be splinted when not exercising.
- No passive flexion should be performed.
- The hand must be kept moist at all times to prevent drying out of the tendons and subsequent rupture. Exercises must therefore be carried out under water or with the dressings intact.
- Full fist making should only be carried out under supervision.
- To reduce the stresses on the tendons while maintaining full joint range, interphalangeal flexion can be performed with the MCPs in extension and interphalangeal extension with the MCPs in flexion.
- A single exposed central slip can be protected with a small gutter extension splint. Surgical fixation of the PIP joint with Kirschner wires may be necessary to allow bridging of the central slip by scar tissue.

Activities of daily living

- Personal independence of patients while on the Burns Unit should be encouraged
- Help with daily living activity will increase the patient's self-esteem and independence
- Enlarged handles may be required while the hand is maintained in plastic hand bags
- Book supports, playing card holders and page turners will assist the patient to start functional use and provide mental stimuli.

Light activity therapy

Attention must be paid to prevent blistering or oedema of the delicate tissues of the hand.
  For example:

- gross pinch – solitaire, dominoes and scrabble
- fine pinch – pick-up sticks, quilling.

Intermediate rehabilitation

Wound healing and skin grafting

If healing does not occur spontaneously within 2–3 weeks, split skin grafts are applied and the area immobilised for 3–5 days until grafts adhere (take). Extensive exposure of tendons on the dorsum of the hand or fingers or excision of deep necrosed tissue can be covered with a skin and subcutaneous tissue flap, e.g. cross finger flap. The flap area is immobilised for 1–2 weeks.

Skin grafts

Split skin grafts are a sheet of skin shaved through the dermis, either laid on in sheet form or cut into strips or squares. Meshing the skin to (Fig. 2.60) expand it allows a larger area of burn to be covered. Split skin grafts do not grow hair and have no sweat or sebaceous glands. They have a tendency to shrink and cause contractures, particularly over joints.

Full-thickness grafts do not contract and have a better texture and colour.

Skin flaps

Skin flaps contain subcutaneous tissue and have their own blood supply. They do not contract.

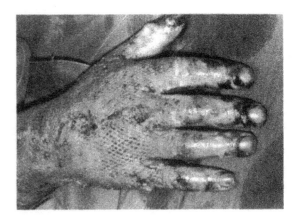

Figure 2.60 Mesh grafted hands post-burn. (Reproduced with permission of Nelson Thornes Ltd from Therapy for the Burn Patient, Leveridge, 1991.)

Exercise

At the first change of dressing, the take and stability of the graft will be assessed before exercises are commenced. With the dressings down, the range of movement can be measured, stresses on the grafted areas seen and exercises performed. Mobilisation will initially be gentle, with assistance at end of range only. Hand holds need to be carefully considered to minimise friction to the newly grafted areas.

Any dressings that need to be reapplied should be as light as possible, and large joints such as the elbow need jointed dressings to allow as full a range of movement as possible. Elevation and positioning, started preoperatively, need to be continued.

Once the scar is stable, treatment can become more vigorous and passive stretches included. During the healing process, the alignment and orientation of collagen fibres can be influenced by the stresses which are applied. Stretches at this stage can therefore influence the range of movement. Active exercises must follow passive stretches to strengthen and maintain any range gained.

Once the patient's general condition allows, endurance, strengthening and general flexibility exercises can be taught to counteract the effects of general anaesthesia, bed rest and hospitalisation. This could include static bike, rowing machines, putty exercises and ball games.

Joint mobilisations

Joint mobilisations are used if limitations to movement are due to joint stiffness as well as scar tissue.

Continuous passive motion (CPM)

The main advantage of CPM (Fig. 2.61) is that it can maintain gentle range of movement in a hand which stiffens very quickly between treatment sessions: e.g. in a less compliant patient CPM can maintain some of the movement gained with treatment. Because of the difficulty of fixing the machine to the fingertips, CPM cannot be applied

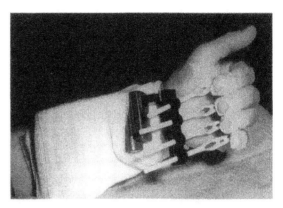

Figure 2.61 CPM on burn patient.

to unhealed burns unless sutures through the nails are used. In order to achieve a stretch at stiff joints it may be necessary to block mobile joints with a small splint.

Oedema management

Should oedema persist and the burn surface is sufficiently healed, a tubigrip, lycra glove, finger stall or compression wrap can be used as a compression measure. The hand must be closely observed to ensure that circulation is not occluded. This method should not be used when oedema is due to infection or inflammation.

Splinting

Deep partial-thickness and full-thickness burns are most likely to develop thick scar tissue and subsequent contractures.

Static splints. The thumb web is particularly prone to contracture and if a paddle splint is not being worn, a thermoplastic first web night splint can be provided. Cupping of the palm with the inability to open the hand to grasp objects may develop, secondary to palmar scarring. A dorsally placed halo splint may be required.

Dynamic splints. Dynamic splinting exerts a steady force to increase the range of motion of a joint. It is often used to correct finger contractures, e.g. by increasing MCP joint flexion or IP joint extension or in maintaining the thumb web.

Serial static splints. Serial splinting to correct contractures does not increase range of movement, but maintains that gained through exercise.

Activity programme

The light activity programme should be continued. The Microprocessor Upper Limb Exerciser (MULE) can be used for the restoration of functional grip (Fig. 2.62).

As the graft area settles, length of activity can be increased as patient tolerance and needs dictate.

Contraindicated activities include constant immersion of the hand in water, toxic dyes and abrasive movements of the skin. Graded activity can be extended to include desensitisation of grafted areas – tactile games and 'sensitivity boxes' containing lentils, polystyrene chips and marbles.

Scar management

As the scar matures, the patient needs to be shown how to massage the scars with an aqueous cream where hair follicles and sweat glands have been destroyed. This is particularly important following deep dermal burns.

Hypertrophic scarring develops in 70–80% of all burn scars and can cause gross deformity with joint contractures. Subjectively, the scars are often hypersensitive, itchy and tight, red and thickened. Burnt skin must be protected from strong sunlight.

The skin should be covered with total block sun lotion when exposed to sun, for at least 1 year after burn.

Compression garments

Larsen has shown that mechanical pressure with a corresponding stretch applied to a hypertrophic scar will eventually remodel it. A lycra glove, designed to put effective pressure on a hypertrophic scar, may be ready-made or made to measure. Accurate sizing is important. The scar should be completely healed before the glove is fitted because of the vulnerability of skin in the early stages of wound healing. If necessary, the glove should be fitted with a zipper to help application. The fit should ensure good contact with web spaces. Open tips make dexterity easier.

Inserts

To enhance the constant and controlled pressure of garments, silastic or foam inserts may be indicated to provide extra pressure on a particular scar area. The areas that commonly benefit are the web spaces, palmar surface and lateral aspect of the little finger. The type of insert is based on skin condition, functional needs and the amount of pressure required (Fig. 2.63). It can be incorporated with a splint, bandaged or taped into place or used under a lycra glove, providing a firm

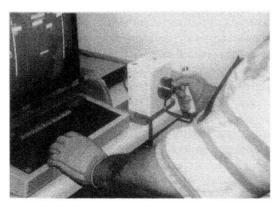

Figure 2.62 Burn patient using MULE upper limb exercise.

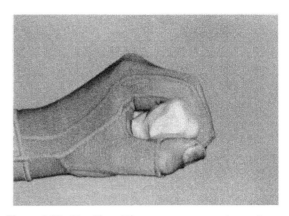

Figure 2.63 Hand in anti-burn scar pressure glove using silicone putty.

pressure that is non-abrasive to the skin, non-toxic, non-irritant and non-sensitising. The skin must be checked regularly for maceration or breakdown. Inserts can limit motion or function. For this reason, it may be necessary to use softer, less restricting inserts during the day and more rigid ones at night.

Hygiene is important with the use of pressure garments and silastics. Careful instruction for the patients and their relatives is of utmost importance.

Sensory re-education

Often patients complain of sensory alterations in the burnt hand, including hyperaesthesia, hypoaesthesia and temperature intolerance. Accurate sensory interpretation is essential for function and safety; patients must be instructed how to protect themselves from further injury. In addition to daily activity, a programme of sensory retraining will help.

Progression and upgrading of activities

More resisted activity such as printing and horticulture, heavy workshop activity and BTE (Baltimore Therapeutic Equipment) work stimulator can be programmed. Attention should be given to equate activity to the patient's skills and employment needs.

Hand burns in children

With children, close contact with the parents is essential. Parents will be taught stretches and educated about the importance of continued play and functional activities throughout their child's rehabilitation. Passive physiological movements may be performed on a child that is too young to cooperate with exercises.

Palmar burns in children can be splinted post-grafting by using 'oyster splints' which maintain the MCP joints in extension and the fingers in abduction and extension. Whereas an adult splinted in this way would lose range of movement, a child's hand is much more flexible and will quickly resume full range. After 3 weeks,

periods of play are initiated out of the splint, which is then only worn during rest periods and at night.

Late rehabilitation

All therapy is directed towards a return to pre-injury activities and treatment does not end on discharge from hospital. A patient with full range of movement will still need regular follow-up for at least the first 4 months, as it is during this phase that scar tissue can become hypertrophic and joint contractures develop, leading to an alteration in functional ability. Due to secondary changes, the position of deformity can become fixed and functionally limiting. Secondary changes include shortening of the collateral ligaments, volar displacement of the lateral bands, adhesions of the volar plates and tightening of Cleland's ligaments.

In some patients with active scar tissue it may be necessary to continue treatment for at least 1 year after healing has occurred.

Late deformities

The 'claw' hand can progress to a boutonnière (buttonhole) deformity if the central slip of the extensor mechanism is involved (Fig. 2.64). At this stage, a Capener splint is an effective

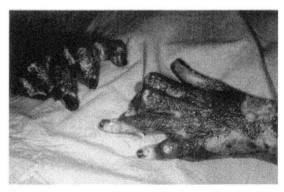

Figure 2.64 Burned hands showing boutonnière deformity of PIP joints. (Reproduced with permission of Nelson Thornes Ltd from Therapy for the Burn Patient, Leveridge, 1991.)

dynamic extension splint. Contracture of the finger and thumb web spaces can lead to a reduction in span and cylinder grasp. Prolonged deformity can result in long flexor and extensor tendon tightness and ultimately tightness of the intrinsic muscles, swan-neck deformities, syndactylies, little finger abduction and lateral rotation and hyperextension of the thumb IP joint.

Psychological problems

The stress of burn injury can induce acute psychological reactions, which can complicate recovery. The patient may face not only problems of his own health but also major life concerns: loss of loved ones or work colleagues, loss of home, inability to work and financial loss.

The therapist must show patience and understanding, gain cooperation and goal set, form rapport and give explanation of procedures. Psychological adjustment to the visual impact and acceptance of the effort required in the rehabilitation process requires full involvement in the treatment programme by the patient.

When the injury affects the patient's ability to return to full employment, a work assessment should be carried out, initially in the sheltered environment of the Unit, and when appropriate, also in the work place.

The goal of hand therapy in burns treatment is to ensure that the hand remains a functional tool with minimal deformity and disfigurement.

FURTHER READING

Clark JA: Classification of burns. Types of burns. In: A colour atlas of burn injuries. London: Chapman and Hall Medical, 1992: 2–24.
Covay MH: Application of CPM Devices with burn patients. JBCR 9(5):496–7, 1988
Kealey GP, Jensen K: Aggressive approach to physical therapy management of the burned hand. Phys Ther 65(5):683–5, 1988.
Larsen DL: The prevention and correction of burn scar contracture and hypertrophy. Texas Shriner's Burn Institute, 1973.
Leveridge AC: Therapy for the burn patient. London: Chapman and Hall, 1991, Chaps 3, 4, 7 and 10.

Nadel E: Rehabilitation of the burned hand. Top Acute Care Trauma Rehab 1(4): 50–61, 1987.
Perkins K et al: Silicone gel, new treatment for burns scars and contractures. Adelaide J Burns 9(3):201, 1982.
Rochester AP, Staite KD, Steele VA: Physiotherapy management following the Bradford City Football Club Fire, May 11, 1985. Physiotherapy 73(1):2–5, 1987.
Salter M, Cheshire L (eds): Hand therapy principles and practice. Oxford: Butterworth-Heinemann, 2000, 196–210.
Wynn Parry CB: The stiff hand. In: Rehabilitation of the hand, 4th edn. London: Butterworth, 1981:254–62.

H. AMPUTATIONS

W Bruce Conolly

INTRODUCTION

Surgical amputation is one of the most commonly and yet poorly performed of all operations. The result to the patient will depend on the experience of the surgeon and of the hand therapist, whose judgement and technical skill can make the difference between a satisfactory or poor outcome.

SURGICAL PRINCIPLES

General principles – indications

Amputations of a digit or digits or part of the hand are indicated if there is:

1. irretrievable impairment of circulation
2. severe uncontrollable infection
3. soft tissue or skeletal malignancy

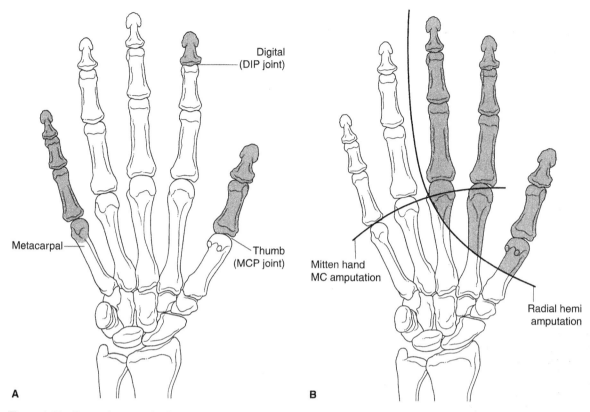

Figure 2.65   Types of amputation in the hand. A: Fingers/thumb. B: Hand.

4. disuse resulting from persisting pain or stiffness.

Types of amputation (Fig. 2.65)

There may be amputation of:

1. a finger or fingers
2. the thumb
3. radial or ulnar hemi-amputation where there is a combination of finger and thumb amputation
4. metacarpal amputation (mitten hand)
5. amputation of the whole hand itself
6. below elbow amputation
7. more proximal amputation, above-elbow, forequarter amputation.

Surgical considerations for elective amputations

An amputation stump should:

1. be painless, but have sensation.
2. have an adequate durable soft tissue pad
3. be of functional length wherever possible. An index finger stump shorter than the PIP joint is often not useful when the patient requires two-point pinch grip.

General technique for amputation
(Fig. 2.66)

1. Skin flaps are carefully planned so that they are closed over the bony stump with no tension. Raising of the skin flaps will expose

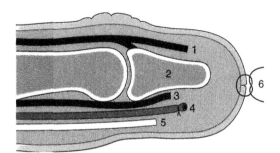

Figure 2.66 Technique for amputation of a digit. The extensor and flexor tendons are cut so that they retract from the stump. The bone is trimmed into a rounded stump. The artery is dissected from the nerve and ligated. The nerve is cut about 1 cm proximal to the stump. The skin is closed loosely with fine sutures.

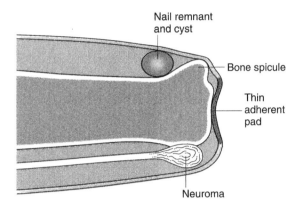

Figure 2.67 Amputation complications may be caused by a thin adherent pad, a bone spicule, a digital neuroma or nail remnant and cyst.

and allow treatment of the underlying bone, flexor and extensor tendon mechanism and the neurovascular bundle.

2. The level of section of the bone is decided according to the amount of soft tissue cover available. The bone end is contoured to avoid bony spicules.
3. Both flexor and extensor tendons are resected away from the stump so they do not adhere to the stump and tether the stump and the adjacent tendon mechanism.
4. The digital vessels are dissected and ligated to avoid haematoma.
5. The digital nerves are dissected very gently and cleanly sectioned or diathermied about 1 cm proximal to the stump to minimise the problem of any neuroma which may form.
6. The skin is then closed without tension over the stump.
7. A non-adherent gentle compression bandage is applied.
8. The wrist and digit are splinted with a volar slab and the hand is elevated for at least 48 hours.

Complications of amputations
(Fig. 2.67)

These include:

1. inadequate skin cover with a thin pad which may be adherent to the underlying bone

2. neuroma and pain in the stump
3. poor circulation
4. stiffness of the joints of the affected or adjacent digit
5. phantom pain
6. reflex sympathetic dystrophy.

FUNCTION AND SIGNIFICANCE OF INDIVIDUAL DIGITS

The thumb

The thumb is the most mobile and important digit of the hand, representing 40% of overall hand function. The essentials of normal thumb function include opposability, stability, length and sensibility.

The index finger

The index finger provides stability and balance in delicate everyday activity such as writing and drawing and the use of precision instruments. Length is vital. As the level of amputation in this digit approaches the PIP joint, pinch of the function is transferred to the adjacent middle finger.

The middle finger

The middle finger contributes to power grip, supports the index finger in pulp-to-pulp pinch and provides a cupping action that prevents small objects from falling through the hand when it is closed.

The ring finger

Together with the little finger, the ring finger is very important for power grip function and also prevents small objects from falling through

the closed hand. This finger is important cosmetically.

The little finger

The little finger is important in power grip, adding to the width of grasp. It also helps in controlling fine movements in activity, such as writing, because it extends the ulnar border of the palm.

I. PROSTHETICS

Judith Davidson

INTRODUCTION

The impact of amputation of a thumb, multiple fingers, a hand or arm is very serious. The loss of fine hand function, sense of touch and proprioception and aesthetic appearance are only partly compensated for by the provision of a prosthesis. Even the loss of one distal part of a single digit is devastating to many individuals due to both functional and cosmetic reasons.

There is an unusually high rejection rate of upper-extremity prostheses throughout the world and it is often very difficult to predict which amputees will be successful users. Successful outcomes are often a mix of physical, psychological and emotional factors.[1] A multidisciplinary rehabilitation team experienced in the rehabilitation of upper limb amputees, is essential to ensure the best chance of a successful outcome.

Even if amputees choose to reject their prostheses, it is important that they are able to achieve self-confidence and a stable independent lifestyle where social and occupational roles have been re-established.

This chapter is intended as an introduction to the principles of rehabilitation of upper limb amputees. For those involved in the rehabilitation of upper limb amputees, the detailed texts of Atkins and Meier,[2] Schantschi[3] and Bowker and Michael[4] are prerequisite readings.

PRINCIPLES OF REHABILITATION OF THE UPPER LIMB AMPUTEE

The aim of rehabilitation of people with upper limb amputations is to:

- develop self-esteem and self-confidence
- regain and maintain a full range of movement in all intact joints
- reduce oedema in the residual limb
- manage the stump pain, phantom pain and possible neuromata
- provide counselling for post-traumatic stress disorder, depression and anger management
- provide the patient directed prosthetic fitting and training
- assist in achieving independence in self-care, domestic and leisure activities using either a prosthesis or modified equipment
- assist the amputee in resuming independent driving
- advise on the selection of modified equipment
- provide advice on vocational options and encourage a return to work.

PRE-PROSTHETIC TREATMENT

Immediate pre-prosthetic treatment is vital. This treatment also continues throughout the rehabilitation process. The prime objectives are considered below.

Provision of psychological counselling

The hands and arms are means of self-expression through affection, self-identity and manual dexterity and are a means of providing for the family as tools of work. The realisation that technology can only offer a limited replacement compounds these fears. Psychological assistance can assist in dealing with the shock of the amputation and the feelings of inadequacy and incapacity. Sabolich[5] is excellent reading for understanding the impact of an amputation.

Pain management

The absence or presence of any type of pain makes an enormous difference to the general level of life satisfaction and to prosthetic use by the amputee. Every amputee should be carefully assessed and monitored for levels of phantom pain, sensitivity and neuromata. Pain levels often increase after discharge from acute care. Opioids are not appropriate for phantom pain, stump pain or neuromata. Medication and/or a TENS machine may be trialled.

Changing hand dominance

Changing one's hand dominance is a very slow process over a 2 year time span. It is often repetitive and monotonous and a wide variety of remedial activities need to be incorporated into treatment programmes. Nearly all amputees will use their intact upper limb as their dominant limb.

Teaching one-handed techniques

The provision of specialised equipment for daily tasks needs to be addressed. The provision of a spinning knob is necessary for driving. Amputees need to be able to perform daily tasks with and without their prosthesis.

Stump bandaging

Interstitial oedema develops subsequent to the cut lymphatics. The aim of stump bandaging is to produce a stump ready for prosthetic fitting in as short a time as possible by reducing the oedema. Effective prosthetic operation requires an intimate socket fit and this requires a stable stump volume.

Preservation of strength and range of movement

Physical therapy aims to maintain a strong shoulder girdle movement, including scapula, shoulder and elbow joint movement. The retention of all available forearm pronation and supination is vital.

Construction of a temporary prosthesis

The construction of a temporary cable-operated prosthesis will assist in reducing oedema, maintaining stump shape and conditioning of the stump as well as encouraging bilaterality. It can assist the patient and his or her family to develop realistic expectations about the functionality and appearance of the prosthesis. Most patients are disappointed with their definitive prosthesis. If the patient is appropriately orientated to the realities of the prosthesis, how it looks and operates, they will be better prepared to accept the limitations of the prosthesis when it is delivered.

PROSTHETIC OPTIONS

Four main prosthetic options are described below. Selection of the right prosthetic option is not easy. It has to made by the whole treatment team and the patient, keeping in mind:

- level of amputation
- phantom and stump pain
- viable muscle sites for myoelectric control
- patient's lifestyle – home, work and leisure
- cosmetic requirements
- goals and expectations of family members and friends
- other medical problems or disabilities.

Many amputees will require more than one type of prosthesis. Due to the differing functions and reliabilities of the cable-operated and externally powered prostheses, both should be prescribed if funding allows. Amputees can then choose their 'preferred' limb; they may well use both for different tasks.

For the high-level amputee, both a cable-operated and a cosmetic prosthesis may be provided. For the partial hand amputee, an orthosis and cosmetic glove may be prescribed.

A passive, cosmetic finger, thumb, hand or arm

The importance of aesthetic appearance cannot be underestimated: this preoccupation can be partly resolved by providing a cosmetic glove for partial hand amputations and a cosmetic limb for more proximal amputations.

Cosmetic fingertips can be provided for single digit amputations but are usually more of a hindrance than a help for functional tasks. For amputees with the loss of a thumb, a cosmetic glove can be provided or, alternatively, a rigid opposition thumb post: both have functional limitations but often meet a need in all amputees to be given an opportunity to achieve their maximum level of functioning.

A cosmetic limb for high above elbow and more proximal amputations is nearly always required, as these levels of amputation are unlikely to be able to achieve sufficient cable excursion and power to operate a cable-controlled body-powered prosthesis. Such limbs include a friction-controlled shoulder joint and a passive lockable elbow joint,

a foam and stocking covering the limb together with a light-weight rigid plastic hand. Forequarter amputees are often provided with a shoulder filler, which allows them to hold their clothes up when not wearing the limb (Figs 2.68–2.70).

A cable-operated body-powered prosthesis

These prostheses utilise the mechanical principles of a control cable attached to a harness that forms a loop encircling the opposite axilla. Tension on this harness and cabling is transmitted to the artificial elbow and terminal device (hand or hook). Poor adjustment of any of the components dramatically decreases the efficiency of the cable operation. These artificial limbs are strong, reliable and relatively inexpensive; they are relatively lightweight.

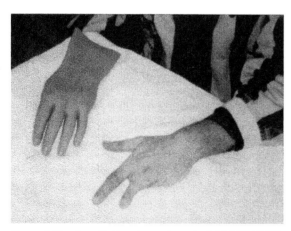

Figure 2.68 A partial hand amputee who had a traumatic amputation of his middle, ring and little fingers was fitted with a cosmetic glove. (Reproduced with permission from Boscheinen–Morrin J, Conolly WB: The hand: fundamentals of therapy. Oxford: Butterworth-Heinemann.)

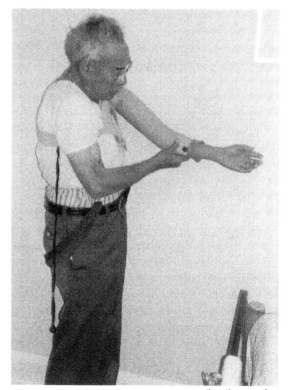

Figure 2.69 A forequarter amputee operating the passive elbow lock of his cosmetic arm.

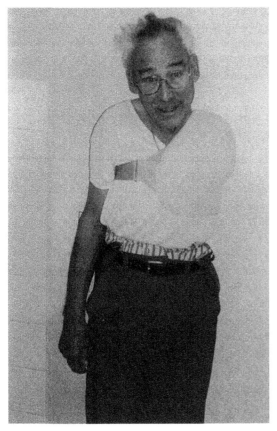

Figure 2.70 A shoulder filler.

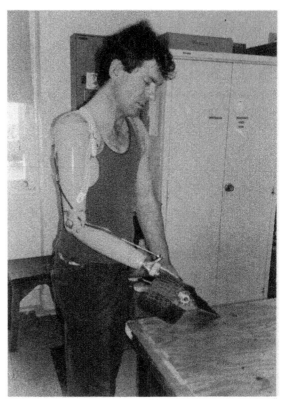

Figure 2.71 An above-elbow amputee using a cable-operated prosthesis with a split hook to hold a piece of leather while using his intact hand to punch holes.

Terminal devices available include either a mechanical hand or a hook. The mechanical hand operates with a cable and can exert a low fixed prehension force in a pincer grip. The most commonly prescribed hooks are voluntary opening split hooks, where pinch force is determined by the number of rubber bands used. These hooks come in various shapes, sizes and weights and need to be prescribed after assessment of each amputee's lifestyle. Wrist and elbow units will also need to be prescribed (Fig. 2.71).

The development of roll-on-silicone sockets has dramatically increased suspension and harnessing options in recent years.[6]

An externally powered artificial limb

Most externally powered artificial limbs are myoelectric controlled. These controls utilise the electrical activity during a muscle contraction to control the flow of energy from a battery to a motor in the prosthetic device, which then operates the terminal device. The control signals come from intact distal muscles in the amputated limb that are not required for any other function.

Myoelectric terminal devices include both hands and hooks and these can provide much greater pinch force than voluntary opening hooks and hands. The Otto Bock electric hand can provide about 10 kg of pinch force. The Greiffer electric hook provides about 20 kg of pinch force.

For the below-elbow amputee, a myoelectric prosthesis requires no harness, because the socket is self-suspending from the epicondyles. The prosthesis provides a simple, direct and efficient form of non-dominant hand function. For

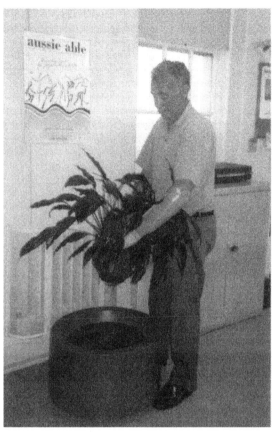

Figure 2.72 A below-elbow amputee with a myoelectric prosthesis with an Otto Bock Greiffer.

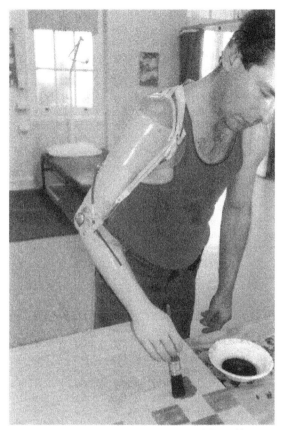

Figure 2.73 An above-elbow amputee training with an electric hand with a body-powered elbow.

the higher levels of amputation where the benefits of external power are more important, the fittings of externally powered prostheses are also far more complex. A combination of myoelectric and switch controls may be required or, alternatively, servo control may be utilised. A combination of body-powered elbow and electric terminal devices may provide much better function than an all-electric limb (Figs 2.72 and 2.73).

Externally powered limbs are far more expensive and are considerably heavier and less reliable than body-powered limbs. However, they offer a stronger grip, absence of harnessing for the below-elbow amputee and a very acceptable aesthetic appearance. For the amputee who does indoor work and requires good cosmesis, an externally powered limb may be the preferred option. For the very high-level amputee, external power may be the only means by which an active terminal device can be utilised.

Orthotic devices for specific tasks

Orthotic devices can provide improved function for specific tasks, especially for the partial hand amputee. Devices can be individually designed to allow for attachment of cutlery, pens, potato peeler or even butchers' knives. An opposition post with an adjustable platform is available for the partial hand amputee. There are also a multitude of sporting devices that can be fitted into the conventional wrist unit of an artificial limb[7] (Fig. 2.74).

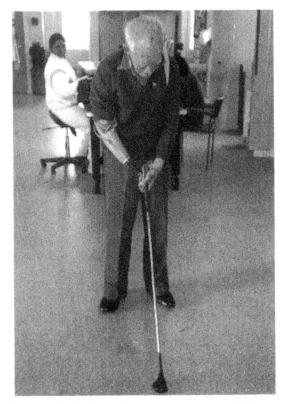

Figure 2.74 A below-elbow amputee using a golf club holding prosthesis.

PROSTHETIC TRAINING

Adequate training is mandatory if an amputee is to use his prosthesis effectively. The following factors will need to be addressed:

- Prosthetic component terminology and care of the artificial limb. The amputee will also need to be independent in putting the prosthesis on and off.
- Care of the residual limb, including regular washing and checking for skin abrasions. If redness of the skin persists, the socket may need modification. In hot weather, amputees perspire more and therefore need to take greater care with their skin.
- Body control motions. Scapular abduction, humeral flexion and elbow flexion are used for terminal device operation. Humeral extension, depression and abduction is used for elbow operation. For use of a myoelectric prosthesis, the amputee needs to learn independent control of viable muscle sites using a biofeedback machine or temporary myoelectric limb.
- Training for manual operation of the wrist unit, shoulder unit and elbow rotation is important. The amputee must learn to use the wrist unit to pre-position the hook before opening.
- Controls training is necessary to develop accurate placement and tension control of the terminal device.[8]
- Functional use training is the most prolonged stage of prosthetic training. Tasks include cutting food, dressing, using scissors, tying shoes, sewing, washing and drying dishes, food preparation, using the telephone, wrapping a package, handling money and putting on gloves and coat. All tasks used for training should be relevant to the patient's lifestyle.[9]
- Schantschi[3] in the *Manual of Upper Extremity Prosthetics* from the University of California provides an excellent explanation of training schedules, as does Atkins and Meier.[2] The video produced by Heinze,[10] who is a bilateral upper limb amputee, is also an excellent reference.

VOCATIONAL TRAINING

Rehabilitation of upper limb amputees must include discussion of vocational issues. While some amputees will be keen to return to their pre-injury work, others will refuse to do so. Anger at the cause of the accident, fear of re-injury and post-traumatic stress may all interfere with a return to the pre-injury workplace.

Amputees may well need vocational training to enable a return to the work force. Many amputees will change from manual work to more clerical-type work.[11] An on-site vocational evaluation by the treating occupational therapist is invaluable.[12]

KEY STATEMENTS

1. Prostheses can only partly compensate for physical loss of multiple fingers, thumb, hand or arm.
2. Psychological counselling will assist the amputee to come to terms with their feelings of shock, inadequacy and incapacity.

3. Amputees need to be taught one-handed methods to manage most of their daily activities.
4. Artificial limbs can be supplied as cosmetic prostheses, orthotic devices, cable-operated limb prostheses or myoelectric prostheses. Early fitting is crucial to the long-term outcome.
5. Training of prosthetic controls and prosthetic function is vital if amputees are to achieve maximal outcomes.
6. Many amputees will require vocational retraining to assist them to return to work.
7. Rehabilitation of an amputee is a long process. The rehabilitation team should aim to develop a working partnership with amputees, where meeting their requests become the prime goal of the team.

REFERENCES

1. Herberts P Korner L Caine K: Rehabilitaion of unilateral below elbow amputees with myoelectric prostheses. Scan J Rehab Med 12:123–8, 1980.
2. Atkins DJ, Meier RH: Comprehensive management of the upper limb amputee. New York: Springer Verlag, 1989.
3. Schantschi WR: Manual of upper extremity prosthetics. Dept. of Engineering, University of California, 1958.
4. Bowker JH, Michael JW: Atlas of limb prosthetics: surgical, prosthetic and rehabilitation principles. American Academy of Orthopaedic Surgeons. St. Louis: Mosby, 1992.
5. Sabolich J: You're not alone. With the personal stories of 38 Amputees. Sabolich Prosthetic & Research Center, Oklahoma City, 1991.
6. Kristinsson O: The Iceross concept: a discussion of a philosophy. Prosth Orthot Int 17:49–55, 1993.
7. Michael JW, Gailey RW, Bowker JH: New developments in recreational prostheses and adaptive devices for the amputee. Clin Orthopaed Rel Res No. 256:64–75, 1990.
8. Hermansson LM: Structured training of children fitted with myoelectric prostheses. Prosth Orthot Int 15:88–92, 1991.
9. Jones L, McGlynn M: Rehabilitation after a letter-bomb attack causing bilateral hand loss and other injuries: case report. Disab Rehab 14(3):152–5, 1992.
10. Heinze A: The use of upper extremity prostheses (a video of a bilateral amputee). Distributed by South Australian Film Corporation.
11. Jones LE, Davidson JH: The long term outcomes of upper limb amputees treated at a rehabilitation centre in Sydney, Australia. Disab Rehab 17(8):437–42, 1995.
12. Fraser C: A survey of users of upper limb prostheses. Br J Occup Ther 56(5):166–8, 1993.

J. THE STIFF HAND

W Bruce Conolly and Rosemary Prosser

INTRODUCTION

Stable coordinated motion requires a balance between mobility and stability. Excessive stiffness disrupts this balance and impinges on hand function. Stiffness in this chapter will refer to excessive stiffness that manifests itself in loss of glide of the mobile tissue structures, e.g. joints and musculotendinous units. A contracture is defined as a fixed shortening of the mobile tissue structures.

Stiffness may complicate any injury, surgical procedure or inflammatory condition. It is the most common cause of disability after hand injury. Stiffness alone may cause a considerable functional loss. Stiffness associated with pain may render the hand almost useless.

CAUSES OF STIFFNESS

Excessive persistent oedema is the most common cause of stiffness. Stiffness may also result from inactivity or disuse from any cause, particularly when pain is a significant factor. Stiffness can occur after injury, as an aftermath of infection or as a part of arthritis. It may also be congenital.

PATHOGENESIS

Oedema is a protein-rich fluid that carries the chemical mediators of lysis and synthesis of new connective tissue. Oedema that follows injury is rich in fibrocytes, producing fibrous tissue which heals the injured connective tissue. This same fibrous tissue can also form adhesions that contract and restrict the full excursion of the capsule, ligaments and tendons.[1,2] Untreated oedema may result in irreversible stiffness. The greater the oedema present, the greater the potential stiffness problem.

Oedema forms due to:

- Mechanical pressure – there is reduction of venous and lymphatic flow without simultaneous reduction of arterial flow. Limb dependency and constriction from tight bandages increase this pressure, thereby increasing oedema.
- Chemical effects – the tissue reaction caused by chemical mediators such as histamine, substance p and bradykinins influences osmotic pressures and thus water infiltration into the tissues.
- Neurogenic influences – pain and sympathetic nervous system activity leads to loss of motion and limb dependency, causing oedema.

The dorsum of the hand and digits has very mobile loose skin. This is an ideal place for oedema to collect. The oedema pulls the skin taut and prevents metacarpophalangeal (MP) joint flexion. If uncorrected, the MP joints will posture in extension or hyperextension and the IP joints in flexion. In this position the MP joint's collateral ligaments and the PIP joint's volar plate are shortened. If untreated, this position will lead to significant tightness and stiffness in these joint structures and, eventually, contracture in this position.

ANATOMICAL STRUCTURES INVOLVED

1. Joints: capsular and ligament fibrosis causes joint contracture. A PIP joint flexion

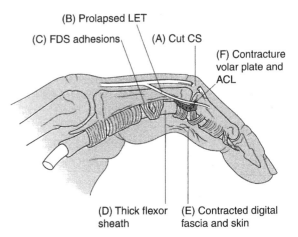

Figure 2.75 Causes of PIP joint flexion contracture. A: Disruption of the central slip (CS). B: Volar subluxation of the lateral extensor tendon (LET). C: Adhesions of the flexor tendon to the proximal phalanx. D: Contracture of the flexor tendon sheath. E: Contracture of the volar digital fascia and skin. F: Contracture of the volar plate and the associated accessory collateral ligament (ACL). There may also be a bony block preventing PIP joint extension.

contracture is the most common contracture encountered. It is due primarily to contracture of the volar plate, check rein ligament, collateral ligaments, and secondary capsule and adjacent connective tissue adhesion[3–5] (Fig. 2.75). Anatomically, the MP joint's volar plate is not so susceptible to contracture. The MP joint is more likely to develop an extension contracture due to contracture of the collateral ligaments when postured in the extended position.

2. Tendons: restriction of tendon glide, both flexor and extensor, may limit motion. This may be due to adhesions at the pulleys or FDS bifurcation, FDS adhesion to FDP, tendon adhesion to bone or adhesion to adjacent connective tissue.

3. Fascia: fascial fibrosis and contracture such as in Dupuytren's contracture.

4. Muscles: constriction of the circulatory system causing muscle ischaemia leads to fibrosis. The muscle may become short and tight as the passive connective tissue component contracts. This may be

accompanied by a weak limited excursion due to the loss of active sarcomeres.[6]

5. Skin: skin and soft tissue web contractures. These contractures may be primary, such as in burns, or secondary, following immobilisation in a shortened position.

CLASSIC CONTRACTURE POSITIONS OF THE HAND

1. Intrinsic plus – MP flexion and IP extension, e.g. intrinsic ischaemic contracture
2. Intrinsic minus – MP hyperextension and IP flexion, e.g. ulnar claw hand
3. Dupuytren's contracture – MP and PIP flexion contracture, and web contractures
4. MP extension contracture
5. PIP flexion contracture.

GENERAL PRINCIPLES OF THE TREATMENT OF STIFFNESS

Conservative

Management of the stiff hand is one of the biggest challenges for the treating hand therapist. Stiff joints and other soft tissues often take many months of well-directed treatment to soften and become pliable.

Prevention

In many cases, hand stiffness can be prevented. If there is a significant risk of stiffness, e.g. severe burns or crushing injuries, the therapist should deal with this as early as possible by anticipation and prevention. This requires:

1. Early oedema control: excessive oedema is the prime cause of excessive scar tissue and adhesion formation. Primarily elevation, compression and massage are used.
2. Rest the hand in a safe position: when stiffness seems unavoidable, as after a severe crush injury, it is important to splint the hand in a safe position. The safe position is wrist slight extension (20–30 degrees) MP joint flexion and IP joint extension with the thumb

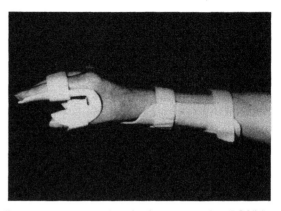

Figure 2.76 The position of safe immobilisation (POSI) is wrist extension 20–30 degrees, MP flexion 50–70 degrees and IP extended 0 degrees. It is important that the splint is applied correctly so that this position is achieved. If the hand is very oedematous and painful, several alterations in the splint position may be required over several days to achieve the appropriate POSI position.

in palmar abduction in the same plane as the index finger (Fig. 2.76). This rests the joint ligament and capsular structures in a lengthened position, limiting joint tightening and contracture.

3. Maintenance of muscle power: muscle strength is maintained by active and resisted exercise and use of the hand.
4. Maintenance of tissue glide: active and passive movements are used to maintain the gliding excursion of the joint structures and musculotendinous unit, which are essential for motion and functional use of the hand.
5. Control of anxiety and pain: pain is a strong inhibitor, both physiologically and psychologically. Analgesia following surgery and painful conditions such as reflex sympathetic dystrophy (RSD) (CRPS I), needs to be appropriate for the condition being treated. This may include analgesics, corticosteroids and regional or sympathetic blocks.

Therapy for the stiff hand

A detailed and precise assessment is necessary to focus treatment on the stiff structures. The stiff structures need to be identified. For example, if poor digit flexion is the problem, is the cause lack of flexor tendon pull through or restriction in passive motion? Differentiation between tight extrinsic extensors as opposed to tight intrinsics is necessary. If IP joint flexion decreases with MP extension, then the intrinsics are tight. If IP joint flexion decreases with MP flexion, then the extrinsic extensor is tight. If IP joint flexion does not change with MP position, the joint itself is tight. This can be confirmed by evaluation of the passive accessory glide of the joint. Oblique retinacular ligament (ORL) length should also be assessed. If DIP joint flexion is decreased by PIP extension, the ORL is tight.

Setting treatment goals and priorities requires patient participation. Often there is stiffness in more than one direction of joint motion. In this situation the treatment needs to be carefully balanced. Initially, digit flexion to enable grip may be the priority. Once a more functional grip is gained, the priority may shift to improving extension while maintaining the gains made in flexion. This is often a delicate balance.

Established stiffness in the hand requires long-term treatment. Treatment techniques are biased toward those which soften the tissues and facilitate length changes. To obtain a long-term gain in changing tissue length, the principle of low tension over a prolonged period is vital.[7-10] For this reason splintage is one of the most, if not the most, effective technique in improving tissue length and pliability.[11] Other techniques used include massage (2–5 min done 4–6 times a day), compression garments and pads, heat in the lengthened position, an exercise programme with a high frequency (4–6 times a day) and functional activities.

Tissue-stretching techniques

Heat and massage. Tissue stretching techniques are generally enhanced by massage and heat. Heat applied before or during stretching will facilitate a greater stretch with less discomfort.

Passive stretching. The tissues are held at their end range for 15–60 seconds. The stretch should be pain-free and specific to those structures involved, e.g. ORL, intrinsics, long extensors.

Active stretching. Active stretching is aimed at the musculotendinous unit and its fibrous attachments. The muscle is worked to its maximum in outer range; this is followed by maximal relaxation, which allows maximum lengthening of the muscle.

Passive joint mobilisation (PJMs). This particular technique is aimed at tight joint structures only. Clinically, it is most beneficial when all other tissue tightness has been dealt with first.

Splinting. The splint design will depend on what structure it is aimed at, e.g. joint only, musculotendinous unit or skin. The splint design must be biomechanically sound and comfortable to wear. Generally, it is agreed that the splint producing the greatest total end range time (TERT) will be the most effective.[12] Therefore, the splint enabling the best patient compliance to wearing time will provide the best TERT and the best result. A serial static splint will provide a longer end range time than a dynamic splint (e.g. rubber band power force) per hour worn; however, a dynamic splint may be tolerated for a longer time during a 24-hour period. TERT must account for both these factors. Splinting duration in terms of weeks or months must also be considered. Collagen and covalent bond turnover takes approximately 6 weeks. An acceptable clinical improvement may take many cycles of collagen turnover. Clinically, authors have recommended from 3 to 6 months of splinting.[3,13] Prosser[14] reports the average splint wearing time for 20 patients with PIP joint flexion contracture to be 6–14 hours per day for 3–5 months.

Oedema and scar management

Compression garments and compression pads aim at softening scar tissue by decreasing fibrous tissue water content and changing the architecture of the fibrous matrix.[1,2] Diligent scar massage done for short periods frequently during the day is clinically very effective in mobilising the skin and subcutaneous tissues.

Muscle strength

Muscle strength should not be forgotten. Joint range cannot be maintained if the muscles are unable to move the joints in their newly gained range. A graded resisted exercise programme is necessary for these patients. Resisted functional use of the hand or a resisted activity programme may fulfill this purpose while enabling the patient to be productive.

OPERATIVE TREATMENT

Operative treatment will depend on the cause of the stiffness (Fig. 2.77). Often multiple tissues are involved, requiring multiple surgical procedures:

Structure: operative treatment

- Skin: excision of scar; skin replacement by grafting or flap transfer
- Fascia: fasciectomy, fasciotomy
- Joint: ligament or capsular release, removal of bony block, joint debridement, implant arthroplasty or fusion
- Tendon: tenolysis, tenotomy.

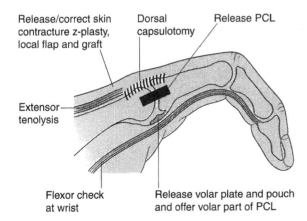

Release/correct skin contracture z-plasty, local flap and graft

Dorsal capsulotomy

Release PCL

Extensor tenolysis

Flexor check at wrist

Release volar plate and pouch and offer volar part of PCL

Figure 2.77 Operative treatment for each structure involved in extension contracture of the MCP joint.

Indications

The patient must want and need improved function. The patient must also be psychologically, socially and economically prepared for the procedure and the necessary aftercare. A period of time off work may be necessary in the early stages.

Adequate conservative treatment must have been tried first. Ideally, the patient's hand should be pain-free and the soft tissues should be as soft and pliable as possible. X-rays are taken before any surgical release to evaluate any joint damage or malunion. A full hand therapy assessment to determine the patient's functional loss and long-term needs will assist in the planning of surgical procedures.

As a general principle, if possible, the surgery should be done under local anaesthesia, so the patient is awake and able to cooperate by moving the tendon and joint during the procedure. The necessity of associated procedures, such as tenolysis or correction of a malunion, can then be determined.

Contraindications

The contraindications to surgical release of contracted tissues include infection, inflammation and RSD, unless there is a diagnosed reversible cause such as neuroma or carpal tunnel syndrome (CTS). An inability to carry out the postoperative therapy programme is also a contraindication.

Postoperative therapy goals

The aims of the therapy programme following any surgical release of contracted or adherent tissues is:

1. To maintain the gains made in surgery.
2. To limit further scar and adhesion formation. Early effective oedema control and early active motion are essential if this is to be achieved.
3. To restore the maximal glide and strength of the musculotendinous unit.
4. To improve and maximise functional use of the hand.

SURGICAL PROCEDURES

Release of MP joint extension contracture

Surgery

Capsulectomy of the MP joint is approached through a longitudinal curved incision for one joint or transverse approach for more than one joint (Fig. 2.77). The extensor tendon is first freed from adhesions from the skin and the underlying metacarpal. The tendon is split longitudinally to expose the capsule of the MP joint, which is then incised transversely and if necessary excised. One or both collateral ligaments are released from the metacarpal head. A transarticular K-wire may be needed to hold the joint in the corrected position for 7–10 days. The extensor tendon is repaired with interrupted non-absorbable sutures. In optimal circumstances a gain of 60 degrees of MP movement can result.

Therapy

The therapy programme aims to maintain the gained MP flexion. If the joints are held by K-wires in flexion, this enables the therapist to concentrate on restoring IP preoperative range before MP joint motion needs to be dealt with. The hand is rested in a POSI splint until the K-wires are removed.

As soon as the K-wires are removed, the therapy programme focuses on active MP joint exercises, with emphasis on flexion. IP isolated exercises are continued and composite flexion and extension is commenced. After removal of sutures at approximately 2 weeks, scar management is commenced. The POSI splint may need to be continued both day and night for a further 4 weeks.

At approximately 3 weeks a graded resisted exercise programme is started. Intrinsic flexion of the MP joints with the wrist in extension is emphasised. This promotes better isolated MP joint motion. Extensor digitorum communis (EDC) glide needs to be checked and monitored throughout the postoperative programme. A dynamic flexion splint worn intermittently during the day may be necessary as early as 3 weeks post-release. Some form of night flexion splinting may be required for 2–5 months to maintain the flexion range while the scar tissue is maturing. Serial static splinting is simple and effective.

Specific tips

1. Distal migration of a dynamic MP flexion splint is a common problem. Laseter[15] recommends a dorsally based splint with a palmar bar. This type of splint design needs careful fitting and application to avoid pressure that may restrict circulation. Clinically, a circumferential splint with reasonable wrist extension (30 degrees) prevents splint migration and provides good distribution of pressure (Fig. 2.78). A 3/4 circumferential splint with a rolled hole for the thumb may also be adequate.

2. Co-contraction can be counterproductive and frustrating for both the patient and therapist. This occurs due to muscle weakness, overexertion by the patient and sometimes from a learned abnormal movement pattern. For example, if the EDC has been used as an accessory wrist extensor, MP flexion with wrist extension will be difficult. Biofeedback, good verbal feedback and strengthening the weak muscles in isolation can be used to address this problem.

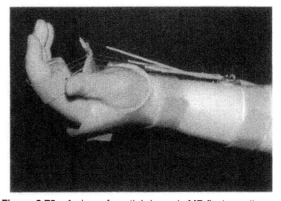

Figure 2.78 A circumferential dynamic MP flexion splint with the wrist in approximately 30 degrees extension gives good pressure distribution to the hand and forearm and prevents splint migration.

Release of PIP joint flexion contracture

Surgery

A volar zigzag approach, raising thick skin flaps, allows exposure and retraction of both neurovascular bundles. A transverse incision is then made in the flexor sheath at the level of the PIP joint. The FDP and FDS tendons are retracted and the volar plate exposed and each check rein ligament exposed and cut. Sometimes the entire volar plate may need releasing from the neck of the proximal phalanx. The articular branch of the digital artery is protected. Division of the posterior flexor sheath as well as the oblique retinacular ligament and any other tight fascia in the area may be necessary. A K-wire may be needed to hold the joint in about 15 degrees of flexion for 4–7 days (Fig. 2.79).

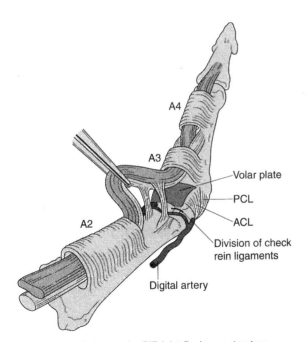

Figure 2.79 Release of a PIP joint flexion contracture. The flexor tendons are exposed between the A2 and A4 pulleys. Each check rein ligament and, if necessary, the entire proximal attachment of the volar plate is sectioned. The attachment of the accessory collateral ligament (ACL) may also need to be cut at this junction to the volar plate. PCL = proper collateral ligament.

Therapy

The goal of the therapy programme is to maintain maximum PIP joint extension. If the joint is held by a K-wire just off full extension, the initial therapy programme is focused on restoring MP and DIP motion. PIP joint flexion contracture causes adaptive shortening of the ORL and lateral extensor bands. When the PIP joint is held extended after a long period in the flexed posture, DIP flexion may be difficult due to the increased extensor tension from this adaptive shortening. DIP flexion can be improved with diligent passive and active flexion exercise. Oedema is controlled by the modalities mentioned previously.

After removal of the K-wires, treatment focuses on maintaining PIP extension while gaining flexion. The extensor tendon may be weak and stretched after a prolonged period in flexion. Extension splinting during the day and night to support the weakened extensor tendon and maintain length of the volar structures is vital. Splintage needs to be prolonged, up to 5 or 6 months according to most clinical reports.[3–5,14]

A static or dynamic splint may be used. The static splint may be hand- or digit-based. The PIP joint is held in extension and the MP joint in flexion if it is included. Dynamic splints utilised include the outrigger splint or a spring wire Capener splint (Fig. 2.80). The spring wire splint is a hand-based and low-profile splint. The outrigger's tension is more adjustable; however, the splint is a little more cumbersome than a spring wire splint. In the later stages, a neoprene sleeve may be adequate for day-time splinting: it provides quite a low tension force, is easy to wear and allows flexion for functional use while still providing a gentle extension force when the hand is at rest. If the joint is very reactive, an outrigger or neoprene sleeve may be more appropriate, as both of these splints can provide low tension forces (150 g or less) to the joint.

PIP exercises are commenced as soon as possible. Active extension and flexion as well as blocked extension are recommended as soon as the wires are removed. Blocked PIP extension with the MP held in flexion enables the tension developed in

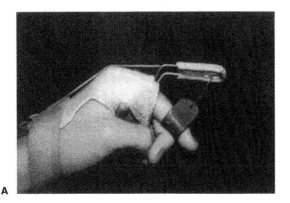

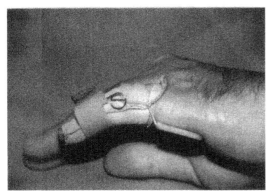

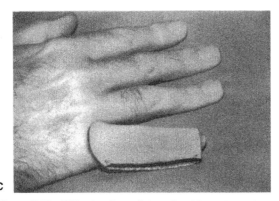

Figure 2.80 PIP extension splintage for at least 4 months is necessary following PIP joint flexion contracture release. A dynamic splint may be preferred as it allows some flexion while maintaining extension. Dynamic splints include:
A: Low-profile outrigger with rubber band traction.
B: Capener spring wire extension splint. C: Neoprene sleeve.

the EDC to be transferred to the PIP joint, thus strengthening the extension force at the PIP joint. A resisted exercise programme is commenced at 6 weeks. At this time there should still be a strong

emphasis on extension. Flexion exercises may need to be discontinued or reduced if extension is being lost.

Release of PIP joint extension contracture

Surgery

A bilateral approach exposes the extensor apparatus and the transverse retinacular ligament and the flexor sheath. The dorsal capsule is exposed and incised transversely, taking care not to damage the central slip. The dorsoproximal attachment of the proper collateral ligament may need releasing from each side of the head of the proximal phalanx. Once passive flexion has been restored, the need for flexor tendon tenolysis is assessed by asking the patient to actively flex the joint.

Therapy

Following PIP extension release, PIP flexion exercises are commenced as soon as possible. A dynamic flexion splint is applied as soon as the tissues will tolerate this. This may need to be alternated with intermittent static extension splintage if an extension lag of more than 20 degrees develops. Oedema control and an active exercise programme is commenced immediately. Exercise, mobilising and resting splintage need to be carefully balanced and will depend on the amount of inflammation, range of motion and glide of the soft tissues.

Intrinsic contracture of the hand

Contracture of the intrinsics, thenar and hypothenar groups may be secondary to ischaemia, Dupuytren's contracture, rheumatoid arthritis, spastic conditions or may follow as a consequence of incorrect splintage. Biomechanically, disruption of one structure in the digit will affect the intrinsic balance and may lead to an intrinsic contracture: e.g. MP volar subluxation and PIP joint dorsal subluxation. Intrinsic muscle fibrosis and contracture may follow severe crush injuries. The ischaemic muscle heals with fibrotic tissue, which contracts pulling the musculotendinous unit into a shortened position. The digits then assume the intrinsic plus posture, MP flexion and IP extension.

There are many different techniques for intrinsic release. The surgical procedure used will depend on what structures are involved. Techniques include:

- distal release by dividing the lateral bands, e.g. for swan-neck deformity
- release of the interossei proximal to the MP joint and division of the ACL of the MP joint, e.g. with MP joint flexion contracture
- release of the interossei from the metacarpal, e.g. for spastic conditions
- release of the intrinsic with crossed intrinsic transfer or lateral band transfer, e.g. in severe crush injuries where the intrinsic muscle itself has been damaged.

Therapy

The aim of the post-surgical therapy is to maintain intrinsic length. Within 48 hours post-release a dynamic intrinsic stretch splint (Fig. 2.81) is fitted. This is worn day and night for the first 6 weeks. Then at night for up to 6 months following release.

The exercise programme commences as soon as possible within the first 2 postoperative days. Extrinsic flexion is practised hourly; i.e. PIP and DIP combined flexion with the MP joints in extension. MP joint range is monitored. Formal MP joint exercises are usually commenced between week 2 and 3. The timing of composite flexion and extension exercise and resisted grip activities will vary from 4 to 8 weeks, depending on the progress of extrinsic flexion. Oedema control and scar management are most important. They are attended to as early as possible using the previously mentioned techniques.

Specific tip

The intrinsic muscles have a strong tendency to tighten as the scar of the surgery matures. To prevent recurrence of the contracture, vigilant night splinting for up to 6 months is essential.

Adduction contracture of the thumb

Surgery

An adduction contracture may develop from various causes, including crushing injuries, infection, burns, Dupuytren's contracture, arthritis or

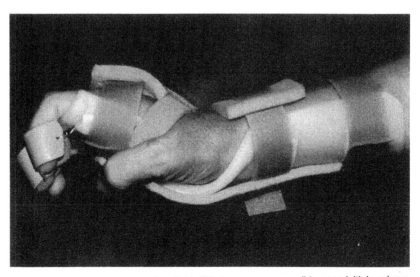

Figure 2.81 An intrinsic stretch splint is fitted as soon as possible once initial oedema has settled. The intrinsic muscles have a strong tendency to tighten as the scar of surgery matures. Vigilant night splinting of up to 6 months is necessary.

nerve palsy. The first web skin and fascia shorten, there may be fibrosis of the adductor pollicis muscle and/or shortening of the ligaments and dorsal capsule of the first CMC joint.

At surgery, contracted superficial fascia and fibrous tissue is removed; the contracted first dorsal interosseous and adductor pollicis are released from the first metacarpal. The dorsal capsule of the first CMC joint may require release and a skin flap may be necessary to fill the secondary defect.

Therapy

Therapy aims at maintaining the gain in the first web span while encouraging function. Splintage is vital. A static splint is worn, maintaining the web span in a palmar abduction position in the day and night for the first 2–3 weeks (Fig. 2.82). Subsequently, the static splint is continued at night for a prolonged period, which may be as long as 6 months. From 3 to 8 weeks, depending on the state of the tissues and the use of the hand,

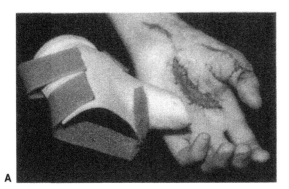 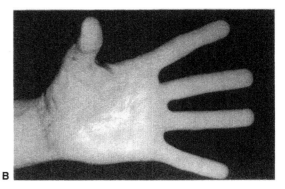

Figure 2.82 A: A hand-based static splint was used to maintain the thumb web space following thumb web release which required Z-plasty and skin grafting. B: Final result at 8 months post-release.

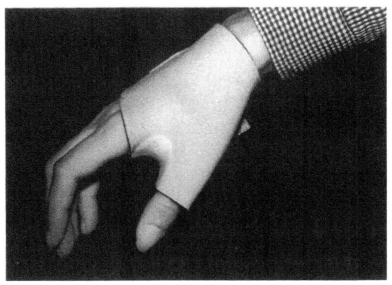

Figure 2.83 A neoprene splint with a thermoplastic strut can be used in the day from 3 weeks postoperative. This allows the thumb to be used while still maintaining some abduction pressure in the web.

a neoprene splint with a thumb web thermoplastic strut (Fig. 2.83) is worn in the day time.

At 2 weeks, the sutures are removed and the usual wound and scar care regime, e.g. massage, compression garments and pads, is commenced. Active and passive exercises are commenced in the first postoperative week. Care not to overstretch the MP joint laterally should be exercised when stretching the thumb web: this should be performed at the CMC joint level. Graded resistive use and exercise can be commenced by the third week.

Tenolysis

Tenolysis is a freeing procedure. The prerequisites for tenolysis are a functional need by the patient, adequate skin and soft tissue cover, a maximal passive joint range of motion and good muscular tone. There may be associated problems such as fracture malunion with deformity or a secondary joint contracture which may need surgical attention at the time of tenolysis if a good result is to be achieved. Local anaesthetic is used with the patient awake and able to cooperate with movements during the procedure. Adequate exposure of the adherent tendon is necessary; the tendon is then mobilised. The mobility of the tendon is checked by asking the patient to fully extend and flex the digit.

POST-SURGICAL MANAGEMENT

Tenolysis requires immediate mobilisation of the freed tendons. The aim of therapy is to preserve maximum tendon glide and range of motion, to prevent rupture and joint stiffness. The most important factor in the postoperative programme is an appropriate balance between rest and exercise.

Flexor tenolysis

The flexor tendons have a normal excursion of 18–25 mm.[16] Injury, infection or surgery can cause adhesions and block flexor tendon glide. Secondary contracture of other tissues including the fascia and joints may follow.

Surgery

Through a volar zigzag incision the tendon is exposed from proximal to distal. The pulleys are preserved and sharp dissection is needed to dissect circumferentially around the tendon, creating a plane between the pulley and the phalanx. One slip of the FDS may need resection. The digital nerves and vessels are protected. Under local anaesthetic, the surgeon can limit the procedure to the area causing the problem.

Therapy

The goals of the therapy programme will depend on several factors at the time of surgery, including tendon integrity, active and passive range of motion after lysis and pulley integrity. Communication with the surgeon regarding the status of these factors is essential for treatment planning.

Passive and active exercises are commenced immediately following surgery. Passive exercises are done first to minimise the resistance to active motion of the tenolysed tendon. Differential flexor tendon gliding exercises as described by Wehbe and Hunter[17] are commenced as soon as possible. The aim is to gain maximal glide with minimal inflammation. This can be a delicate balance. The hand is rested in a POSI splint between exercise sessions. Exercises are done hourly or second hourly with a low repetition rate, e.g. 3 to 5 times per exercise. Frequency and repetition rate will depend on tendon and pulley integrity and the degree of inflammation.

If there has been pulley damage or pulley reconstruction the pulley will need protection. Manual pressure or reinforcement in terms of a Velcro or thermoplastic ring is recommended. Pulley protection for up to 6 months is necessary, particularly if the hand is used for heavy activities.

Specific tip

1. In cases where passive range is poor, CPM can be a useful adjunct to treatment. The CPM is applied intermittently during the day before active exercise sessions. Using CPM to maintain passive range enables the patient to concentrate on active motion and tendon glide during exercise sessions.

2. FES to augment active contraction can be helpful if active range and tendon pull through is poor. The patient is instructed to contract the muscle in time with the muscle stimulation. The muscle stimulator must be set to allow for adequate time for contraction and relaxation. Generally the off/relaxation time is twice that of the contraction time.

Extensor tenolysis

Extensor tendon adhesions often form due to the close proximity of the tendon to the skeleton, the thin flat shape of the tendon and the thin overlying skin and subcutaneous tissues.

Surgery

The incision and exposure must allow for adequate skin and soft tissue dissection. The tendon is freed circumferentially from all adhesions. If there is an associated flexor tendon adhesion or joint contracture a bilateral neutral digital approach provides good exposure to both flexor and extensor aspect. The surgery is done under local block so that maximal voluntary active glide can be checked at the time of surgery. Those anatomical structures maintaining the central position of the extensor tendon must be maintained or repaired.

Therapy

Therapy aims to maintain extensor glide and prevent adhesion reformation. Passive and active exercises are commenced immediately following surgery. Exercises are done with a high frequency and low repetition rate. The tendon may be weak and stretched if it has had a prolonged period of inactivity in a lengthened position over the joint. Extension splintage to rest the tendon in a more advantageous position is usually necessary. The exercise programme should include EDC extension, intrinsic extension and blocked PIP extension. Resisted grip should be delayed until a strong extensor contraction can be achieved.

REFERENCES

1. Akeson W, Amiel D, Woo S: Immobility effects on synovial joints. The pathomechanics of joint contracture. Biorheology 17:95–110, 1980.
2. Frank C, Amiel D, Woo S: Normal ligament properties and ligament healing. Clin Orth Rel Res 196:15–20, 1985.
3. Snell E, Conolly WB: Post-traumatic flexion contracture of the proximal interphalangeal joint, surgical release and post operative therapy – a review of 21 subjects. In: Proceedings of the First Congress of the International Federation of Societies of Hand Therapists, Tel Aviv, Israel, 1989:42.
4. Watson K, Turkeltaub S: Stiff joints. In: Green D (ed.), Operative hand surgery. New York: Churchill Livingstone, 1979:537–52.
5. Young V, Wray R, Weeks P: The surgical management of stiff joints in the hand. Plast Reconstr Surg 62:835–41, 1978.
6. Tabary J, Tabary C, Tardiue C et al: Physiological and structural changes in the cat's soleus muscle due to immobilisation at different lengths by plaster casts. J Physiol 244:231–44, 1972.
7. Brand P, Hollister A: Clinical mechanics of the hand, 2nd edn. St Louis: Mosby, 1985.
8. Fess E: Principles and methods of splinting for mobilisation of joints. In: Hunter J, Schneider L, Mackin E, Callahan A (eds), Rehabilitation of the hand, 3rd edn. St Louis: Mosby, 1990:1101–8.

9. Colditz J: Spring – wire splinting of the proximal interphalangeal joint. In: Hunter J, Schneider L, Mackin E, Callahan A (eds), Rehabilitation of the hand, 3rd edn. St Louis: Mosby, 1990:1109–19.
10. Kottke F, Pauley O, Ptak R: The rationale for prolonged stretching for correction of shortening of connective tissue. Arch Phys Med Rehab 47:345–52, 1966.
11. Kolumban S: The role of static and dynamic splints, physiotherapy techniques and time in straightening contracted interphalangeal joints. Leprosy in India Oct:323–8, 1969.
12. Flowers K, LaStayo P: Effect of total end range time on improving passive range of motion. J Hand Ther 7:150–7, 1994.
13. Weeks P, Wray R, Kuxhause M: The results of non-operative management of stiff joints in the hand. Plast Reconstr Surg 62:58–63, 1978.
14. Prosser R: Splinting in the management of proximal interphalangeal joint flexion contracture. J Hand Ther 9:378–86, 1996.
15. Laseter G: Postoperative management of capsulectomies. In: Hunter J, Schneider L, Mackin E, Callahan A (eds), Rehabilitation of the hand, 3rd edn. St Louis: Mosby, 1990:364–70.
16. Simmons B, De La Caffiniere J: Physiology of flexion of the finger. In: Tubiana R (ed.), The hand, 1981:384.
17. Wehbe M, Hunter J: Flexor tendon gliding in the hand. Part I, differential gliding. J Hand Surg 10A:575, 1985.

K.   DUPUYTREN'S CONTRACTURE

W Bruce Conolly and Rosemary Prosser

DEFINITION AND PATHOLOGY

Dupuytren's disease is a proliferative fibroplasia of the fascial bands (Dupuytren's cords). These cords displace the neurovascular bundles. Secondary involvement of the skin and joints causes soft tissue and skeletal contractures, which is a biologically reactive process in certain genetically susceptible individuals. The pathological new tissue comprises immature collagen and fibroblasts. There may be extrapalmar ectopic deposits, manifesting as knuckle pads, plantar nodules and Peyronie's disease (Fig. 2.84).

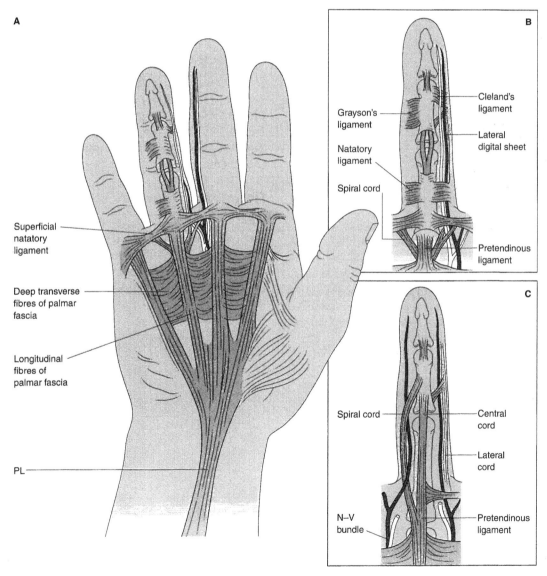

Figure 2.84   Anatomy of the palmar and digital fascia (A) and cords in the fingers (B, C) which may cause MP and PIP joint contracture and digital nerve displacement.

INDICATION FOR OPERATION

The aim of surgery is to regain or restore hand function. It is not possible to cure the disease. Surgical treatment is not then a radical excision but a release of tension to stabilise the biology. Operation is indicated, then, if the patient has a functional disability from a flexion contracture of any or all of the three finger joints (MP, PIP or DIP) or from a web contracture. The timing and type of procedure will depend on three sets of factors:

- the individual patient's circumstances (Dupuytren's diathesis, age, family history, general history)
- the type of hand (thick, stiff, arthritic or sweaty hands may not get the result hoped for)
- the type and extent of contracture – whether it be local or diffuse in the digit, involving single or multiple digits (Fig. 2.85)

CONTRAINDICATIONS

If there is associated skin excoriation or infection in the web, or arthritis in the hand likely to be exaggerated by the surgery, or if the patient is thought unlikely to follow a postoperative exercise programme, then surgery is probably contraindicated, at least for the present. Preoperative loss of digit extension should not be exchanged for a postoperative loss of flexion.

OPERATIVE PROCEDURES FOR DUPUYTREN'S CONTRACTURE

Fasciotomy

Fasciotomy may be open (where one dissects the neurovascular bundle) or closed (percutaneous).

Fasciotomy is indicated if there is a discrete pretendinous cord and mobile overlying skin causing an MP joint contracture. Fasciotomy may be a preliminary to fasciectomy in severe contractures or as an elective procedure in older people. Recurrence after this technique is common.

Regional fasciectomy

In this operation, the Dupuytren's disease fascia, nodules and cords are resected from the proximal palm to the distal extent in the digits. This may require extensive dissection, with particular attention to preserving the neurovascular bundles (Fig. 2.86).

Dermo-fasciectomy

After fasciectomy, resection of skin may be carried out to prevent local recurrence, especially where there is a Dupuytren's diathesis or to replace skin which is itself heavily involved with the disease or where the skin lacks sufficient circulation after fasciectomy for adequate healing.

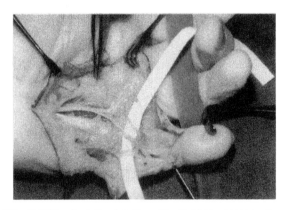

Figure 2.86 An extensive dissection is often necessary to remove the diseased fascia. Neurovascular structures are identified and preserved. Skin grafting (Wolfe graft) may be necessary in areas of dense Dupuytren's disease. Grafting also ensures no recurrence of Dupuytren's disease under the graft.

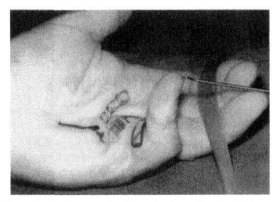

Figure 2.85 Preoperative Dupuytren's contracture. Note the cord and nodule involvement in the palm and digit.

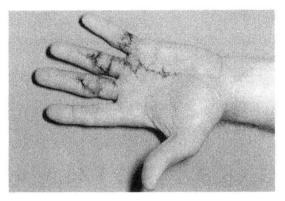

Figure 2.87 Appearance of the hand at 2 weeks, showing healing of the two Z-plasty flaps and skin graft (Wolfe graft) of the little finger.

Mostly, it is the skin over the proximal pulp or the distal palm which is excised and then covered by a full-thickness (Wolfe) graft,[1] taken either from the upper inner arm or the groin (Fig. 2.87). There must be an intact flexor tendon sheath to accept such a graft.

TYPES OF WOUND CLOSURE AFTER OPERATIONS FOR DUPUYTREN'S CONTRACTURE

This may be a Z-plasty (after a longitudinal approach), V–Y plasty, Wolfe graft (see dermo-fasciectomy) or split skin grafting.

Some wounds are left open to heal spontaneously, e.g. the open wound technique. Quite extensive transverse wounds in the palm, and occasionally the digit, heal over a 2–5 week period by the process of wound contraction. This process of contraction and marginal epithelialisation results in a transverse scar with normal adjacent skin and underlying soft tissue.

Early exercises can begin without the risk of haematoma or infection (Fig. 2.88).

Associated procedures to fasciectomy

PIP joint release

In cases of long-standing PIP flexion contracture in Dupuytren's disease, the PIP joint may remain in a

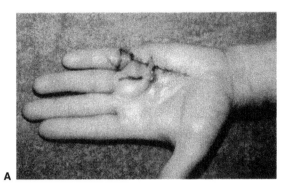

A

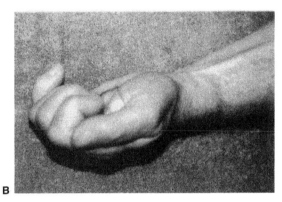

B

Figure 2.88 Range of motion at 2 weeks following Dupuytren's excision with open palm technique.

state of flexion. In these cases the surgeon may, after dividing the digital fascia, divide Cleland's ligament and occasionally the fibrosed flexor sheath. If the joint remains flexed, the check rein ligament may be divided. It is rare to perform an open PIP joint capsulotomy because these patients may develop considerable postoperative stiffness. In most cases after fasciectomy a gentle manipulation of the PIP joint in conjunction with postoperative extension splintage provides reasonable PIP joint extension. In these long-standing flexion contracture cases, the extensor apparatus may become attenuated.

Amputation

Amputation at the PIP or the MP joint level may be indicated for irreversible contracture of the recurrent disease, especially in older people, and on occasions where the finger does not remain viable after extensive fasciectomy.

Complications of surgical procedures for Dupuytren's disease

Surgical complications:

- Intraoperative:
  ischaemic digit
  haematoma.
- Postoperative:
  ischaemic skin necrosis
  scar contracture
  joint stiffness
  reflex dystrophy.

Overall, the recurrence rates after fasciotomy and localised fasciectomy are about 70% and after regional, fasciectomy 10–15%, although only 15% of these patients may require revision surgery.[1]

General comment

Many of the patients presenting for surgery are of the older age, some need treatment for diabetes and alcoholism and others have underlying arthritis and are prone to stiffness.

The surgery of fasciectomy is quite extensive, representing quite a significant injury to the hand.

In long-standing cases of Dupuytren's contracture with severe flexion deformities, the neurovascular bundles may be tight and with release of the contracture and stretching of these bundles many patients experience a period of digital numbness. This does, however, resolve eventually.

POSTOPERATIVE MANAGEMENT PRINCIPLES

- Maintain the digital extension gained in surgery with appropriate splintage
- Regain the digital flexion while maintaining extension
- Prevent wound complications and excessive inflammation
- Soften the surgical scar
- Prevention/control of pain, flare reactions or reflex sympathetic dystrophy (RSD)

Splinting

- Patients with severe flexion contracture may require splintage for the first 7–14 days; after this time, night splintage is usually adequate.
- If the patient loses extension during the day, then periods of extension splintage during the day may be necessary. This may range from 2 to 8 hours/day plus night splintage.
- Hands with slow healing grafts or prolonged wound inflammation may also require splintage during the day for a longer period.
- Night extension splintage may need to be prolonged 4–6 months.[2]

Type of splint

Static

A thermoplastic splint with wrist in neutral or slight extension, MPs neutral 0 degree and IPs in maximal extension gained by the surgery is used to maintain correction. The DIP joint should not be hyperextended. A forearm-based splint may be necessary initially, if there is considerable swelling and/or wound reaction. A hand- or digit-based splint may be all that is required if there is minimal wound reaction (Fig. 2.89).

Once the wound has healed, a compression pad alone may be adequate to maintain extension.

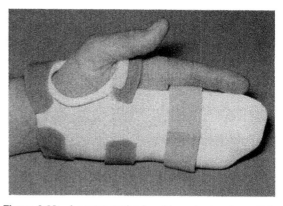

Figure 2.89 A postoperative hand-based extension splint is used to maintain the correction gained in surgery. It is worn at night and intermittently during the day for the first 7–14 days. After this time, it may be required at night only for 3–6 months.

Dynamic

Dynamic outrigger splintage can be considered for those patients with preoperative contractures of the MP and PIP joints greater than 60 degrees, if the surgeon reports a 'springy end feel' or if it is thought that a static splint will require many adjustments.

Wound care

Dressings and debridement

- As many of these patients have had considerable surgical dissection, the wound can be quite extensive and take some time to settle. The hand should be rested until the acute inflammation has settled.
- Early wound care involves cleaning of the wound with saline and a simple Vaseline gauze and cotton gauze dressing.
- If the wound is sloughy, appropriate cleaning and debriding agents can be used, e.g. hydrogen peroxide.[3] Improved dressing materials, e.g., alganates and colloids, also assist in gaining wound closure.
- Once the inflammation has settled, and this may take 5–10 days, warm lux soaks or whirlpool treatment may commence. This helps debride any thick eschar and softens the incision line to facilitate exercise. If there is any concern regarding the wound, the surgeon should be contacted.
- Compression wrap applied early and gently will help to decrease swelling and inflammation, thereby decreasing the likelihood of a thick scar. If there is any vascular compromise, this should be delayed until both surgeon and therapist are satisfied with the vascular status. The compression wrap is applied for 15 min and then removed and vascular return checked before continuing compression wrap over an extended period. The patient can be taught to check his/her own circulation.
- Skin grafts: these are usually Wolfe grafts and have tie-over sutures with a small foam pressure pad. This should not be disturbed for 5–7 days; during this time the hand is rested. Once the tie-over sutures are removed, provided the graft has taken and the wound settled, short lux soaks can be commenced. Whirlpool treatment should not be commenced until 10–14 days, as the turbulence may lift the edges of the graft.

- Open wound technique: it is our experience that these wounds heal very quickly (approximately 14–21 days) with very few, if any, problems.
- The open wound can be treated like a normal suture line. It will require a simple Vaseline gauze/cotton gauze dressing until it heals.
- Lux soaks and whirlpool can be commenced early (5–10 days).
- Prosthetic foam can be used to give compression to the wound early (approximately 5–7 days) if necessary, as it allows the wound to be ventilated.[4]

Scar care

Massage. This technique should be done at least four times per day for 2–3 min. Massaging should apply firm but gentle pressure and should gently move the subcutaneous tissues. If the tissues become red or swollen following massage, the massaging is too firm. A cold pack should be applied to decrease the inflammation.

Compression silicone pads. The pads can be applied as soon as the wound has healed to soften the scar (Fig. 2.90). Prosthetic foam compression pads can be applied if there is an open area.[2,5]

The compression pad is usually worn at night and evening, leaving the hands free during the day to be used.

Ultrasound. It is our experience that diligent massaging and the use of compression wraps and pads is most effective for softening the scar. The ultrasound literature reports that heating is the most desirable effect to be obtained from ultrasound.[6–8] It is our clinical experience that ultrasound is beneficial for those scars that are excessively tender or painful; heating of the tissues can be achieved by other modalities that do not require as much of the therapist's time.

Exercise and functional activities

- Exercise is commenced early, at approximately 3–5 days postoperative. Initially, the unoperated digits are exercised actively through the full range. On the operated digits, DIP active isolated flexion/extension exercises are commenced. This is particularly important following the release of a long-standing flexion contracture, as the lateral bands of the extensor mechanism and oblique retinacular ligament have often become tight. Once the flexion contraction has been corrected, these structures are even tighter and can restrict DIP flexion considerably.

• At 7–10 days, isolated PIP flexion/extension and intrinsic MP flexion/extension (that is MP flexion with IPs extended) is commenced, along with gentle gross/composite flexion and extension. The patient is encouraged to use his/her hand for light, pain-free ADL when not wearing the splint.

• At 2–3 weeks, passive stretching techniques can be added for flexion, such as passive flexion exercises, isolated and gross, or bandaging into flexion and heat (warm water, wax or a hot pack).

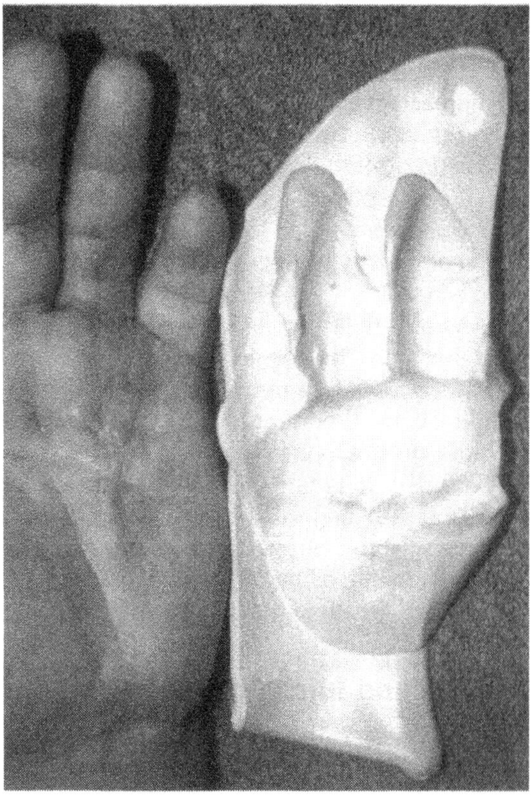

Care should be taken with wax and hot packs that they are not too hot and increase the oedema in the early stages. Also:

1. light resistance is added to the exercise programme
2. functional activities are introduced into the exercise programme.

• From 3–6 weeks, the exercise programme is upgraded to include moderate resistance, e.g. contract/relax, and heavier functional activities.

• After 6 weeks, each individual is progressed as quickly as possible back to full resistance activities and sport.

Specific tips

Splinting

DIP hypertension can be prevented by using a small roll of splinting material under the DIP joint, or moulding the splint into some flexion at the DIP joint while maintaining PIP extension (Fig. 2.91).

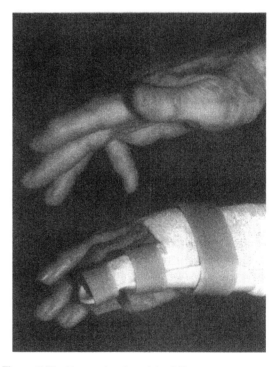

Figure 2.90 A compression silicone pad forms a perfect impression of the scar. This enables contact and pressure to soften all parts of the scar.

Figure 2.91 Hyperextension of the DIP joint can be corrected with a splint which rests or gently stretches the DIP joint into flexion while maintaining PIP extension. The splint is shown on the left hand which had a similar degree of contracture to the right preoperatively.

PIP flexion contracture

Persistent PIP flexion contracture or an early recurring PIP flexion contracture may require more specific splinting. Early dynamic splintage, either a hand-based outrigger or a Capener splint, can be made to apply the extension force specifically to the PIP joint.[5,9] This type of splintage also allows motion, thus helping to reduce stiffness. Specific attention must be given to controlling swelling with dynamic splints. A pressure garment or pressure wrap under the splint is essential in the first 3–4 weeks postoperatively. In the later stages, 4–5 weeks onward, a night static or dynamic splint in combination with a neoprene sleeve in the day may be adequate.

Be aware of those patients with underlying osteoarthritis: complete reduction of a flexion contracture in these circumstances may not be possible.

Inflammation

If the hand has inflammation that is taking a long time to settle, be patient – *Don't* press on. Some of these patients require 7–10 days of relative rest for the inflammation to settle, as the surgical dissection is very extensive.

Use cold packs and compression wraps early, as long as there are no contraindications.

Alcohol

Ingestion of alcohol, especially more than 1 or 2 drinks per day increases swelling, due to the vasodilation effect of alcohol: this may be a factor in prolonged swelling and inflammation.

Granulomas

Granulomas may resolve with pressure alone – ventilated adhesive tape, such as hypafix or fixamil, over the granuloma will often be enough. Otherwise, the application of a caustic pencil (silver nitrate) to the granuloma will resolve it (Fig. 2.92).

Pain

If there is prolonged or excessive pain following surgery, first check the dressing and splint, which should be released if they are tight. Transcutaneous electrical nerve stimulation (TENS) can be helpful.[10,11] It should be applied proximally in the forearm or arm to the peripheral nerves or stellate ganglion.

If, on examination, the pain is due to an irritable brachial plexus from the regional block anaesthetic, gentle brachial plexus mobilisation techniques and TENS will often resolve this. Therapy should not be painful.

Reflex sympathetic dystrophy

If an RSD develops, the usual post-fasciectomy programme should be adjusted and treatment should be aimed at the RSD. The wound will still need wound care and a compression garment is also beneficial in controlling swelling. Passive

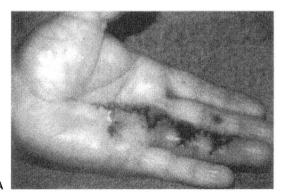
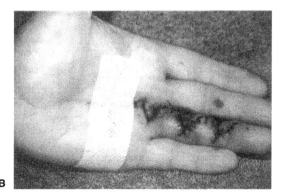

A   B

Figure 2.92 A palmar granuloma has developed on the suture line. Application of hypafix in this case resolved the granuloma in 2–3 weeks.

range of movement is contraindicated and for this reason extension splintage may need to be discontinued temporarily until the RSD symptoms are controlled. The stress loading programme[12] can be instituted early on. The patient is encouraged to use his hand, as long as it is pain-free activity.

Therapy should not be painful – splinting and formal exercises can be recommended once the pain has settled.

REFERENCES

1. Hueston J: Limited fasciectomy for Dupuytren's contracture. *Plast Reconstr Surg* 27:569–85, 1961.
2. Fietti VG, Mackin EJ: Open palm technique in Dupuytren's disease. In: Hunter JM, Schneider LH, Mackin EJ, Callahan AD (eds), Rehabilitation of the hand. St Louis: Mosby, 1990.
3. Smith KL: Wound care for the hand patient. In: Hunter JM, Schneider LH, Mackin EJ, Callahan AD (eds), Rehabilitation of the hand. St Louis: Mosby, 1990.
4. Stewart KM: Therapist's management of the mutilated hand. In: Hunter JM, Schneider LH, Mackin EJ, Callahan AD (eds), Rehabilitation of the hand. St Louis: Mosby, 1990.
5. Boscheinen-Morrin J, Davey V, Conolly WB: The hand – fundamentals of therapy. Oxford: Butterworth Heinemann, 1992:167–78.
6. Wadsworth H, Chanmugan APP: Electrophysical agents in physiotherapy. Marrickville: Science Press, 1980:139–202.
7. Taylor Mullins PA: Use of therapeutic modalities in upper extremity rehabilitation. In: Hunter JM, Schneider LH, Mackin EJ, Callahan AD (eds), Rehabilitation of the hand. St Louis: Mosby, 1990.
8. Cannon NM, Taylor Mullins P: Modalities. In: Malick MH, Kasch MC (eds), Manual on management of specific hand problems. Pittsburgh: American Rehabilitation Educational Network, 1984.
9. Colditz J: Dynamic splinting of the stiff hand. In: Hunter JM, Schneider LH, Mackin EJ, Callahan AD (eds), Rehabilitation of the hand. St Louis: Mosby, 1990.
10. Lee VH, Reynolds CC: Clinical application of transcutaneous electrical nerve stimulator in patients with upper extremity pain. In: Hunter JM, Schneider LH, Mackin EJ, Callahan AD (eds), Rehabilitation of the hand. St Louis: Mosby, 1990.
11. Wells P, Frampton V, Bowsher F: Transcutaneous electrical nerve stimulation and 'chronic pain'. In: Pain management by physiotherapy. Oxford: Butterworth Heinemann, 1994:115–40.
12. Watson HK, Carlson L: Treatment of reflex sympathetic dystrophy of the hand with an active 'stress loading' programme. J Hand Surg 12A:779–85, 1987.

L. VASCULAR DISORDERS

James A Masson

COMPARTMENT SYNDROME

Compartment syndrome occurs when there is increased pressure within a confined osseofascial space, producing a decrease in tissue blood flow, oxygenation and, ultimately, function. If unrelieved, there is vascular compromise and, ultimately, ischaemic necrosis of muscle and nerves.

Anatomy

The forearm contains three distinct muscle compartments: the volar compartment, containing the flexor muscles; the dorsal compartment, containing the extensor muscles; and the radial mobile wad, which contains the brachioradialis and the radial wrist extensors. The hand contains 10 discrete fascial compartments: four dorsal interosseous spaces, three palmar interosseous spaces, spaces for the thenar and hypothenar muscles respectively, and the adductor space. Any one of these spaces may be involved in a compartment syndrome.

Aetiology

There are many causes of compartment syndrome, but the most important are:

1. fractures (forearm, distal radius) and their surgical management, whether closed or open
2. arterial injury (supracondylar fracture, blunt or penetrating trauma)
3. tight casts or dressings following surgery or fracture reduction

4. crush injury
5. burns
6. intra-arterial drug injection
7. lying on the limb for extended periods of time in an unconscious patient (e.g. drug overdose).

Clinical

A high index of suspicion must be maintained in any patient with an injury that may give rise to a compartment syndrome.[1] Persistent pain is the *sine qua non* of a compartment syndrome. In fact, some hand surgery units will not prescribe intramuscular narcotic analgesia in the postoperative period for fear of masking just this problem. Passive stretching of the muscles involved will exacerbate the pain, and this alone should be sufficient clinical indication to proceed to fasciotomy. The affected muscles will also become weak. Diminished sensibility in the distribution of the nerve or nerves that pass through the affected muscle group (usually the median nerve and sometimes the ulnar nerve in the forearm) can occur, due to nerve ischaemia and compression. Although proximal arterial occlusion could produce the same spectrum of symptoms and signs, in compartment syndrome, the arterial pulses are still usually palpable. Therefore, compartment syndrome should be suspected in the presence of the six P's – pain, pressure, pain with stretch, paresis, paraesthesiae and pulses present.

An obvious compartment syndrome is easy to diagnose and treat. However, the symptoms and signs can progress insidiously. Frequent, repeat clinical examinations will unmask the trend. Occasionally, it may be necessary to resort to some invasive method of measuring intracompartmental pressure to confirm the diagnosis. The unconscious patient is such an indication. Traditionally, a Wick catheter[2] or the Whitesides' infusion method[3] have been used. However, there are now commercially available hand-held units which are much more 'user-friendly': 30 mmHg is usually recommended as the threshold above which fasciotomy should be performed. However, it cannot be emphasised enough that clinical suspicion

alone should be sufficient indication to proceed to fasciotomy.

Surgical treatment

The appropriate treatment for a diagnosed compartment syndrome is fasciotomy of the involved space.[4] In the forearm, this may involve both volar and dorsal fasciotomies. In a volar forearm fasciotomy, it is necessary to release the flexor muscle group throughout its entire muscular length, i.e. from the medial epicondyle to the wrist. The median and ulnar nerves should also be decompressed at the wrist. The usual principles of incision planning are adhered to by avoiding crossing flexion creases at right angles, and skin flaps are elevated to avoid subsequent exposure of the median nerve at the wrist and the ulnar nerve at the elbow. The extensor compartment and mobile wad of the forearm can be released through a single longitudinal incision (Fig. 2.93).

Parallel incisions on the dorsum of the hand between the second and third, and fourth and fifth metacarpals will allow decompression of the dorsal and volar interossei as well as the adductor compartment. The thenar compartment can be released through a longitudinal incision along the radial border of the first metacarpal while the hypothenar muscles can be released through a similar incision along the ulnar border of the fifth metacarpal.

No attempt is made to close the skin at the time of the initial decompression. The wounds are dressed and the forearm and hand are splinted in the position of safe immobilisation. Delayed primary closure or split-thickness skin grafting can be performed 72–96 hours later when most of the swelling has subsided. If the wound requires grafting, the grafts can be removed subsequently by serial excision, as there is usually no actual skin loss.

If sufficient muscle has necrosed, rhabdomyolysis occurs and myoglobin is released into the bloodstream. Myoglobinuria can produce acute renal failure, from both direct nephrotoxicity and tubular obstruction. A high urine output must be

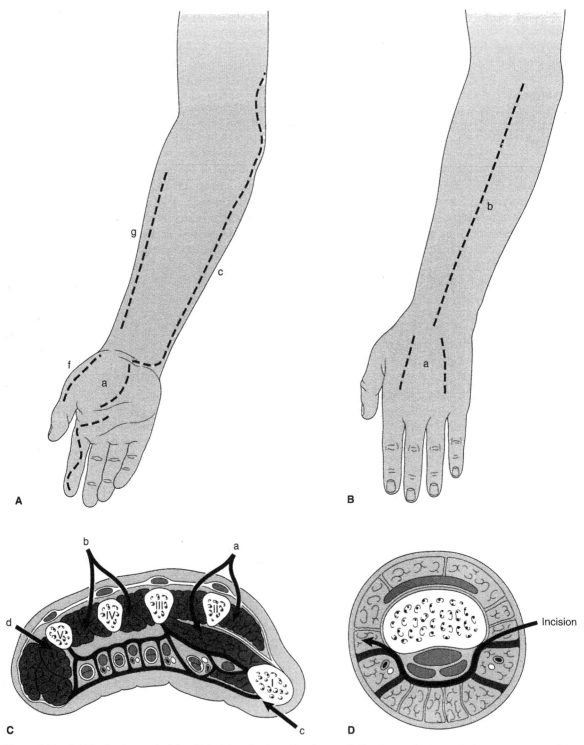

Figure 2.93 A: Volar fasciotomy incision. B: Incisions for dorsal fasciotomy. C: Fasciotomy for the intrinsic compartments of the hand. D: Fasciotomy for the digit.

obtained in these patients, often necessitating pharmacological diuresis.

POSTOPERATIVE MANAGEMENT

Immediately following surgery, the hand and wrist are splinted in the position of safe immobilisation (POSI). Once the patient's general medical condition and surgical wounds have settled, which may be anywhere from 2 days to 1 week, gentle assisted active and passive range of movement (ROM) exercises are commenced for the shoulder, elbow, wrist and hand.

The two most common problems for the patient and therapist following decompression are scar adhesion and prolonged neurogenic pain. The incision required to decompress the forearm is extensive. When this is combined with the oedema which results from the compartment syndrome itself, the scarring can be significant. Gentle compression wraps and garments must be used judiciously and monitored carefully. The tissues must not be aggravated further by more pressure. Elevation and massage are the two safest and most effective modalities. Early active mobilisation also promotes fluid mobilisation and drainage.

Persistent pain can be a difficult problem to treat. Early intervention with pain-relieving modalities is essential to gain control before lasting changes in the anterior horn cells occur. Treatment techniques may include electrotherapy modalities (TENS, heat, interferential), relaxation techniques, behaviour modification and improvement in general body fitness. TENS is a very effective, well-documented modality. It is portable, easy to use, and also enables the patient to take control of the problem.

Once the acute stage has passed, the patient must be re-assessed. Any residual problems, such as PIP joint flexion contractures, weakness of grip or diminished nerve function, need to be addressed.

VOLKMANN'S CONTRACTURE

Volkmann's ischaemic contracture is the end result of a compartment syndrome where muscles and nerves have died and been replaced by fibrous scar. Vascular compromise of the muscle is most severe towards the centre of the muscle bellies adjacent to the bone and around the anterior interosseous artery. The periphery of the muscle is relatively spared, probably due to better collateral circulation. Therefore, those muscles which are most severely affected are the deep flexor group, i.e. flexor digitorum profundus (FDP) and flexor pollicis longus (FPL). The next most affected group is one layer more superficial, i.e. flexor digitorum superficialis (FDS) and pronator teres. The wrist flexors and the dorsal forearm musculature are relatively spared. The nerves which pass through the area of muscle infarction are also damaged, initially by ischaemia and then by compression. The median nerve passes in the plane between the FDS and the FDP and is most commonly and severely affected. The ulnar nerve is more protected, lying medial to the area of most severe damage. However, it can also be badly damaged in an extensive contracture. Muscle and nerve recovery is dependent on the ischaemic time. If compression is relieved before irreversible changes occur, spontaneous recovery may ensue. However, once the muscles and nerves have infarcted, they will be replaced by scar.

The appearance of the upper limb in a patient with a full-blown Volkmann's contracture is therefore forearm pronation, wrist flexion, MP joint hyperextension and IP flexion. The palmar surface of the hand and fingers will also be insensate from ischaemia and compression of the median and ulnar nerves. These severe contractures are most commonly seen in mismanaged supracondylar fractures where there is forearm ischaemia from compression of the brachial artery.

Treatment

This condition is one where prevention is certainly better than cure. If a compartment syndrome is diagnosed early enough, and a decompressive fasciotomy performed, the ischaemic changes may well be reversible. However, if the ischaemic insult persists much beyond 48 hours, there will be permanent damage, which can range from mild to severe.

Post-injury therapy

The initial treatment in an established contracture is non-surgical. Recovery is slow in this condition, and great patience must be exercised, especially in nerve recovery. Once the scar has matured and the maximal benefits from therapeutic measures have been realised, surgery may be appropriate.

The major problems are:

1. joint and muscle contractures
2. poor muscle function (length and strength) due to muscle infarction and loss of nerve function
3. poor nerve function due to ischaemic damage.

Therapy is directed at improving all of these problems.

Joint and muscle contracture

The primary treatment technique for this problem is splinting or casting. Serial casting, serial static splinting or dynamic splinting have all been used to deal with this difficult problem. Serial casting tends to be more effective with very stiff joints with a firm end feel. Total end range time is the most significant factor in splinting efficacy. Perhaps this is why serial casting is more effective in resistant joints.

Contracted muscles require splinting or casting the entire length of the muscle–tendon unit. Following a Volkmann's contracture, both extrinsic and intrinsic muscles require splinting or casting.

Poor muscle function

The residual muscle requires exercise both to glide and strengthen the musculotendinous unit. All modes of exercise can be used – active, passive, and different forms of resisted exercise, such as contract–relax or repeated contractions. Use of the hand and arm in everyday activity is strongly encouraged. A strengthening activity programme is also beneficial. If there has been significant muscle infarction, there is usually significant fibrosis and scarring within the residual muscle. Very

dense and fibrotic tissue may not respond well to therapy. Even serial casting may prove fruitless. These cases require surgical intervention.

Poor nerve function

The therapist needs to monitor nerve function and its progression by muscle charting and sensibility evaluation (see Chapter 7A). A maintenance programme of passive joint exercise to prevent further contracture and an appropriate exercise programme for muscles that have been reinnervated are prescribed. If the patient has loss of protective sensibility, instruction with regard to prevention of injury or burns is necessary.

Surgical treatment

In mild cases, excision of the muscle infarct may allow release of the contracture. Fractional lengthening or a formal tendon lengthening may be required to restore optimal tone. In more extensive contractures, however, this will not suffice. There are two main surgical options for moderately severe contractures, both of which include neurolysis of the median and ulnar nerves as appropriate. In the first procedure, a flexor slide, the origins of the flexor muscles are released from the humerus, radius and ulna as required, and the entire flexor-pronator mass is slid distally down the forearm until satisfactory tone is returned to the fingers and thumb.[5] This procedure involves a very extensive dissection of the forearm, including the area of infarction.

Therapy following flexor slide

Postoperative therapy includes protective splintage that maintains the muscle–tendon length obtained in the surgery. Routine oedema, wound and scar management is carried out. Gentle passive and assisted active exercises are commenced immediately. The therapy programme is graduated slowly. Light resistance can be started at 4–6 weeks. Full resistive work is not commenced before 12 weeks.

The other surgical option is to ignore the infarct, transect the flexor tendons distal to it and restore flexor tendon function through tendon transfers. Commonly employed transfers use the brachioradialis to power the FPL and the ECRL can be transferred into all four profundus tendons (see Chapter 7D).

In the most severe contractures, not only does extrinsic flexor function need to be restored but one must also consider the requirements for thumb opposition and intrinsic function in the fingers. These can be restored by selective tendon transfers at a later stage. Although the tendon transfers mentioned above can still be used in severe contractures, in selected cases where donor motor units are unavailable, free muscle transfer may be indicated. Gracilis and the medial head of gastrocnemius have been the most popular muscles transferred and can provide mass grip function of fingers and thumb in appropriately selected cases.

Raynaud's phenomenon

Raynaud's phenomenon is a vasospastic disorder, characterised by episodic digital ischaemia with white, blue and, finally, red discolouration of the fingers.[6] The ischaemic pallor results from vasoconstriction; cyanosis ensues from the subsequent venous dilatation and pooling of deoxygenated blood; and finally, reactive hyperaemia produces the red flush. Raynaud's phenomenon may be associated with digital ulceration and tissue necrosis. Raynaud's phenomenon occurs in areas rich in arteriovenous anastomoses, such as the fingers, but the thumb is often spared. It can also affect the toes, ears and nose. It is usually precipitated by cold exposure, but may also be induced by vibration, stress or vasoconstrictive drugs.[7] It is estimated to affect 5–10% of the general population and usually occurs in young and middle-aged women. Raynaud's phenomenon may occur independently (primary) or be associated with an underlying disease (secondary), of which the most common is scleroderma (systemic sclerosis). In primary Raynaud's, the patient tends to be younger, and has bilateral symmetrical colour changes following a defined precipitating event, e.g. cold. Secondary Raynaud's tends to have a later onset, with asymmetrical finger involvement, and tends to be associated with trophic changes and gangrene.

Pathophysiology

The mechanisms behind the attacks of vasospasm remain speculative. Original theories suggested sympathetic overactivity. More recent theories suggest that there is an intrinsic fault in the digital artery which makes it more sensitive to cold. There is a diffuse small vessel vasculopathy, with persistent vasospasm, thickened vessel walls from endothelial cell changes, increased blood viscosity and low digital artery blood pressure distal to obstructions. There appears to be increased sensitivity of alpha$_2$-adrenoreceptors and serotonin receptors.

Treatment

The treatment of Raynaud's phenomenon is usually conservative (Table 2.2). Avoidance of precipitating factors is crucial. For mild cases, reassurance, the wearing of gloves, cold avoidance, and cessation of tobacco and caffeine all help. Biofeedback may be beneficial. The calcium channel blocker nifedipine is the first line in drug therapy. Other calcium channel blockers or ACE (angiotensin-converting enzyme) inhibitors are also used. Pentoxifylline improves red blood cell deformability, and may be useful, especially in cases of ulceration. Topical nitrates work for some patients.

Surgical sympathectomy is of variable benefit. When performed at stellate ganglion level, it is of little or no use. However, digital sympathectomy has had more promising results, especially when a preoperative digital nerve block shows an improvement in the Doppler arterial waveform: whether it acts by localised sympathectomy or adventitial decompression is not really known. The exact extent of digital sympathectomy is also contentious, with some authors decompressing only the proper digital arteries over a period of 1 cm, whereas others recommend a much more extensive operation, including the radial and ulnar arteries at the wrist, the superficial palmar arch, the common digital arteries and the proper digital arteries well out into the fingers.

Table 2.2 Preventive measures and treatments of Raynaud's phenomenon (Reproduced with permission from Browne et al.[6])

Cold protection	Avoid exposure to cold temperatures and to abrupt temperature changes Wear warm clothing – multi-layered, hat, scarf, mittens Special material – down, Gore-Tex, Thinsulate Electric mittens and socks
Minor treatment	Warm water soaks, hand shaking, arm whirling
Behaviour modification	Avoid emotionally stressful situations Stress management training Biofeedback Avoid certain medications and drugs, e.g. caffeine Stop smoking
Occupational modification	Avoid or modify use of vibratory machines Consider changing jobs
Vasodilatation	Calcium channel blockers Nitrates Prostaglandins and prostacyclins Serotonin antagonists Alpha-adrenergic blocking agents Sympatholytics
Miscellaneous	Platelet aggregation inhibitors Plasmapheresis Fibrinolysis Increased red cell deformability Volume expanders Anabolic steroids
Surgery	Sympathectomy Correction of anatomical abnormality

REFERENCES

1. Mabee JR: Compartment syndrome: A complication of acute extremity trauma. J Emerg Med 12:651, 1994.
2. Mubarak SJ et al: The Wick catheter technique for measurement of intramuscular pressure. A new research and clinical tool. J Bone Joint Surg 58A: 1016, 1976.
3. Whitesides TE Jr et al: Tissue pressure measurements as a determinant for the need of fasciotomy. Clin Orthop 113:43, 1975.
4. Rowland SA: Fasciotomy: the treatment of compartment syndrome. In: Green DP (ed.), Operative hand surgery, 3rd edn. Edinburgh: Churchill Livingstone, 1993:661.
5. Tsuge K: Management of established Volkmann's contracture. In: Green DP (ed.), Operative hand surgery, 3rd edn. Edinburgh: Churchill Livingstone, 1993:593.
6. Browne BJ, Jotte RS, Rolnick M: Raynaud's phenomenon in the emergency department. J Emerg Med 13:369, 1995.
7. Coffman JD: Raynaud's phenomenon. Hypertension 17:593, 1991.

3

The wrist

A. FUNCTIONAL ANATOMY AND ASSESSMENT

Paul LaStayo

The purpose of this chapter is to review the functional anatomy of the wrist complex and describe clinical provocative manoeuvres that can be used to help identify the cause of wrist pain.

THE ARTICULATIONS OF THE WRIST

Wrist complex range of motion

Functional wrist movement is a result of interactions at the radiocarpal articulation, within and between carpal bones, at the carpal–metacarpal level and at the junction between the distal radius and the ulna/triangular fibrocartilage complex.[3] When functioning properly, the wrist is capable of attaining 120 degrees of flexion and extension, 100 degrees of combined radial and ulnar deviation and 150 degrees of forearm rotation.[5] Functional range of motion (ROM) requirements, however, are significantly less, with 40 degrees of flexion and extension and a 100 degree arc of forearm rotation required for activities of daily living.[38]

The distal radius and extrinsic ligaments of the wrist

The distal articular surface of the radius is angulated palmarly 10–15 (mean 11) degrees

109

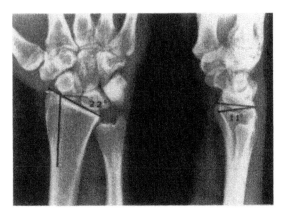

Figure 3.1 The AP film on the left illustrates normal radial inclination and the lateral film on the right illustrates normal volar tilt of the articular surface of the distal radius. (Reproduced with permission from Palmer AK.[31])

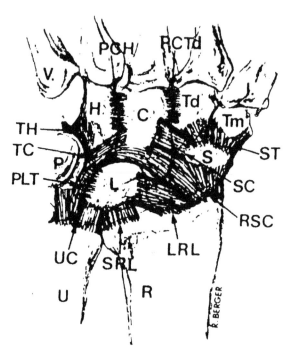

Figure 3.2 Ligamentous anatomy of the wrist from a palmar perspective with the underlying bony elements. Bones: R = radius, U = ulna, S = scaphoid, L = lunate, P = pisiform, Tm = trapezium, Td = trapezoid, C = capitate, H = hamate, I = metacarpal I, V = metacarpal V. Ligaments: RSC = radioscaphocapitate, LRL = long radiolunate, SRL = short radiolunate, UC = ulnocarpal (ulnolunate, ulnotriquetral and ulnocapitate), PLT = palmar lunotriquetral, TC = triquetrocapitate, TH = triquetrohamate, SC = scaphocapitate, ST = scaphotrapezium-trapezoid, PCTd = palmar trapeziocapitate, PCH = palmar capitohamate. (Reproduced with permission from Berger RA: Anatomy and basic biomechanics of the wrist. In: Manske PR (ed.), Hand surgery update. Englewood, CO: American Society for Surgery of the Hand, 1994.)

and inclinated ulnarly 15–25 (mean 22) degrees (Fig. 3.1).[31] Restoring these normal osseous angles is imperative after distal radius fractures, as accurate reductions have been shown to correlate with improved outcomes.[18,21,26,42] Malunited fractures, with dorsal angulation and shortening of the radius, the most debilitating deformities, can lead to limited ROM,[19] midcarpal instability,[44] alterations in the transmission of axial forces[40] and reduced grip strength.[46]

From the palmar aspect of the distal radius arise the distinct extrinsic ligaments of the wrist (Fig. 3.2). From radial to ulnar they are:

- The radioscaphocapitate (RSC), which is the most radial of these ligaments and functions as a radial collateral ligament.
- The long radiolunate (LRL) ligament, just ulnar to the RSC, connects the radius and lunate, but also supports the proximal pole of the scaphoid.
- The short radiolunate (SRL) ligament, arising from the palmar margin of the lunate fossa and attaching to the lunate, is the principal stabiliser of the lunate.[3]
- Located ulnarly are the ulnolunate, ulnotriquetral and ulnocapitate ligaments (known collectively as the ulnocarpal ligament), with attachments as their names imply. These ligaments are stabilisers of the ulnar carpus and thus compliment the

function of the triangular fibrocartilage complex (TFCC).[31]
- There is one relatively weak extrinsic ligament dorsally, the dorsal radiocarpal (DRC) ligament, which inserts on to the triquetrum and into the region of the lunotriquetral joint.[3]

The distal radioulnar joint (DRUJ)

DRUJ

The anatomy of the DRUJ promotes both rotational and sliding movements between the radius

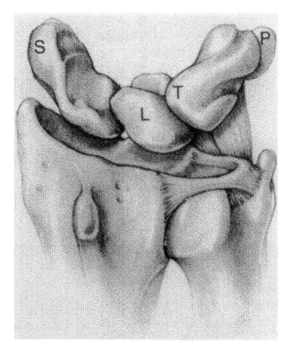

Figure 3.3 The distal radioulnar articulation in neutral or zero rotation with the ulnar head seated within the sigmoid notch and the proximal row of carpal bones (S = scaphoid, L = lunate, T = triquetrum, P = pisiform) distally. The triangular fibrocartilage and the ulnocarpal ligament are represented by the two equilateral triangles perpendicular to one another. (Reproduced with permission from Bowers WH: The distal radioulnar joint. In: Green DP (ed.), Operative hand surgery, 3rd edn. New York: Churchill Livingstone, 1993.)

and ulna, resulting in forearm rotation.[9] This movement is controlled largely by the TFCC (Fig. 3.3). When the wrist complex is axially loaded, as in gripping, the radius, through its articulation with the lateral carpus, absorbs approximately 80% of the force through the forearm while the ulna, through its articulation with the medial carpus and the TFCC, carries 20% of the load.[31] When the normal articular relationship between the distal radius and ulna is disrupted, as seen with malunited distal radius fractures and DRUJ incongruity, loads through the radius and ulna can exceed physiological limits.[33] Reproducing a patient's symptoms with palpation of the DRUJ, and/or compression of the DRUJ while rotating the forearm should make an examiner suspicious of DRUJ malalignment or degenerative

changes.[17,28] Ulnar variance, the distance that the ulnar head extends below (negative) or above (positive) the articular surface of the radius, can also effect this force distribution markedly with the latter increasing ulnar-sided forces and the former increasing radial-sided forces.[33] Ulnar variance changes in a positive direction with forearm pronation and grasping.[12,32] This combined forearm rotation and gripping can adversely impact ulnar-sided structures such as the TFCC, lunate and lunotriquetral ligament.[17]

TFCC

The TFCC, a compilation of fibrocartilage, ligaments, meniscus homologue and an articular disk, serves to stabilise the DRUJ and separate the DRUJ from the carpus and distal radius.[5] A common traumatic tear of the articular disk occurs approximately 1–2 mm ulnar to the TFCC's attachment to the radius (Fig. 3.4).[8,9] The central portion of the articular disk, where degenerative perforations occur, does not contribute to joint stability, yet is well-suited for compressive and tensile stresses.[8,9] The central 80–85% of the articular disk is avascular, which often renders this region incapable of healing.

Assessing the articular disk region of the TFCC with the forearm pronated, wrist ulnarly deviated and hand fisted increases ulnar variance and often reproduces pain in patients with ulnocarpal abutment and TFCC articular disk lesions.[48] Another assessment technique, the TFCC shear test (Fig. 3.5), which produces shearing forces across the TFCC has been found to have a sensitivity of 66%, specificity of 66%, positive predictive value of 58% and a negative predictive value of 69% in identifying TFCC lesions.[22]

Unlike the central portion of the TFCC, the dorsal (DRUL) and palmar (PRUL) radioulnar ligaments of the TFCC serve a stabilising function and are well vascularised, thus improving their healing capabilities.[8,11,39] It is generally agreed that portions of the PRUL and DRUL become taut at the end ranges of forearm rotation.[9] If excessive DRUJ volar or dorsal translation is detected in full pronation or supination, a tear of the DRUL and/or PRUL might be suspected.[11,27]

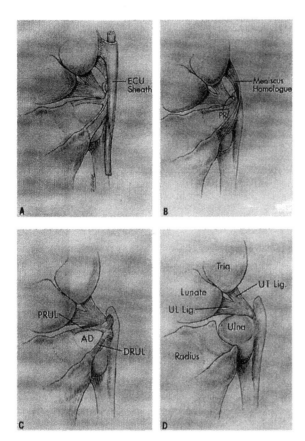

Figure 3.4 The triangular fibrocartilage complex (TFCC) viewed from the dorsal side of the wrist. A: Intact TFCC. The extensor carpi ulnaris (ECU) sheath extends farther than drawn, all the way to the fifth metacarpal, with connections to the triquetrum and hamate. B: The ECU sheath has been removed along with its thickened floor (also referred to as the ulnar collateral ligament). The meniscus homologue (MH) originates from the dorsal margin of the radius and sweeps palmar and ulnar to insert into the palmar/ulnar aspect of the triquetrum. Along its course it has fibres inserting into the ulnar styloid. As the MH sweeps past the styloid and the palmar radioulnar ligament (PRUL), it forms the dorsal roof of the prestyloid recess (PR), a synovial-lined recess that variably connects to the palmar aspect of the ulnar styloid. C: The MH has been removed so the entire TFC proper (articular disk (AD)), PRUL and dorsal radioulnar ligament (DRUL) can be seen. There are two insertion sites into the ulna – the fovea at the base of the ulnar styloid and the styloid itself. D: The TFCC has been removed. The ulnolunate (UL) and ulnotriquetral (UT) ligaments extend from the palmar aspect of the respective carpal bones and the lunotriquetral interosseous ligament to the ulna, inserting into the foveal area and the base of the ulnar styloid. (Reproduced with permission from Jaffe R, Chidgey LK, LaStayo PC: The distal radioulnar joint: anatomy and management of disorders. J Hand Ther 9:129–38, 1996.)

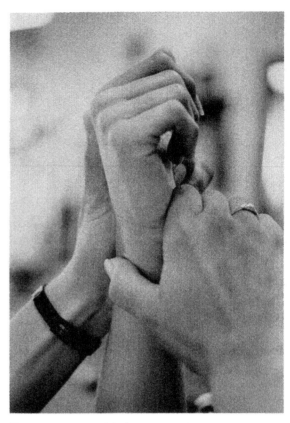

Figure 3.5 The TFCC shear test or ulnomeniscotriquetral dorsal glide test requires the examiner to stabilise the patient's radius with one hand and glide the piso-triquetral complex dorsally (with radial side of PIP joint) and the ulna volarly (with the thumb). A positive test is when this shearing manoeuvre reproduces the patient's symptoms.

The radiocarpal and midcarpal joints

The radiocarpal joint is formed by the articulation of the proximal carpal row (scaphoid, lunate, triquetrum and pisiform) and the articular surface of the radius and the TFCC. The midcarpal joint is the articulation between the proximal carpal row and distal carpal row (trapezium, trapezoid, capitate, hamate) (see Figs 3.1 and 3.2). Motion occurs not only between the carpal rows (intercarpal motion) but within the carpal rows (intracarpal motion). There is some discrepancy regarding the contribution of each wrist joint to specific wrist motions. Functionally, however, it is safe to say that both the radiocarpal and midcarpal joints contribute to flexion, extension and deviations of the wrist and, clinically, both of these joints need to be addressed when attempting to restore wrist motion.[50]

Common carpal fractures, instabilities and degenerative changes

The scaphoid bridges the two carpal rows, making the entire carpus more capable of stabilising itself against compressive forces.[14] Unfortunately, the stabilising attributes of the scaphoid are often compromised, as scaphoid fractures and nonunions are not uncommon.[2] Painful palpation into the snuff box region of the wrist, limited wrist ROM and decreased grip strength should raise the clinician's index of suspicion that a scaphoid fracture may be present.[2,34] Localised tenderness over the lunate may be indicative of Kienböck's disease.[2]

Radial-sided wrist pain may be the result of instability and/or degenerative arthritis at the trapezium and first carpometacarpal (CMC) joint. Grinding the thumb metacarpal into the trapezium may reproduce symptoms if degenerative arthritis is present (Fig. 3.6). If the joint is hypermobile laterally and/or dorsally, the ligaments at the CMC joint may be lax.[10] A similar compression test which may detect degenerative changes at the pisotriquetral joint has the examiner 'rock' or push the pisiform against the surface of the triquetrum.[24]

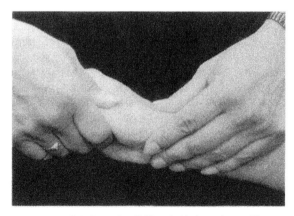

Figure 3.6 Grind test for CMC arthritis is performed by grinding the patient's first metacarpal into the trapezium.

The wrist intrinsic ligaments (scapholunate and lunotriquetral)

Between the carpal bones there are numerous intrinsic ligaments (see Fig. 3.2). The scapholunate (SL) and lunotriquetral (LT) ligaments, which are arguably the most critical ligaments of the wrist, can, when disrupted, cause common forms of carpal instability.[3,30,43] Disruption of the dorsal and palmar aspects of either the SL and LT ligament results in altered kinematics within the proximal row, pain, impairment and disability.[16,37]

Scaphoid shift test (scaphoid instability and/or SL disruption)

The scaphoid shift test is used to assess the stability of the scaphoid (Fig. 3.7).[47] A positive test, which would indicate that the scaphoid is unstable, is described as a resounding 'thunk' or reproduction of symptoms. Since a high incidence of positive scaphoid shift tests are seen in the uninjured wrist, clinicians should be cautious when interpreting a test result as positive if the test did not reproduce the patient's pain. When used to assess for the presence of an SL ligament tear, the scaphoid shift test has a sensitivity of 69%, specificity of 66%, positive predictive value of 48% and a negative predictive value of 78%.[22]

Ballottement test (lunotriquetral joint stability)

The ballottement test stresses the LT ligament and evaluates the stability of the LT joint (Fig. 3.8).[35] A positive finding for the ballottement test is a reproduction of the patient's pain and or excessive laxity. Regarding LT ligament tears, the ballottement test is 64% sensitive, 44% specific and has a positive and negative predictive value of 24% and 81%, respectively.[22]

Palpation

Tenderness in the SL or LT interval with palpation may also indicate ligamentous pathology;[41] however, there is some question as to the ability to identify specific ligamentous lesions by palpation alone.[29]

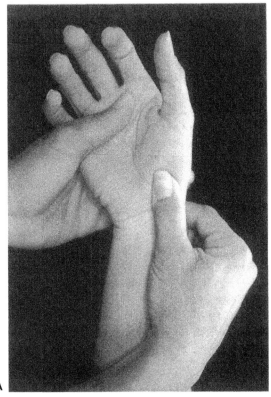 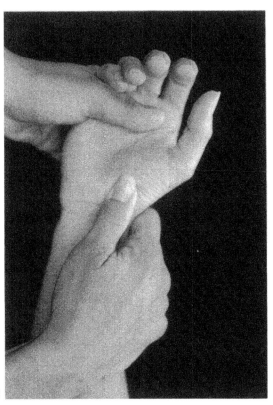

Figure 3.7 The scaphoid shift test is performed by having the examiner attempt to prevent the scaphoid from moving into its normal palmar flexed position by applying pressure, via their thumb, over the scaphoid tubercle while the wrist is passively brought from ulnar (A) into radial deviation and some flexion (B). A positive test is one that reproduces the patient's symptoms and/or a painful clunk.

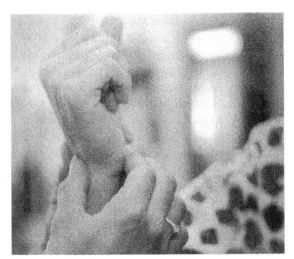

Figure 3.8 The ballottement test stresses the LT ligament by passively translating the pisotriquetral complex volarly and dorsally while stabilising the lunate. A positive test is when excessive laxity is noted and/or a reproduction of symptoms.

Midcarpal instability

Ligaments which cross the midcarpal joint, such as the triquetrocapitate fascicle of the ulnar arcuate ligament complex, which is a supportive ligamentous sling for the capitate, is the main stabiliser of the midcarpal joint.[15]

Assessment techniques that help identify midcarpal instability include passive deviation of the actively clenched fist, passive volar and dorsal translation of the triquetrum on the hamate or passive circumduction of the wrist. If any of these movements produce an audible, palpable or painful 'clunk', midcarpal instability should be considered.[15,48,49] Pain and/or clunking with passive translation of the proximal carpal row on the distal radius may be associated with carpal instability non-dissociative (CIND). Snapping and clicking at the midcarpal (capito–lunate interface) with passive translation between the proximal and distal carpal rows may be indicative of a central carpal instability wrist (CLIP).[15]

TENDONS AND RETINACULAR SYSTEM OF THE WRIST
Volar fascia and carpal tunnel

The forearm fascia becomes thicker at its distal margins where, at the level of the proximal row, it forms the volar carpal ligament, which attaches laterally on the scaphoid and medially on the pisiform. Further distal, the fibres of the flexor retinaculum become thicker to form the transverse carpal ligament, which connects to the hook of the hamate and the palmar ridge of the trapezium. This fibrous compartment, known as the carpal tunnel, contains the long finger and thumb flexor tendons and the median nerve (Fig. 3.9).

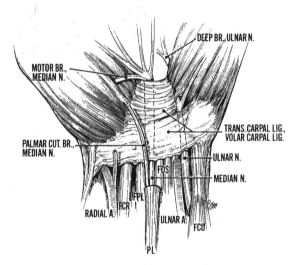

Figure 3.9 The volar carpal ligament and transverse carpal ligament serve as the roof to the carpal tunnel. The contents of the carpal tunnel are the median nerve and the long finger flexors (flexor digitorum superficialis (FDS) and flexor digitorum profundus (not shown) and thumb flexor FPL). The wrist flexors (flexor carpi radialis (FCR), palmaris longus (PL) and flexor carpi ulnaris (FCU)) are shown crossing the wrist. The median nerve with its palmar cutaneous branch and motor branch are shown as well as the ulnar nerve, deep branch of the ulnar nerve and the radial artery. (Reproduced with permission from Eversmann WW: Entrapment and compression neuropathies. In: Green DP (ed.), Operative hand surgery, 3rd edn. New York: Churchill Livingstone, 1993.)

Volar tendons and compartments

The flexor carpi radialis (FCR), which has a separate fibrous tunnel near its insertion on the trapezium, is a primary wrist flexor.[6] The flexor carpi ulnaris (FCU) attaches to the pisiform which, in turn, is connected to the hook of the hamate via the pisohamate ligament and to the fifth metacarpal by means of the pisometacarpal ligament.[3] The FCU flexes and ulnarly deviates the wrist. This muscle is an important muscle in heavy manual labour, as it is the muscle which powers an axe and hammer type of stroke.[6] The palmaris longus (PL) is an inconsistent (absent in 10% of hands) and variable pure wrist flexor, inserting on the palmar aponeurosis.[6]

Extensor tendons and dorsal retinaculum compartments

Originating from the deep aspect of the supratendinous layer of fascia are six longitudinal fibrous compartments for synovial sheaths and extensor tendons that cross the wrist (Fig. 3.10).

Wrist extensors

The second compartment contains the extensor carpi radialis longus (ECRL) and brevis (ECRB), and the sixth compartment, houses the extensor carpi ulnaris (ECU); these are the three primary wrist extensors. The ECRL, inserting on the base of the second metacarpal, actually has a larger moment arm for flexion of the elbow and for radial deviation of the wrist. It is, however, most effective as a wrist extensor when radial deviation is balanced by the primary ulnar deviator (the ECU) and when the elbow is extended.[6]

The ECRB, although smaller in mass than the ECRL, is a more effective wrist extensor due to its insertion on the base of the third metacarpal, its larger moment arm for wrist extension and it is uninfluenced by elbow position.[6]

The ECU is unique amongst the wrist extensors as it changes its relationship to the axis of wrist movements and rests on the medial side of the ulnar head during pronation, where it is a strong ulnar deviator. In supination, the ECU is

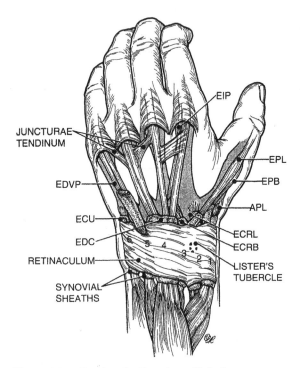

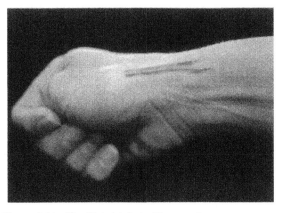

Figure 3.11 The Finkelstein test is an active manoeuvre where the patient places the thumb within the hand and holds it tightly with the other fingers while ulnarly deviating the wrist. An intense pain over the course of the first dorsal compartment at the radial styloid would indicate the presence of de Quervain's disease.

Figure 3.10 The dorsal retinaculum with its five fibro-osseous and one fibrous (fifth dorsal compartment) compartments. The first compartment contains the abductor pollicis longus (APL) and extensor pollicis brevis (EPB); the second houses the extensor carpi radialis longus (ECRL) and extensor carpi radialis brevis (ECRB); the third is the extensor pollicis longus (EPL), which angles around Lister's tubercle; the fourth is the extensor digitorum communis (EDC) to the fingers as well as the extensor indicis proprius (EIP); the fifth is the extensor digiti quinti proprius (EDQP); and the sixth is the extensor carpi ulnaris (ECU). (Reproduced with permission from Doyle JR: Extensor tendon acute injuries. In: Green DP (ed.), Operative hand surgery, 3rd edn. New York: Churchill Livingstone, 1993.)

positioned dorsally to maximise its moment arm for wrist extension.[36] The ECU tendon, which inserts on the base of the fifth metacarpal, is firmly stabilised in its groove on the ulnar head by a collar of synovium-lined deep fascia. This fascial housing may rupture with subluxation of the ECU from its groove during forearm rotation, resulting in ulnar wrist pain.[36] Stress-induced tenosynovitis with partial tendon rupture is another source of chronic problems on the ulnar side of the wrist.[36] To assess for ECU instability, the clinician must supinate the forearm with one hand while palpating the ECU tendon with the other. The patient then actively ulnarly deviates his wrist against clinician-provided resistance. Visible or palpable subluxation of the ECU with this manoeuvre indicates instability.[7]

Primary thumb extensor/abductor and secondary wrist mover

The first compartment, located laterally, contains the abductor pollicis longus (APL) and the extensor pollicis brevis (EPB) tendons. Unlike standard anatomical depictions, the APL is often present in multiple tendinous forms.[20] Although named as a mover of the thumb, the APL can also radially deviate the wrist and flex the wrist when it is located volar to the wrist flexion/extension axis.[6] The EPB is more commonly comprised of a single tendon, although duplications have been noted.[20] The EPB is smaller and weaker than the APL, but its actions at the wrist are similar to that of the APL. Within the first dorsal compartment these tendons may be separated by septations (fibrous or osseofibrous divisions), which create separate compartments and potential sites of compression as in de Quervain's disease.[20] The Finkelstein's test is commonly used to assess for the presence of de Quervain's disease (Fig. 3.11).[13] The third compartment where the extensor pollicis longus

(EPL) tendon turns laterally at Lister's tubercle is a potential site of tendon rupture with rheumatoid arthritis and/or fractures of the distal radius.[36]

Finger extensors

Blending with the dorsal wrist capsule are the floor of the fourth and fifth compartments, which contain the extensor digitorum communis (EDC),

extensor indicis proprius (EIP) and the extensor digiti quinti (EDQ), respectively. These digital extensors can assist wrist extension. They become primary wrist extensors when extension of the wrist follows digital extension in an obligate fashion. This is an unnatural functional sequence as it limits the spatial positioning of the hand and grasping power and is often seen as a problem during the rehabilitation of wrist fractures.[36]

REFERENCES

1. Agee JM: Mechanics of tendons that cross the wrist. In: Brand PW, Hollister A (eds), Clinical mechanics of the hand. St Louis: Mosby Year Book, 1993:371–8.
2. Amadio PC, Taleisnik J: Fractures of the carpal bones. In: Green DP (ed.), Operative hand surgery. New York: Churchill Livingstone, 1993:799–860.
3. Berger RA, Garcia-Elias M: General anatomy of the wrist. In: An KN, Berger RA, Cooney WP (eds), Biomechanics of the wrist joint. New York: Springer-Verlag, 1991:1–22.
4. Berger RA, Blair WF: The radioscapholunate ligament: a gross and histologic description. Anat Rec 210:393–405, 1984.
5. Bowers WH: In: Green DP (ed.), Operative hand surgery. New York: Churchill Livingstone, 1982:743–69.
6. Brand PW, Hollister A: Clinical mechanics of the hand. St Louis: Mosby Year Book, 1993:254–352.
7. Burkhalter SS et al.: Post-traumatic recurrent subluxation of the extensor carpi ulnaris tendon. J Hand Surg 7A, 1982.
8. Chidgey LK: Histologic anatomy of the triangular fibrocartilage. Hand Clin 2:249–62, 1991.
9. Chidgey LK: The distal radioulnar joint: problems and solutions. J Am Acad Orthop Surg 2:95–109, 1995.
10. Eaton RG, Littler JW: A study of the basal joint of the thumb. Treatment of its disabilities by fusion. J Bone Joint Surg 51A:661–8, 1969.
11. Ekenstam F, Hagert CG: Anatomical studies on the geometry and stability of the distal radioulnar joint. Scand J Plast Reconstr Surg 19:17–25, 1985.
12. Epner RA, Bowers, Guilford WB: Ulna variance: the effect of wrist positioning and roentgen filming technique. J Hand Surg 7:298–305, 1982.
13. Finkelstein H: Stenosing tendovaginitis at the radial styloid process. J Bone Joint Surg 12A:509–40, 1930.
14. Gilford WW, Bolton RH, Lambrinudi C: The mechanism of the wrist joint with special reference to fractures of the scaphoid. Guy's Hosp Rec 92:52–9, 1943.
15. Green DP: Carpal dislocations and instabilities. In: Green DP (ed.), Operative hand surgery. New York: Churchill Livingstone, 1993:861–928.
16. Horii E, Garcia-Elias M, An KN et al.: A kinematic study of lunotriquetral dissociations. J Hand Surg 16A:355–62, 1991.
17. Jaffe R, Chidgey LK, LaStayo PC: The distal radioulnar joint: anatomy and management of disorders. J Hand Ther 9:129–38, 1996.
18. Kaukonen JP, Karaharju EO, Porras M et al.: Functional recovery after fractures of the distal forearm. Analysis of radiographic and other factors affecting the outcome. Ann Chir Gynaecol 77:27–31, 1988.
19. Kazuki K, Kususnoki M, Yamada J et al.: Cineradiographic study of wrist motion after fracture of the distal radius. J Hand Surg (Am) 18:41–6, 1993.
20. Kirkpatrick WH: De Quervain's disease. In: Hunter JM, Schneider LH, Mackin EJ et al. (eds), Rehabilitation of the hand: surgery and therapy. St Louis: CV Mosby, 1990:304–7.
21. Laseter GA, Carter PR: Management of distal radius fractures. J Hand Ther 9:114–28, 1996.
22. LaStayo PC, Howell J: Clinical provocative tests used in evaluating wrist pain: a descriptive study. J Hand Ther 1:10–17, 1995.
23. Lewis OJ, Hamshere RJ, Bucknill TM: The anatomy of the wrist joint. J Anat 106:539–52, 1970.
24. Lipshietz T, Osterman AL: New methods in the evaluation of chronic wrist pain. Univ Penn Orthop J 20–4, 1990.
25. Mayfield JK, Williams WJ, Erdman AG et al.: Biomechanical properties of human carpal ligaments. Orthop Trans 3:143–4, 1979.
26. McQueen M: Colles fracture: Does the anatomical result affect the final function? J Bone Joint Surg (Br) 70:649–51, 1988.
27. Mino DE, Palmer AK, Levishon EM: The role of radiography and computerized tomography in the diagnosis of subluxation and dislocation of the distal radioulnar joint. J Hand Surg 8:23–31, 1983.
28. Nagle DJ: Arthroscopic treatment of degenerative tears of the triangular fibrocartilage. Hand Clin 10:615–24, 1994.
29. North ER, Meyer S: Wrist injuries: correlation of clinical and arthroscopic findings. J Hand Surg 15A:915–20, 1990.
30. Nowak MD: Material properties of ligaments. In: An KN, Berger RA, Cooney WP (eds), Biomechanics of the wrist joint. New York: Springer-Verlag 1991:139–56.
31. Palmer AK: Fractures of the distal radius. In: Green DP (ed.), Operative hand surgery, 3rd edn. New York: Churchill Livingstone, 1993:929–71.

32. Palmer AK, Glisson RR, Werner FW: Ulnar variance determination. J Hand Surg 7:376–9, 1982.
33. Palmer AK, Werner FW: Biomechanics of the distal radioulnar joint. Clin Orthop 187:26–35, 1984.
34. Prosser R, Hebert T: Management of carpal fractures and dislocations. J Hand Ther 9:139–47, 1996.
35. Regan DS, Linscheid RI, Dobyns JH: Lunotriquetral sprains. J Hand Surg 9A:502–14, 1984.
36. Rosenthal EA: The extensor tendons. In: Hunter JM, Schneider LH, Mackin EJ et al. (eds), Rehabilitation of the hand: surgery and therapy. St. Louis: CV Mosby, 1990:458–91.
37. Ruby LK, An KN, Linscheid RL et al.: The effects of scapholunate ligament section on scapholunate motion. J Hand Surg 12A:767–71, 1987.
38. Ryu J, Cooney WP, Askew LJ et al.: Functional ranges of motion of the wrist joint. J Hand Surg 16A:409–19, 1991.
39. Schuind F, An KN, Berglund L et al.: The distal radioulnar ligaments. A biomechanical study. J Hand Surg 16A:1106–14, 1991.
40. Short WH, Palmer AK, Werner FW et al.: A biomechanical study of distal radial fractures. J Hand Surg (Am) 12:523–34, 1987.
41. Skirvin T: Clinical examination of the wrist. J Hand Ther 9:96–107, 1996.
42. Solgaard S: Function after distal radius fracture. Acta Orthop Scand 59:39–42, 1988.
43. Taliesnik J: Scapholunate dissociation. In: Strickland JW, Steichen JB (eds), Difficult problems in hand surgery. St. Louis: CV Mosby, 1982:341–8.
44. Taliesnik J, Watson HK: Midcarpal instability caused by mal-united fractures of the distal radius. J Hand Surg (Am) 9:350–7, 1984.
45. Taliesnik J: Pain on the ulnar side of the wrist. Hand Clin 1:51–68, 1987.
46. Villar RN, Marsh D: Three years after Colles' fracture. A prospective review. J Bone Joint Surg (Br) 69:635–8, 1987.
47. Watson HK, Ashmead D, Makhlouf MV: Examination of the scaphoid. J Hand Surg 13A:657–60, 1988.
48. Whipple TL: Arthroscopic surgery: the wrist. Philadelphia: JB Lippincott, 1993.
49. Wright TW, Michlovitz SL: Management of carpal instabilities. J Hand Ther 9:148–57, 1996.
50. Youm Y, McMurtry RY, Flatt AE et al.: An experimental study of radio-ulnar deviation and flexion–extension. J Bone Joint Surg 60A:423–31, 1978.

B. KINEMATICS OF THE WRIST AND MOBILISATION TECHNIQUES

Deirdree McGee

Anatomical and functional characteristics of the carpals have made kinematic research of the wrist difficult and controversial. The carpals are small, irregularly shaped and have multiaxial rotary movements, which are very difficult to measure. Accurate examination of their relative movements during active physiological movements would require three-dimensional analysis during active movement with intracortical plates inserted into the carpal's periostium. Research so far has involved the use of biplanar X-rays[12,14,34,35] and three-dimensional studies of cadavers, dissected to the ligaments and *passively* moved or positioned.[3,5,9,15,26] Hence our understanding of carpal movements and mobilisations may alter as further research is completed.

The muscles that move the wrist insert beyond the carpal bones on to the metacarpals.[8] Movement of the carpals is achieved passively via bone on bone compression and ligament tension.[30] The palmar and dorsal radiocarpal and interrosseous ligaments are crucial to this force transference. These are capsular ligaments;[2] hence, mobilisation techniques are joint glides as well as capsular and ligamentous stretches. This is achieved by tractioning the involved bones at the same time as one glides. All glides to increase range of motion should be performed at the end of the available range.

FLEXION

During flexion, both the radiocarpal joint (RCJ) and midcarpal joint (MCJ) flex. The relative contributions of the MCJ and RCJ to flexion/extension range of motion is debated in the research,[3–5,9,15–17,26,27,29,31] though the predominance of one joint's contribution over the other found in flexion is reversed in extension.[24] The discrepancies are understandable considering the inherent difficulties associated with measuring carpal kinematics. Active flexion is created by the combined forces of flexor carpi radialis (FCR) and flexor carpi ulnaris (FCU). The osteokinematics of the MCJ and RCJ can be described following the forces created by each of these muscles. FCR inserts on to metacarpals 2 and 3 (MC2, MC3). These metacarpals are firmly wedged to the distal carpal row (DCR) by both the interlocking of articular surfaces and the dense ligamentous connections between the DCR and the bases of the metacarpals. They are described as a fixed unit of the hand[2,6,22,24,26,28,34,35] and so negligible gliding movement occurs here. The active force of FCR pulls MC2 and MC3 together with capitate and trapezoid,[2] causing them to flex (roll volar) at the MCJ.[5,9,16,17,23,27,34,35] In terms of arthrokinematics, this can be described as a dorsal glide of the proximal pole of capitate on scaphoid and lunate.[15,29] This midcarpal articulation has been described as a condyloid joint.[22]

The compressive force is transferred from capitate on to scaphoid and lunate and, together with the tensile force of the dorsal intercarpal ligament,[2,4,9,16,17,23,27,34,35] causes scaphoid and lunate to flex (roll volar) at the RCJ. Arthrokinematically, the proximal poles of scaphoid and lunate glide dorsally on the radius (Fig. 3.12). This flexion movement of scaphoid, shortens the proximal–distal distance of the proximal carpal row (PCR), which relaxes the tension of the palmar radiocarpal and intercarpal ligaments, allowing further gliding movements at the midcarpal joint (MCJ).[23] The scaphoid has been found to move through a greater arc than triquetrum, and triquetrum more than lunate.[15,29]

The joint axes of the radioscaphoid and radiolunate joint, as with all the carpal joints, are not in pure anatomical planes. Therefore conjunct rotation occurs, with flexion and extension. De Lange[7] described these as 'out of plane movements'. As scaphoid flexes it has been found to also pronate and lunate supinate.[3,7,12,15,29] Capitate in one study was found to supinate in extension and pronate in flexion relative to lunate.[15]

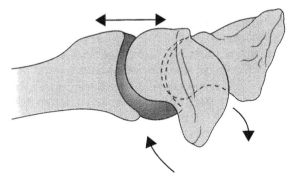

Figure 3.12 During flexion, the proximal poles of scaphoid and lunate glide dorsally on the radius, along with flexion movement of the scaphoid.

FCU forces the fifth metacarpal (MC5) to flex (roll volar) on hamate and hence arthrokinematically forces the proximal pole of MC5 to glide dorsally on hamate. Approximately 30 degrees of flexion/extension movement is possible at this joint.[6] The movement of hamate and triquetrum is a helical spiral rather than a translational glide.[2,30] The transferred force of FCU causes hamate to roll or rotate anteriorly on triquetrum,[23,33] causing the distal pole of hamate to move volar. As it rolls volar, it also glides proximally relative to triquetrum (Fig. 3.13). The transference of this force from triquetrum to the triangular fibrocartilage complex (TFCC) has not been documented in the research. The author proposes that triquetrum also flexes relative to the TFCC and, hence, arthrokinematically the proximal pole of triquetrum glides dorsally on the TFCC (Table 3.1).

The MCJ and the RCJ both flex during wrist flexion. Mobilisations to increase flexion range of motion (Table 3.2) should involve both the MCJ, RCJ and ulna aspect carpometacarpal joint (CMCJ) with simultaneous traction of the opposing joint surfaces: at the CMCJ, a dorsal glide of the proximal pole of MC5 on hamate; at the MCJ, a dorsal glide of the proximal pole of capitate on scaphoid and lunate, and an anterior rotation (roll)/proximal glide of hamate on triquetrum (Fig. 3.13); at the RCJ, a dorsal glide of the proximal pole of scaphoid into pronation on the radius, and a dorsal glide of the proximal pole of lunate into supination on the radius.

EXTENSION

During extension, both the MCJ and RCJ extend. The active forces creating this movement are extensor carpi radialis longus and brevis (ECRL/ECRB) and extensor carpi ulnaris (ECU). ECRL/ECRB pull MC2 and 3 in a dorsal direction. As negligible movement occurs between the MC2 and 3 and the DCR,[2,4,6,22,23,26] the force is transferred to the capitate and trapezoid. Capitate is forced extend (roll dorsal) on scaphoid and lunate.[2–5,9,24,26,27,29,34,35] This increases the tension on the palmar interosseous ligaments, which then pulls scaphoid and lunate into extension also.[2–5,15,26,27,29,35] Scaphoid and lunate have been

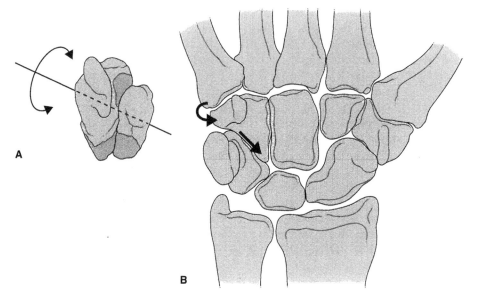

Figure 3.13 During flexion, the hamate rolls anteriorly on the triquetrum and glides proximally relative to the triquetrum.

Table 3.1 Carpal movements (osteokinematics) during wrist flexion

Muscles active	
FCR	FCU
2MC and 3MC compress capitate and trapezoid, minimal movement	Proximal pole 5MC glides dorsal on hamate
Capitate flexes on scaphoid and lunate, i.e. MCJ flexion	Hamate anteriorly rotates on triquetrum, i.e. MCJ flexion
Scaphoid flexes and pronates on the radius; lunate flexes and supinates on the radius, i.e. RCJ flexion	Proximal pole of triquetrum flexes on the TFCC, i.e. RCJ flexion

For abbreviations, see text.

Table 3.2 Mobilisations to increase flexion

CMCJ 5: Glide proximal pole of MC4 & 5 dorsally on hamate

MCJ: Glide proximal pole of capitate dorsally on scaphoid and lunate; anteriorly rotate/proximal glide of hamate on triquetrum

RCJ: Glide proximal pole of scaphoid dorsally and into pronation on the radius; glide proximal pole of lunate dorsally and into supination on the radius

For abbreviations, see text.

measured to experience 'out of plane movements', i.e. conjunct movements during extension, scaphoid into supination, and lunate into pronation.[3,7,12,15,29] Arthrokinematically, the proximal pole of capitate glides volar on scaphoid and lunate, the proximal pole of lunate glides volar and into pronation on the radius, and the proximal pole of scaphoid glides volar and into supination on the radius. The extension of scaphoid (Fig. 3.14B), lengthens the proximal–distal distance of scaphoid in the PCR and further tenses the palmar ligaments.[24,32] This effectively locks the MCJ, limiting any further movement to occur there. Extension from this point occurs at the RCJ only.[23,27] It is proposed that extension initially occurs at the MCJ and then continues at the RCJ. The conjunct rotation of scaphoid and lunate into extension/supination and extension/pronation further tenses the palmar interosseous ligaments, assisting in the stablisation of the wrist in this position.[3,7,15,29,32]

The active force of ECU pulls on to MC5, causing it to extend (roll dorsal). Arthrokinematically, the

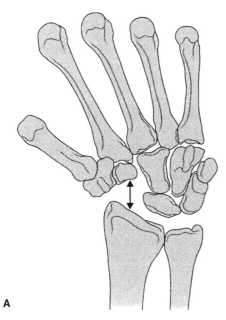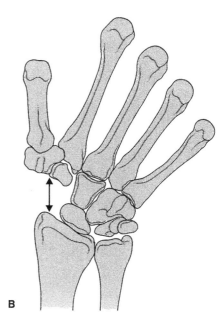

A   **B**

Figure 3.14   During extension the scaphoid and lunate extend. The extension of the scaphoid lengthens the proximal–distal distance of the scaphoid in the PCR.

proximal pole of MC5 glides volar on hamate. Via both bone on bone compression and interosseous and palmar ligament tension, the moving force would be transferred from MC5 to hamate and from hamate to the triquetrum. Hamate would posteriorly rotate (extend) on triquetrum,[32] and glide distally simultaneously relative to triquetrum (see Fig. 3.13). Triquetrum may extend on the TFCC, which arthrokinematically would be a volar glide of the proximal pole of triquetrum on the TFCC (Table 3.3).

Mobilisations to increase extension range of motion (Table 3.4) should involve mobilisations of both the CMCJ of MCJ and RCJ, with simultaneous traction of the opposing joint surfaces: at the CMCJ, a volar glide of the proximal pole of MC5 on hamate; at the MCJ, a volar glide of the proximal pole of capitate on scaphoid and lunate, and a posterior rotation (roll)/distal glide of hamate on triquetrum (Fig. 3.13); at the RCJ, a volar glide of the proximal pole of scaphoid into supination on the radius, and a volar glide of the proximal pole of lunate into pronation on the radius.

Table 3.3   Carpal movements during extension

Muscles active	
ECR	ECU
2MC and 3MC compress capitate and trapezoid, minimal movement	Proximal pole 5MC glides volar on hamate
Capitate extends on scaphoid and lunate, i.e. MCJ extension	Hamate posteriorly rotates on triquetrum, i.e. MCJ extension
Scaphoid extends and supinates on the radius; lunate extends and pronates on the radius, i.e. RCJ extension	Proximal pole of triquetrum glides volar on the TFCC, i.e. RCJ extension

For abbreviations, see text.

Table 3.4   Mobilisations to increase extension

CMCJ 5: Glide proximal pole of MC5 volar on hamate

MCJ: Glide proximal pole of capitate volar on scaphoid and lunate; posteriorly rotate/distal glide of hamate on triquetrum

RCJ: Glide proximal pole of scaphoid volar and into supination on the radius; glide proximal pole of lunate volar and into pronation on the radius

For abbreviations, see text.

RADIAL DEVIATION

During radial deviation (RD), both the MCJ and RCJ deviate radially with conjunct movements particularly found at the RCJ. ECRL/ECRB, FCR, and to a lesser extent abductor pollicis longus (APL), pull the DCR as a unit with the hand into RD (Table 3.5).[15,17,29] Kobayashi[15] found the DCR to also pronate in RD and supinate in ulna deviation (UD); however, Short et al.[29] found these movements to be negligible. Compression of the distal pole of scaphoid causes it to flex at the RCJ[2,16,17,19,23,26,31,32] (see Figs 3.12 and 3.14) and, via the PCR interosseous ligaments, this flexion torque is transferred to lunate and triquetrum, causing them to flex at the RCJ.[2,16,17,19] At the MCJ, triquetrum rolls volar and glides in a proximal direction relative to hamate[3] (see Fig. 3.13).

Table 3.5 Carpal movements during radial deviation

Muscles active: ECRL/B, APL, FCR

MC1–3 compress trapezium and trapezoid and capitate; minimal movement at carpometacarpal joint

Capitate with the DCR and hand RD at the MCJ

Scaphoid and lunate primarily flex with conjunct RD, i.e. RCJ flexion/RD

Triquetrum pulled into flexion at the RCJ, which effectuates an anterior roll and proximal glide relative to hamate at the MCJ

For abbreviations, see text.

This effectively separates hamate and triquetrum, lengthening the ulna side of the carpus,[3,23,32] while the flexion of scaphoid effectively shortens the radial side[2,19,23] (Fig. 3.14).

During this flexion of the PCR, there is also conjunct RD[7,15,23,24,29] (Fig. 3.15). De Lange[7] described these as 'out of plane' movements and further stated that the DCR could also be described to extend relative to the PCR at the MCJ. Due to the concave/convex rule,[8] the arthrokinematics of the RCJ is a combination of a dorsal glide of the PCR to produce flexion and an ulna glide to produce UD[2] (Fig. 3.15). The ulna glide is a small range of movement limited by the carpal ridge on the articular surface of the radius.[2,4,26,35] The relative contributions of the MCJ and the RCJ in RD and UD have also been disputed.[3,26]

Mobilisations to increase RD range of motion should involve primarily the MCJ and RCJ (Table 3.6), with simultaneous traction of the opposing joint surfaces. Due to the sinusoidal

Tabel 3.6 Mobilisations to increase radial deviation

MCJ: Glide proximal pole of trapezium and trapezoid radial on scaphoid; glide proximal pole of capitate ulna on scaphoid and lunate; glide triquetrum in anterior rotation/proximal glide relative to hamate

RCJ: Glide proximal pole of scaphoid and lunate dorsal/ulnar on radius

For abbreviations, see text.

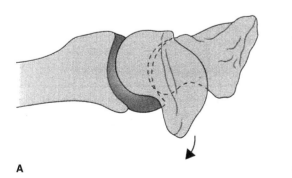
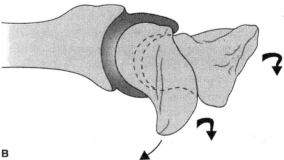

A **B**

Figure 3.15 During radial deviation there is flexion of the proximal carpal row, also conjunct radial deviation.

shape of the MCJ line,[24] RD glides of the DCR as a unit would be difficult and should be addressed as isolated intercarpal joint glides. Due to the concave/convex rule, trapezium and trapezoid would glide radially on scaphoid, and capitate would glide ulna on scaphoid and lunate. Triquetrum would roll anteriorly and glide proximally relative to hamate (see Fig. 3.13). At the RCJ, the proximal pole of scaphoid and lunate would glide dorsal and ulna on the radius, within the limitations of the carpal ridge (see Fig. 3.12).

ULNAR DEVIATION

During UD, the opposite is thought to occur as in RD. That is, UD at the MCJ with extension and conjunct UD at the RCJ. The muscles creating the UD force are FCU and ECU. Together, they pull MC5 into UD, arthrokinematically forcing the proximal pole of MC5 to glide in a dorsal/radial direction on hamate. The transferred force on to hamate causes it to UD and glide proximally relative to triquetrum at the MCJ[1,3,16,17,23,24,32] (see Fig. 3.13), in effect shortening the ulna side of the carpus (see Fig. 3.14).[23,32] Tension is created in the palmar interosseous ligaments of the PCR, which pull lunate and then scaphoid into extension at the RCJ.[2,14,16,17,19,26,28,31,32] The compressive force of the MCJ as it moves into UD, especially capitate, push the PCR into UD simultaneously. Arthrokinematically, the proximal pole of lunate and scaphoid glide volar and radial on the radius.[7,15,29] The extension of scaphoid lengthens it in the PCR and locks the MCJ, further transferring the UD of the DCR to the RCJ (Fig. 3.14).[23]

Table 3.7 Carpal movements during ulna deviation

Muscles active: FCU, ECU
5MC ulna deviates and rolls dorsally on hamate
Hamate UD and glides proximally relative to triquetrum UD of the DCR as a unit
Lunate and scaphoid primarily extend with conjunct UD

For abbreviations, see text.

Table 3.8 Mobilisations to increase ulna deviation

CMCJ5: Glide proximal pole of MC5 radial/volar on the radius
MCJ: Glide proximal pole of capitate radial on scaphoid and lunate; glide hamate radial/proximal relative to triquetrum
RCJ: Glide proximal pole of scaphoid and lunate radial/volar on the radius

For abbreviations, see text.

Hence, at the RCJ extension with conjunct, UD occurs (Table 3.7).[31]

Mobilisations to increase UD (Table 3.8) should involve the CMCJ5, MCJ, and RCJ, with traction of the opposing joint surfaces produced simultaneously: at the CMCJ5, a dorsal/radial glide of the MC5 on hamate; at the MCJ, a radial/proximal glide of hamate on triquetrum, which could also be described as a posterior roll and distal glide of triquetrum on hamate. The relative movements are described as to which bone may move first (see Fig. 3.13): a radial glide of the proximal pole of capitate on scaphoid and lunate; at the RCJ, a volar/radial glide of the proximal pole of scaphoid and lunate on the radius.

REFERENCES

1. Atkinson B: Real biomechanics of the wrist. *AOIMT Newsletter.*
2. Berger RA: The anatomy and basic biomechanics of the wrist joint. J Hand Ther April–June:84–93, 1996.
3. Berger RA, Crowninshield RD, Flatt AE: The three dimensional rotational behaviors of the carpal bones. Clin Orthop 167:303, 1982.
4. Berger RA, Blair WF: The ligament: a gross and histologic description. Anat Rec 210:393–405, 1984.
5. Brumfield RH, Champoux, JA: A biomechanical study of normal functional wrist motion. Clin Orthop 187:23, 1984.
6. Chase RA: Anatomy and kinesiology of the hand. In: Hunter et al. (eds), Rehabilitation of the hand. 1995.
7. de Lange A, Kauer JMG, Hoiskes R: Kinematic behaviour of the human wrist joint. A roentgen stereophotogranunetric analysis. J Orthop Res 3:56–64, 1985.
8. Gray's anatomy, Br. edn 36. Philadelphia: WB Saunders, 1980:436–8.
9. Jackson WT, Hefzy MS, Guo H: Determination of wrist kinematics using magnetic tracking device. Med Eng Phys 16(2):123–33, 1994.

10. Johnston HM: Varying positions of the carpal bones in the different movements at the wrist. J Anat Phys 41:109, 1907.
11. Johnston HM: Varying positions of the carpal bones in the different movements at the wrist. Part II. A. palmar and dorsal flexion. B. Radical and ulnar flexion combined with palmar and dorsal flexion. J Anat Phys 41:280, 1907.
12. Kauer JM: The interdependence of the carpal articulation chains. Acta Ant 88:481, 1976.
13. Kauer JMG: The functional anatomy of the wrist. Clin Orthop 149:9, 1980.
14. Kauer JMG: The interdependence of carpal articular chains. Acta Anat Scand 88:481, 1974.
15. Kobayashi M, Berger RA, Linscheid RL, An KN: Intercarpal kinematics during wrist motion. Hand Clin 13(1):143–9, 1997.
16. Linscheid RL, Dobyns JH, Beckenbaugh RD, Cooney WP, Wood MB: Instability pattern for the wrist. J Hand Surg 8:682, 1983.
17. Linscheid RL: Kinematic considerations of the wrist. Clin Orthop 202:27–39, 1986.
18. Lichtman DM (ed.): The wrist and its disorders. Philadelphia: WB Saunders, 1988.
19. Mayfield JK: Pathogenesis of wrist ligament instability. In: Lichtman DM (ed.), The wrist and its disorders. Philadelphia: WB Saunders, 1988.
20. Mayfield JK: Wrist ligamentous anatomy and pathogenesis of carpal instability. Orthop Clin North Am 15:209–16, 1984.
21. Mayfield JK: Wrist ligamentous anatomy and pathogenesis of carpal instability. Orthop Clin North Am 15:209, 1984.
22. Neylon L: Functional anatomy of the wrist. 1984.
23. Neylon L: Wrist motion in relation to grip and hand motion. 1994.
24. Norkin CC, Levanie PK: Anatomy and biomechanics, 'The wrist complex' 1992:264–70.
25. Radonjic F, Long C: Kinesiology of the wrist. Am J Phys Med 50:57, 1971.
26. Ruby LK et al.: Relative motion of selected carpal bones. J Hand Surg Am 13(1):1–10, 1988.
27. Sarafian SK, Melamed J, Goshgarian FM: Study of wrist motion in flexion and extension. Clin Orthop 126:153, 1977.
28. Savelberg HHCN, Otten JDM, Kooloos JGM, Huiskes R, Kauer JMG: Carpal bone kinematics and ligament lengthening studied for the full range of joint movement. J Biomech 26(12):1389–402, 1993.
29. Short WH, Werner FW, Fortino MD, Mann KA: Analysis of the kinematics of the scaphoid and lunate in the intact wrist joint. Hand Clin 13(1):93–108, 1997.
30. Taleisnik J: Current concepts review: carpal instability. J Bone Joint Surg 70A:1262–8, 1988.
31. Volz RG, Lieb M, Benjamin J: Biomechanics of the wrist. Clin Orthop 149:112–17, 1980.
32. Weber ER: Concepts governing the rotational shift of intercalated segment of the carpus. Orthop Clin North Am 15:193, 1984.
33. Weber ER: Wrist mechanics and its association with ligamentous instability. In: Lichtman DM (ed.), The wrist and its disorders. Philadelphia: WB Saunders, 1988.
34. Youm Y, Flatt AE: Kinematics of the wrist. Clin Orthop 149:21, 1980.
35. Youm Y et al: Kinematics of the wrist. I: An experimental study of radial-ulnar deviation and flexion-extension. J Bone Joint Surg 6A:423, 1978.

C. WRIST INVESTIGATION PROCEDURES – IMAGING

Mark Perko

History and physical examination are prerequisites in the assessment of any disorder of the wrist. The clinician's findings and provisional diagnosis will dictate the course of investigation that is taken. There is no general pathway of investigative procedures but, rather, each situation must be tailored appropriately and investigations chosen accordingly.

RADIOGRAPHS

Plain radiographs remain the first line of investigation. Routine examination includes a posteroanterior, lateral and oblique view.

Initial review of the bone morphology is carried out. Fracture lines are sought. In the initial post-traumatic film, undisplaced fractures can be difficult to identify. In the posteroanterior view, Gilula's lines are assessed.[1] These are the contours of the proximal and distal rows of carpal bones. A step in the normally smooth contour denotes a rupture of one or more of the intercarpal ligaments. An increase in the scapholunate joint width of 3 mm or more is a sign of scapholunate ligament rupture. In this case the scaphoid may appear end on, demonstrating a cortical ring shadow or 'ring' sign (Fig. 3.16). The lunate silhouette is trapezoidal in neutral alignment but will appear triangular with an extension deformity or rhomboidal with a flexion deformity which accompanies a proximal row interosseous ligament disruption. The presence of soft tissue swelling, obliteration of fat planes, or periarticular enlargement can be a valuable clue to underlying injury. Inflammatory or joint disease is evidenced by periarticular swelling, uniform joint space narrowing, periarticular erosions and osteopenia, while, in degenerative arthritis, osteophytes, cysts, subchondral sclerosis and irregular joint space loss are seen.

The zero rotation posteroanterior view is required to correctly assess ulnar variance. This is taken with the patient seated and the hand resting on the cassette with the shoulder in 90 degrees of abduction and the forearm in neutral rotation. The term variance is used to refer to the lengths of the radius and ulna with the forearm in neutral rotation. A positive variance denotes a long ulna and is commonly seen in cases of ulnar carpal impingement, and negative variance is often seen in avascular necrosis of the lunate, given the eponymous name Kienböck's disease.

In a good lateral view the wrist should be in neutral position. This has the axis of the metacarpals and radius colinear. The radius and the ulna overlap. On a normal lateral view the axis of the radius, lunate and capitate should be colinear. The angle between scaphoid and lunate is normally between 30 and 60 degrees. Fixed dorsal rotation of the lunate is termed a DISI deformity and volar rotation a VISI deformity. These terms stand for dorsal or volar intercalated segment instability. After rupture of the scapholunate ligament, the lunate will adopt a DISI or dorsally rotated position (Fig. 3.17) or, in the case of a lunatotriquetral ligament rupture, a VISI or volarly rotated position.

MOTION SERIES AND DYNAMIC VIEWS

Dynamic patterns of wrist instability are often not appreciated on static radiographs. Fixed deformity is usually a late stage of ligament injury or, if present acutely, indicates a more severe disruption. If suspected, clinically additional

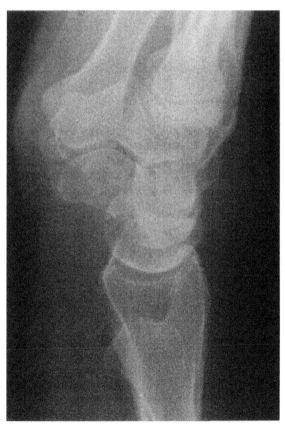

Figure 3.17 Lateral view showing dorsal angulation of the lunate.

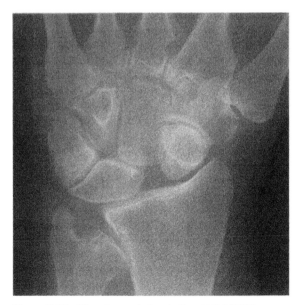

Figure 3.16 Chronic scapholunate ligament rupture. Note the fixed flexion posture of the scaphoid or 'ring' sign appearance.

posteroanterior views in full radial and ulnar deviation and a clenched fist posteroanterior view are taken to place restraining ligaments under stress. A series of the opposite wrist, taking care to use comparable positioning and imaging techniques, is also necessary, as there is considerable variation in the normal population.[2] These views may demonstrate widening of the scapholunate joint on ulnar deviation or on clenched fist views. It may show reduced scaphoid rotation from arthrofibrosis or malunion, which can be a sequel to scaphoid fracture. In cases of ulnar impingement, the clenched fist view may show abutment of the ulna against the lunate. Patients who exhibit unusual clicks or clunks may require fluorography to provide a more detailed analysis of carpal motion, which can be recorded on video for later review.

SPECIFIC CARPAL BONE VIEWS

Views to highlight specific carpal bones can be useful. Scaphoid or trapezium views may demonstrate fractures or scapho–trapezial–trapezoid joint pathology. Carpal tunnel projections provide a tangential view, demonstrating the palmar aspect of the trapezium, tuberosity of the scaphoid, trapezoid, capitate, hook of hamate, triquetrum and pisiform. An off-lateral view with the wrist in radial deviation can provide a good view of the hamate hook, which may not otherwise be seen on standard views (Fig. 3.18).

At this stage, if the radiographs are normal or the diagnosis is not confirmed, it may be necessary to proceed with further investigations such as technetium bone scans, ultrasonography, computed tomography (CT) scanning, magnetic resonance imaging (MRI) or arthrography. The choice of test will be determined by the provisional diagnosis. If bone pathology is being sought, then either bone scanning and/or CT may be considered. Soft tissue lesions such as occult ganglia or tumours can be identified by ultrasonography or MRI. Arthrography is often able to demonstrate ligament tears and perforations but their presence is also seen in normal or asymptomatic wrists. In many cases bilateral arthrography

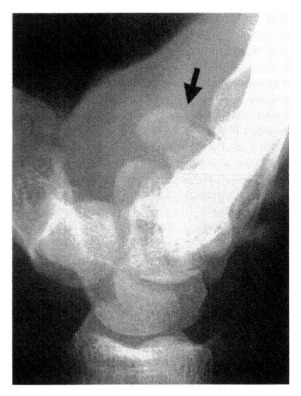

Figure 3.18 Fracture of the base of the hamate hook is clearly visible.

will demonstrate similar findings. This makes interpretation of this investigation difficult and confusing.

ULTRASONOGRAPHY

Although still being evaluated, this modality is very useful for demonstrating soft tissue abnormalities.[3] Improvements in transducer design and image processing technology specifically for musculoskeletal purposes have greatly enhanced the resolution and accuracy of ultrasonography. Scanning is readily available, low cost and has very good patient acceptance. Small ganglia, especially those on the dorsum of the wrist, are well shown, as are the dorsal fibres of the scapholunate joint (Fig. 3.19). Widening can be demonstrated dynamically by maintaining visualisation of the interosseous ligament as the wrist

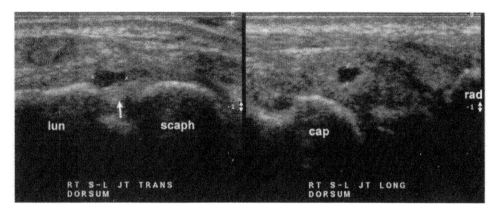

Figure 3.19 Ultrasound view in the transverse plane showing the dorsal surfaces of the scaphoid and lunate with the transverse fibres of the scapholunate ligament. The cystic swelling on the dorsal surface is a ganglion.

is moved from radial to ulnar deviation. Small areas of calcification or avulsion fractures which are difficult to demonstrate on radiographs are well visualised by this method. It is very useful in the identification of soft tissue tumours about the hand and wrist and also for detecting foreign bodies that are not radiopaque.[4] Foreign bodies as small as 1 mm can be detected. The technique is operator-dependent and requires some skill in interpretation. Ultrasound can also be used as a therapeutic aid to guide injection of small or deep-seated ganglia and in specific joint injections.

BONE SCANS

Technetium bone scanning using a three-phase study is a valuable screening investigation. Although its images do not provide great detail, it is an aid in cases of wrist pain where symp-toms are not well localised and plain radiographs are not diagnostic, such as in the early stages of joint inflammatory, degenerative or infective disorders. It is also helpful in the early detection of undisplaced fractures such as the scaphoid, stress fractures or in cases of stage 1 or 2 (Lichtman grading) avascular necrosis of the lunate.[5] The changes seen on bone scan are diagnostic in cases of reflex sympathetic dystrophy (RSD).

COMPUTED TOMOGRAPHY

This radiographic investigation is primarily used to demonstrate bone detail. If a fracture is not obvious on plain films or is suspected on technetium bone scan, then this modality can provide excellent detail; e.g. in single carpal bone fractures or distal radial fractures with an impacted fragment. Union in scaphoid fractures can be difficult to assess with plain radiographs and can be aided with CT scanning. In general terms, CT scans are not helpful in the assessment of wrist pain or carpal instability where the diagnosis is not at least suspected on the plain films or a lesion identified on bone scan.

MAGNETIC RESONANCE IMAGING

MRI is a sophisticated imaging modality which utilises a magnetic field and radiofrequency energy to create an image. It provides good anatomical detail and pathology is often conspicuous due to excellent contrasting detail. Soft tissue structures surrounding the wrist are well imaged and it is excellent for soft tissue tumours and can easily identify vascular malformations with detail equivalent of angiography. A great strength is its ability to assess changes in bone marrow, especially the early detection of avascular necrosis in proximal pole scaphoid fractures and in Kienböck's disease of the lunate where radiographs or bone scans are equivocal. It can identify some tears or disruptions of the triangular fibrocartilage complex (TFCC) or carpal ligaments. Ligament ruptures may be difficult to identify due to the complex structure and variations in orientation of the intercarpal ligaments. Unfortunately, this investigation is expensive and is not readily available in many countries. It is best reserved for cases where specific information is required, such as viability of bone or soft tissue tumours, or where other imaging modalities do not provide sufficient information.

ARTHROSCOPY

The value of arthroscopy is clearly established in both diagnosis and treatment of wrist disorders: many articular, synovial and ligamentous pathologies are beyond the capability of other imaging techniques and are only obvious with direct observation. The development of small-diameter arthroscopes with improved lighting provide comparable visualisation to large-diameter arthroscopes and permit the evaluation of small joints. The use of 1.7 mm or 2.7 mm athroscopes enables visualisation of radiocarpal, midcarpal and distal radioulnar joints. The smaller-diameter instruments allow inspection of the metacarpophalangeal and thumb carpometacarpal joints as well.

The procedure is usually carried out under regional or general anaesthesia with joint distraction achieved by overhead finger trap traction. The instruments are introduced via small incisions on the dorsal, ulnar and radial sides of the wrist, depending on the area of investigation. In the radiocarpal joint the articular surfaces of the scaphoid lunate triquetrum and radius are well seen. The interosseous ligaments as well as the volar radiocarpal ligaments and TFCC can be identified and manipulated by a probe to assess integrity. The presence of a TFCC perforation will expose the head of the ulna and distal radioulnar joint (DRUJ). The midcarpal joint surfaces, including the scaphotrapezial trapezoid (STT) joint, are also well seen and here scapholunate or lunotriquetral instability can best be appreciated from joint malalignment or excessive joint widening.

The distal radioulnar joint can be visualised through separate portals created over the joint.

The value of arthroscopy has been critically assessed in a number of recent reviews[6–8] of both diagnostic and surgical procedures. In patients in whom the cause of wrist pain was uncertain even after other investigations, arthroscopy was able to provide a diagnosis in over 90% of cases. In those in whom the diagnosis is known preoperatively, the arthroscopy provides the ability to assess pathology, perform arthroscopic surgical procedures or allow planning for further surgical procedures after assessing or staging joint pathology.

Standard arthroscopic procedures as applicable to other joints can also be carried out in the wrist. This more advanced area of treatment remains contentious and in most cases the techniques used are still under evaluation and development. Treatment of TFCC pathology is

Table 3.9 Summary of investigations for wrist disorders

Investigation	Condition investigated
Radiographs	
• Standard views	Bone morphology (fractures)
	Joint alignment (dislocations)
	Arthritis, bone lesions
• Dynamic views	Carpal instability
	Ulnar impaction syndrome
• Specific views	Individual carpal bones (hamate hook)
Bone scan	Fractures
	Joint disorders (inflammatory, infective, arthritic)
	Bone vascularity
	Osteopenia (RSD)
	Tumours
Ultrasound	Soft tissue lesions (ligaments, cysts, tumours)
	Foreign bodies
	Tendons, neurovascular structures
CT scanning	Precise bone detail
MRI	Soft tissue lesions
	Bone vascularity
Arthroscopy	
• Diagnostic	Joint lesions, ligament injuries, TFCC lesions
• Therapeutic	Debridement, fracture treatment, ligament repair, ulnar resection

RSD = reflex sympathetic dystrophy, TFCC = triangular fibrocartilage complex.

often most appropriately done with this technique. Debridement of TFCC tears or central perforations with unstable flaps and partial interosseous ligament tears can be accomplished.[9,10] Resection of the distal ulna through the defect in the TFCC can achieve a limited shortening, but if there is an ulna plus variance then formal osteotomy is usually necessary. Peripheral detachments with DRUJ instability can be treated with arthroscopically assisted techniques passing sutures under arthroscopic view. Extracapsular structures are exposed by a small incision for tying of sutures. Partial

carpal bone excision as for osteochondral fragments or with avascular necrosis is possible. Even proximal row carpectomy has been performed in this manner. Undisplaced scaphoid fractures can be internally fixed *in situ* using cannulated screws with radiographic control, and some displaced fractures can also be treated. Distal radial fractures can also be assessed and, in some cases, displaced fragments reduced and secured with percutaneous pins.

A summary of investigations for wrist disorders is given in Table 3.9.

REFERENCES

1. Gilula LA: Carpal injuries: analytical approach and case exercises. AJR 133:503–17, 1979.
2. Schernberg F: Roentgenographic examination of the wrist: a systematic study of the normal, lax and injured wrist. Parts 1&2. J Hand Surg 15B:210–19, 1990
3. Read JW, Conolly WB, Lanzrtta M et al.: Diagnostic ultrasound of the hand and wrist. JHS 61A:1004–10, 1996.
4. Wheen DJ, Conolly WB, Read JW: Ultrasound imaging of occult glomus tumours of the fingertip. Hand Surg 1:1–6, 1996.
5. Lichtman DM, Alexander AH, Mack GR et al.: Keinböck's disease – update on silicone replacement arthroplasty. J Hand Surg &:343–7, 1982.
6. Kelly EP, Stanley JK: Arthroscopy of the wrist. J Hand Surg 15B:236–42, 1990.
7. De Smet L, Dauwe D, Fortems Y, Zachee B, Fabry G: The value of wrist arthroscopy. J Hand Surg 21B:210–12, 1996.
8. Jones WA, Lovell ME: The role of arthroscopy in the investigation of wrist disorders. J Hand Surg 21B:442–5, 1996.
9. Minami A, Ishikawa J, Suenaga N, Kasashima T: Clinical results of treatment of triangular fibrocartilage complex tears by arthroscopic debridement. J Hand Surg 21A:406–11, 1996.
10. Ruch DS, Poehling GG: Arthroscopic management of partial scapholunate and lunotriquetral injuries of the wrist. J Hand Surg 21A:412–17, 1996.

FURTHER READING

Buchler U (ed.): Wrist instability. London: Martin Dunitz, 1996.
Litchman DM (ed.): The wrist and its disorders. Philadelphia: WB Saunders, 1988.
Poznanski AK (ed.): Hand clinics imaging of the hand: 7:1, 1991.

Stanley J, Saffar P: Wrist arthroscopy. London: Martin Dunitz, 1994.
Talesnik J: The wrist: Edinburgh: Churchill Livingstone, 1985.

D. DISTAL RADIAL FRACTURES

Bryce M Meads and Rosemary Prosser

Distal radial fractures are one of the most common fractures in adults. They are frequently seen

in the elderly but can occur at any age. Such fractures can range from simple undisplaced to complex comminuted intra-articular fractures also involving other soft tissue structures.

They cause significant morbidity, with one study finding that only 2.9% of Colles' fractures had no permanent disability.[1]

ANATOMY

The articular aspect of the distal radius is triangular in shape, with the radial styloid as the apex and the base of the triangle the distal radioulnar articulation. The articular surface is biconcave in the radioulnar plane and the dorsal–volar plane. The metaphyseal flare of the distal radius begins about 2 cm proximal to the radiocarpal joint. The metaphyseal cortex is thinner than the diaphyseal region. The distal volar margin of the radius flares, whereas the dorsal radius has a flatter surface.

The distal radius articulates with the scaphoid and the lunate. Approximately 80% of the axial load of the hand is applied through the distal radius, with the remaining 20% through the ulna. A slight prominence between the scaphoid and the lunate articulations on the radius leaves two corresponding fossae.

The extrinsic ligaments of the wrist on the dorsum and volar cortices connect the carpal bones to the distal radius and are often injured with a fracture. The volar ligaments originate from the radius, passing in a distal ulnar direction to prevent ulnar translation of the carpus. They consist of the radioscaphocapitate as well as the long and short radiolunate ligaments that act to stabilise both the radiocarpal and midcarpal joints. The radiotriquetral ligament and the radioscaphocapitate ligaments are the most important dorsal ligaments attaching the carpus to the radius.

The distal radial cortex extends more distally on a neutral posteroanterior (PA) view and has a wavy appearance due to the prominence of Lister's tubercle,[2] around which the extensor pollicis longus (EPL) tendon is drawn. The volar cortex is more prominent ulnarly and has a smooth regular appearance and overlaps with the prominent subchondral aspect of the central aspect of the distal radius (Fig. 3.20).

The distal radius is typically longer than the distal ulna or ulnar minus; however, this does vary between patients and also decreases with age.[3]

The distal radioulnar joint is essentially perpendicular to the radiocarpal joint. This is primarily a rotational joint, allowing for pronation and supination of the forearm. A small amount of translation occurs with full rotation due to the

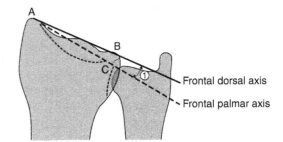

Figure 3.20 The dorsal and volar margins of the radius can be distinguished on a posteroanterior (PA) X-ray, with three different profiles. With care they can be distinguished also in a fractured distal radius. (Reproduced with permission from Sennwald G: The wrist. Berlin: Springer-Verlag, 1987:52.)

sigmoid notch on the radius having a larger arc than the corresponding surface of the distal ulna.

The triangular fibrocartilage covers the distal end of the ulna, extending the smooth congruent appearance of the wrist joint over the distal ulna as it articulates with the proximal carpal row. The triangular fibrocartilage complex (TFCC) consists of the triangular fibrocartilage, the volar and dorsal radioulnar ligaments, the meniscoid complex, the extensor carpi ulnaris (ECU) sheath, ulna capsule and the ulnotriquetral and ulnolunate ligaments.[4]

MECHANISM OF INJURY

The mechanism of injury can be a combination of bending, compression, shearing and rotational forces.

A Colles' fracture, a dorsally displaced fracture within an inch of the distal radius, is thought of as a bending fracture, resulting with initial tension of the palmar cortex and the axial load and causing compression dorsally, resulting in comminution at this point. The distal end of the radius finishes in a supinated position as the hand is fixed and the forearm pronates.

The Smith's type fracture is usually sustained with the wrist volarly flexed, resulting in the palmar displacement and the fracture displaced palmarly.

Shear fractures usually involving a variable extent of the radial styloid are unstable and require operative restoration of the articular surface.

The energy involved in the traumatic episode determines the extent of damage. Seemingly innocuous falls can lead to severe comminution: stress risers can contribute to this, such as old malunions or bone cysts. An osteoporotic distal radius is unable to absorb the energy involved and leads to a more comminuted fracture.

IMAGING

PA, lateral and oblique views of good quality must be taken. Much of the treatment will be decided on these views.

PA and lateral views of the uninvolved side should be taken to act as a template where operative management is being considered, as the

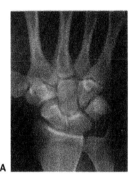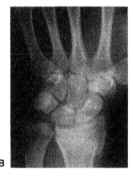

Figure 3.21   X-rays of both sides are essential in difficult fractures, as the uninjured side (A) can be used as a template for preoperative planning, as a guide for anatomical restoration of the wrist articulation following fracture (B). (X-rays with permission from PJ Scougall.)

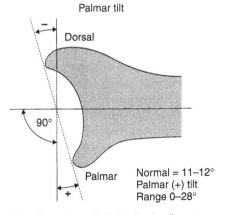

Figure 3.22   The palmar tilt of the distal radius averages 11°, but is variable. (Reproduced with permission from Fernandez DL, Jupiter JB: Fractures of the distal radius. A practical approach to management. New York: Springer Verlag, 1996.)

differences from left to right are small[5] (Fig. 3.21). The comparison PA views must be taken with the shoulder abducted 90 degrees, the elbow flexed 90 degrees and the wrist in neutral so as to assess ulna length. Ulnar variance is typically 0 mm and radial inclination 23 degrees. Values for palmar tilt of the distal radius are from 11 degrees on the lateral view (Fig. 3.22).

Computed tomography (CT) scans are useful in a comminuted fracture to allow for determination of intra-articular comminution and displacement for preoperative planning. It helps to determine the separation of fragments at the articular level of the radiocarpal and distal radio-ulnar joints.

Postoperatively, the reduction is checked by further X-rays, with a PA, lateral and an articular lateral view. An articular lateral view is taken at an angle of 22 degrees from the perpendicular and is ideal for assessing the reduction of the articular surface of the lunate fossa.[6]

CLASSIFICATION

There are a number of classification systems of distal radial fractures based upon the plain X-rays. The most commonly used ones are those of Melone, A.O. Frykman and the Mayo classification (Fig. 3.23). These systems are determined by the intra-articular involvement and the extent of comminution and are useful for comparing treatment methods for similar fractures; however they are not prognostic of final outcome.

MANAGEMENT
Indications

The most important factors that have been identified as determining the outcome are:[7,8]

- shortening of the radius less than 2 mm
- radial inclination greater than 15 degrees
- dorsal angulation greater than 10 degrees
- articular steps 1–2 mm
- articular gaps greater than 1 mm.

In a clinical study, axial shortening of the distal radius by 3–5 mm resulted in an unsatisfactory result in 25% of patients.[9] Radial shortening causes

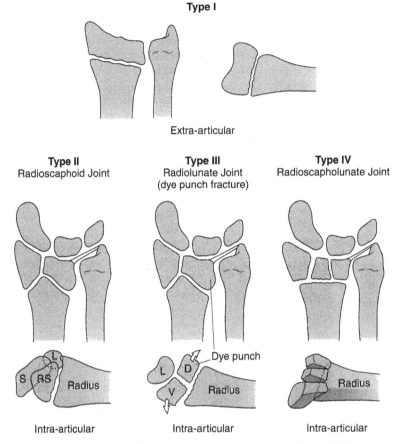

Figure 3.23 The Mayo classification: type I = extra-articular radiocarpal joint, intra-articular radioulnar joint; type II = radioscaphoid joint; type III = radiolunate joint (+/−radioulnar joint); type IV = radioscapholunate, radioulnar joint (complex fracture). (Reproduced with permission from Missakian ML, Cooney WP, Amadio PC et al.: Open reduction and internal fixation for distal radius fractures. J Hand Surg 17:745–55, 1992.)

impingement of the TFCC, causing this to become excessively tight and restricting rotation.[10] Loss of radial inclination has also been shown to be a factor leading to poor results and leads to radial inclination of the hand.[11] Radial inclination of only 10 degrees causes an alteration in the loading of the distal radius.

Fracture union with dorsal inclination restricts palmar flexion. A dorsally angulated fracture has been found to reduce rotation due to alteration of the mechanics of the distal radioulnar joint.

Articular steps of greater than 2 mm[12] were found to lead to degenerative changes in the radiocarpal joint. Steps of 1 mm have also been found

to correlate with increased pain, decreased range of motion and grip strength.[8]

Contact stresses at the distal radius rise with increasing fracture displacement. With a 2 mm step, the mean stress rose 27% and, with a 51% increase in maximum stress above normal values.[13] The ability of cartilage to withstand an increase in stress long term is unknown.

Articular gaps were noted as the most significant factor in functional outcome.[8] Intra-articular gaps can change the congruency of the radiocarpal articulation. A significant reduction in the functional results occurred with a gap of greater than 1 mm on postoperative X-ray films.

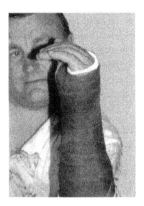

Figure 3.24 The cast should allow full MP flexion; the patient is encouraged to exercise second hourly or hourly if necessary. Both isolated and gross flexion/extension exercises are done.

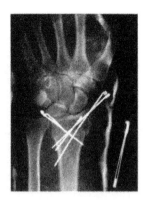

Figure 3.25 Percutaneous pinning used in conjunction with cast immobilisation. (X-ray with permission from Dr D Wheen.)

CLOSED REDUCTION

Fractures with only a minor degree of comminution of the metaphysis and a minimal intra-articular component can be treated with a closed reduction. Elderly patients with contraindications to prolonged anaesthesia and low demands can be treated in this manner.

The fracture is reduced by reversing the mechanism of injury: thus, the deformity is increased to unlock the ends of the bone; distraction is then applied to restore length and then reduced by flexion and ulnar deviation.

The fracture is then held reduced by a well-moulded cast with slight flexion and ulnar deviation of the wrist. Concerns with swelling under circumferential casts in the initial period have made an indication for holding the fracture with padded volar and dorsal plaster slabs.

It is important to ensure the cast ends short of the distal palmar crease to allow full flexion and extension exercises of the metacarpophalangeal (MCP) joints (Fig. 3.24). The palm of the hand must not be crowded when applying the cast, as this compresses the transverse carpal arch of the hand and is very uncomfortable.

Closed reduction is best applied to extra-articular fractures which are relatively stable after reduction: i.e. a fracture with only a small degree of dorsal comminution and where some cortical contact remains.

Percutaneous pinning can easily be added to a closed reduction to provide additional stability to the reduced fragments (Fig. 3.25). This can be performed by transfixing the fracture fragment directly with a wire and securing this by passing the wire through a region of intact cortex. A different technique is to use an intrafocal wire, which is introduced into the fracture site and prevents the fragment from displacing.

The superficial radial nerve can be injured in up to 25% of percutaneous wire insertions. Insertion via a stab incision and a cannula or a tissue protector may reduce this complication.

Therapy following closed reduction

Therapy aims to maximise range of motion, strength and function without compromising fracture healing.

Treatment during cast immobilisation

At this stage therapy aims at maintaining range at the unimmobilised joints, and controlling oedema and pain. Knowledge of the patient's past medical history such as oesteoarthritis, previous injury, diabetes and sympathetic conditions (Raynaud's disease or sweaty palms) may alert the therapist to potential problems and help tailor the therapy programme.

Pain may be an indication of a tight cast, compression or injury to the nerves or an extensive soft tissue as well as a bony injury. Pain levels can be recorded on a visual analogue scale. Pain from soft tissue injury and fracture can usually be relieved with local measures such as cryotherapy and gentle compression to control inflammation and analgesics.

Injury to the median nerve in the carpal tunnel may result from a high-velocity injury in which the median nerve is stretched over the radial fragments or compression caused from pressure resulting from oedema under the cast. A tight cast may cause or contribute to a carpal tunnel syndrome or compression of the superficial radial nerve. A tight cast needs to be removed or at least split to relieve pressure.

Burning pain and vasomotor changes may indicate an impending chronic regional pain syndrome (CRPS) or reflex sympathetic dystrophy (RSD). The cause of the pain needs to be established, so that treatment can be directed to the appropriate structures. Transcutaneous electric nerve stimulation (TENS) applied to an irritable peripheral nerve, or to the nerve and stellate ganglion, can be helpful for those patients with a neurological or sympathetic component to their pain.

Oedema collects in the looser tissues of the dorsum of the hand. This allows the MPs to posture in extension and the IPs in flexion. Active exercise, elevation and compression wraps are all important in oedema management. The application of a Cryocuff™ over the cast and hand in the early stages can be very effective. The Cryocuff combines cold therapy with gentle compression. Elevation is a first-line treatment technique for the control of swelling. If a sling is used, it should be applied so that the hand is elevated higher than the elbow. Care should be taken with slings, as they encourage proximal joint stiffness: for most patients slings should be reserved for when the patient is outside or in public places. Active shoulder flexion combined with finger flexion and extension hourly or second hourly acts as an active pump on the venous and lymphatic systems, pumping oedema proximally out of the hand.

Range of motion exercises improve oedema drainage, prevent tendon adherence and maintain joint mobility in the unimmobilised joints.

The cast should allow full MP flexion, IP extension and enough thumb trapezial metacarpal (TMC) motion to maintain the thumb web space. Blocked joint exercises, tendon gliding exercises and passive range of motion exercises can be used if the joints and tendons are becoming stiff despite active exercises. Intrinsic stretching may also be necessary if the intrinsics are tight.

Therapy after cast removal

The patient often feels vulnerable and weak after removal of the cast. A light elasticised wrist support worn for a couple of weeks often helps to encourage the patient to use the hand and gain confidence.

The focus of the therapy programme is now on restoring wrist range of motion, stability and strength. There are three important factors to consider when setting range of motion goals:

- the anatomical position of the joints seen on X-ray
- the functional wrist range required and desired
- the functional interaction between wrist position and grip strength.

Altered anatomical alignment caused by the fracture will influence motion.[14] Distal fragment angulation may cause loss of extension/flexion range. Radial shortening may disrupt the distal radioulnar joint (DRUJ) and triangular fibrocartilage complex (TFCC), resulting in loss of rotation and ulnar-sided wrist pain.

Therapy will not alter a mechanical block but is very effective in resolving soft tissue restrictions.

Fracture position may ultimately determine range. Several authors have shown[15,16] that most daily activities can be done with 30–40 degrees of both extension and flexion (60–80 degree arc of motion) and 50 degrees of both supination and pronation (100 degree arc of motion).

It is imperative to restore independent wrist extension. This may be particularly difficult if the wrist has been immobilised in flexion. There is a tendency for the finger extensors to be activated when the wrist extensors are weak and the wrist is in a flexed position[17] (Fig. 3.26). A weak grip

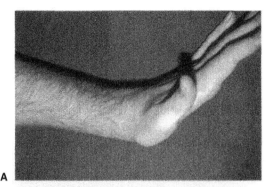

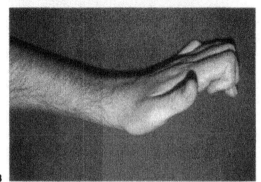

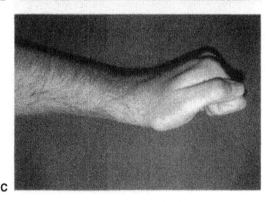

Figure 3.26 Wrist extension using the finger extensors (EDC) sets up an abnormal motor learning pattern. Independent isolated wrist extension is vital for hand function. The patient may have difficulty performing isolated wrist extension (A), even after this has been explained (B). It is usually easier for the patient if a tenodesis action of wrist extension with finger flexion (C) and wrist flexion with finger extension is tried.

with a flexed wrist posture will result if the wrist extensors are not independently activated and strengthened. The tenodesis action of wrist extension with finger flexion and finger relaxation and extension with wrist flexion is practised.

Active exercises for deviation and rotation are also commenced at this time. Rotation exercises can be commenced while still in the cast if the fracture reduction is stable in a short arm cast. Rotation exercises are done with the elbow by the side in order to isolate rotation to the forearm. The patient is instructed to sustain the end range position for each exercise for 5 seconds for all wrist exercises.

Passive exercises, passive joint mobilisations (PJMs), stretching techniques and graded strengthening exercises all begin once the cast is removed. The use of some type of heat in association with passive stretching techniques enhances the stretching achieved.

The effectiveness of Maitland[18] and Kaltenborn[19] style PJMs has been questioned in the literature. Kay et al.[20] showed in a study of distal radial fractures that patients who did not receive PJMs did just as well in the long term as those who did receive them. Clinically, patients report considerable improvement immediately after treatment in range of motion after PJMs. PJMs should be physiological, as discussed in Chapter 3B. Passive motion and PJMs should be followed up with active and resisted motion if the joint range gained with these techniques is to be maintained.

Clinical experience has shown that wrist exercises should not be upgraded until the wrist is able to maintain stability in extension with light to moderate gripping activities. The strengthening programme involves grip strengthening with the wrist in approximately 30 degrees of extension, or small-range wrist extension exercises (10–30 degrees) while gripping. Once this is achieved through range wrist extension, strengthening with a weight can be commenced.

Functional use of the hand to improve strength and set up normal grip patterns cannot be underestimated. Use of the hand is not a substitute for specific exercises; it does, however, increase enormously the amount of muscle contraction required during the day, thereby increasing the demand and strength of the muscles.

There are many different techniques for treating stiffness; they range from manual stretching techniques to continuous passive motion (CPM) and serial static and dynamic splinting (Fig. 3.27). A balance exists between range of motion and muscular strength. Range cannot be maintained unless there is adequate strength in the muscles for the available range. Stretching techniques should be balanced with the strengthening programme. Further information on the treatment of stiffness can be found in Chapter 3H.

Specific tips

If wrist extension is very weak, a lightweight elasticised wrist support with the wrist in extension will encourage a more normal neurological motor pattern during grip strengthening and functional use of the hand. The splint is an adjunct to treatment; it is worn intermittently and is not a substitute for wrist exercises. As soon as light activities of daily living can be done with the wrist in extension, the patient can be weaned from the splint.

The line of force which produces a radial styloid fracture may also pass through the scapholunate ligament. For this reason the scapholunate ligament should be assessed for stability following all radial styloid fractures.

If MP flexion is poor in the early stages, use of a dorsal blocking splint at night in maximal comfortable MP flexion or gentle MP flexion loops/ straps can be applied while in the cast.

OPEN REDUCTION

The benefits of open reduction are to allow stable fixation of unstable fractures for early movement and anatomical restoration of intra-articular fragments.

A volar plate is applied through Henry's approach. The pronator quadratus can be removed from between the fracture fragments. A precontoured plate provides a buttress effect. These are ideal for those intra-articular fractures that have the volar cortex disrupted, such as a Barton's type fracture or the extra-articular Smith's fracture. The volar cortex, as the compression cortex, is thicker and often easier to reduce due to less comminution. A poorer view of the intra-articular component is the compromise from this approach.

Dorsal plating is typically approached via a longitudinal incision through the third compartment and elevating the second and fourth compartments. The EPL tendon is usually left out of the repaired extensor retinaculum. The dorsal approach gives a good view of the articular component of the fracture. The dorsal plate is on the tension surface of the distal radius (Fig. 3.28).

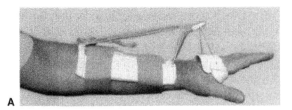

A

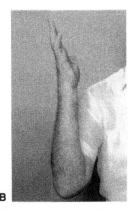

B

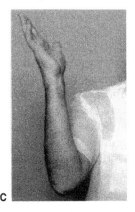

C

Figure 3.27 Wrist stiffness into extension can be addressed with a dynamic wrist extension splint (A). Extension before splintage (B) and motion gained (C) from this type of splinting by this patient can be seen here.

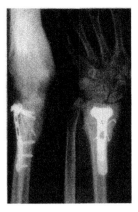

Figure 3.28 Dorsal plating of a difficult fracture; this required bone grafting with extra stabilisation of the graft with K-wires. Anteroposterior view (A) and lateral view (B).

Bone graft can be packed in through comminuted areas to support articular fragments. A block of iliac bone graft can also be inserted to reduce the chance of the fracture settling. Careful surgical technique should be observed in order to avoid the complications of nerve irritation and pain at the graft site. Bone graft substitutes can be utilised for their osteoconductive effect. The addition of growth factors such as bone morphogenetic protein (BMP) may provide clinically useful osteoconductive effects, an alternative in the near future.

A dorsal approach may cause scarring that reduces postoperative wrist flexion with a median range of 40 degrees of flexion with dorsally plated fractures.[21] At an average of 38 months postoperatively, the range of motion of the wrist was 75% of the uninjured side.[8] The grip strength was also lower than the contralateral side, at 69%.

Extensor tendon irritation can occur with a dorsal plate and even lead to rupture on occasions. Therefore removal of these plates should be performed.

Arthroscopic reduction is a new procedure, particularly useful for fractures with intra-articular comminution. It is best delayed for 2–7 days to allow the haematoma to consolidate. There is no doubt that this method will change how we interpret X-rays and assess the results of gapping at the fracture site. The reduction can be held with either K-wires to splint the fracture or percutaneous screw fixation to add compression between fracture fragments.

Arthroscopy can also assess other soft tissue involvement that can occur in 68% of cases.[22] Diagnosis of scapholunate ligament injuries was reported in 32% and TFCC tears in 43%. Once identified, these can be treated appropriately at an early stage.

Therapy following open reduction

Fracture stability and restoration of anatomical alignment of the bones and joint surfaces by open reduction with internal fixation (ORIF) enables the therapist to commence early motion immediately following reduction. Early motion reduces stiffness and assists in the repair of the cartilage following intra-articular fracture. Greater attention can also be given to oedema reduction.

The ORIF is supported with a thermoplastic splint, which is worn for 6 weeks until the fracture is united. Pain control, oedema control and range of motion exercises for the digits and proximal joints are similar to that following closed reduction.

ORIF of high-energy injuries which result in highly comminuted and displaced fractures usually also have considerable soft tissue damage. Early restoration of digit motion and tendon glide is essential if these patients are to obtain a good outcome. There is usually a significant amount of oedema that limits joint range and tendon glide of both the digits and wrist. Cryotherapy in combination with compression is applied intermittently; a gentle compression garment or wrap is worn between sessions to maintain control of the oedema. Care should be taken to monitor circulation, particularly if the circulatory system has been injured. The healing tissues need adequate circulation for tissue repair. In addition, compression garments or wraps should not limit or impede exercises.

The exercise programme is commenced the day after surgery. Appropriate pain control is necessary. Active and passive exercises should be prescribed for the individual patient, depending on their status. Finger wriggling is not good enough. Isolated IP and MP exercises are usually necessary. EDC and flexor tendon gliding exercises are important for maintaining tendon glide. The extrinsic extensors lie immediately over the fracture site and are particularly prone to being caught or limited by adhesion in the healing tissues. If joint range of the digits cannot be maintained, a static splint in the position of safe immobilisation should be used at night and intermittently in the day if necessary.

Wrist exercises can be commenced a few days after fixation. Small-range exercises for extension/flexion and supination/pronation are started first. Isolated wrist extension using a tenodesis motion is emphasised. There should be no EDC action with isolated wrist extension. As the patient improves, range can be increased; deviation exercises can be added later. The exercise programme should focus on four or five specific exercises that are prescribed for the patient. The patient must be able to do the exercises correctly, regularly and frequently during the day, i.e. hourly or second hourly. Too many exercises can be too confusing and tiring for the patient and, as a result, often don't get done correctly.

Once the fracture is united, at approximately 6 weeks, therapy is continued on the same lines as after cast removal.

EXTERNAL FIXATION

External fixateurs are selected for unstable fractures with significant metaphyseal comminution. The fixateur is applied as a neutralisation device and is best at helping to correct the radial length when comminution is severe and the chance of obtaining a satisfactory stable reduction with operative intervention is low. Restoration of the articular surface was found less likely to occur with more than 4–5 intra-articular fragments.[7]

The external fixateur acts via ligamentotaxis and distraction. Even fragments that no longer have an attachment may be able to be reduced by a vacuum effect. The appearance of a large void in the metaphysis after reduction can be bone grafted to reduce the chance of fracture settling and the length of time that the fixateur will be needed.

Distraction alone will not correct the palmar tilt. Palmar translation through the midcarpal joint acts back through the proximal carpal row to tilt the distal radius palmarly.[23] Flexion can be added to the distraction through the fixateur, but wrist flexion also increases the incidence of carpal tunnel syndrome from 13% with 20 degrees to 43% with 40 degrees of wrist flexion.[24] Additional fixation using K-wires can be inserted to stabilise fragments, eliminating the need for wrist flexion.

However, if too much distraction is applied, then increasing stiffness may result. Increasing distraction increases the strain in the dorsal ligaments.[25] It is not known whether the stiffness results from ischaemia of the stretched ligaments or microfailure of the fibres.

The overdistraction of the wrist corresponds to increased extrinsic extensor tendon tightness, which reduces the ability of the fingers to flex into the distal palmar crease and gives rise to a claw hand with hyperextension of the MCP joints.[23] Overdistraction may also lead to delayed union or nonunion of the fracture.

The fixateur is applied for 4–8 weeks. If additional bone graft is inserted, then the fixateur can often be safely removed at 4 weeks. This should reduce the extent of stiffness that is seen after the application of these devices.

Therapy after external fixateur application

Therapy following the application of an external fixateur is similar to that following ORIF. A splint is fabricated to fit around the fixateur, while still providing support to the wrist and forearm (Fig. 3.29). Routine pin site care is necessary.

If pin placement restricts tendon glide, the exercise programme may need to be modified. This commonly occurs in the index finger where pin sites in the second metacarpal may impede distal extensor tendon glide. Particular attention to both active and passive flexion exercises is necessary, especially for the MP joint (Fig. 3.30). The early use of prolonged very gentle flexion stretching using a modified serial static or dynamic splint can be helpful.

Some fixateurs can be unlocked to allow small-range wrist extension and flexion. The surgeon should be consulted prior to any wrist exercises to ascertain the safe wrist range which will not compromise the reduction of the fracture.

Once the fixateur is removed at 4 to 8 weeks, a thermoplastic wrist extension splint is fitted. The splint supports the fracture until it is fully healed on X-ray; this may take a further 4 weeks. At this time, digital and DRUJ motion exercises are upgraded and light graded grip strengthening commenced. Wrist motion is also commenced if it has not been done so already.

DISTAL RADIOULNAR JOINT

The involvement of this joint in distal radial fractures is often forgotten or left as an afterthought. Injuries to the DRUJ can be classified into either stable, unstable or potentially unstable injuries.[10]

Stable injuries can be treated with early active forearm rotation exercises. Unstable DRUJ dislocations can be treated with reduction and immobilising in a supinated position. Rarely, it can be unstable after being reduced. In severe cases a temporary 2 mm K-wire can transfix the radius and ulna; this must be removed later to prevent breaking. It is important to ensure that no soft tissues, such as extensor tendons, are blocking the reduction of this joint prior to this, which may give the misleading impression that the joint is unstable.

Unstable injuries demonstrate subluxation or dislocation of the ulnar head. This can be due to large TFCC tears, disruption of the secondary DRUJ stabilisers as well as to fractures of the base of the ulnar styloid or ulnar head.

Restoration of the sigmoid notch and radial length is essential to address before the distal radioulnar joint.

An unstable DRUJ with a fracture at the base of the ulnar styloid should be fixed, due to the attachments of the TFCC at the base. It can be stabilised using a tension band wire technique or a mini Herbert screw.[10]

Fractures of the neck of the ulna can be internally fixed if it is amenable. Many of these fractures, however, are highly comminuted and do not lend themselves to easy internal fixation. In this instance the results with initial splintage and early rotation exercises have been satisfactory.

Therapy following DRUJ disruption

DRUJ subluxation or dislocation can be a very difficult problem to deal with. An acute injury requires at least 6 weeks of splinting in the reduced position to allow the soft tissues to heal at an appropriate length. In mild cases of subluxation an ulnar carpal support splint may be all that is needed. In the case of dislocation, a sugar tong splint (Fig. 3.31) holding the forearm in supination and preventing rotation may be necessary for at least 6 weeks or until the joint is stable. At 6 weeks this can be exchanged for an ulnar carpal support for a further 4 weeks.

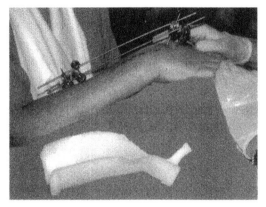

Figure 3.29 A splint to support the hand and wrist can be fabricated around the external fixateur. This provides protection and support of the fracture for the patient.

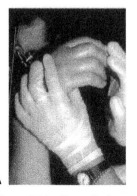 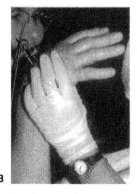

A   **B**

Figure 3.30 Finger flexion and extension exercises are vital to maintain joint range and tendon glide (A). Flexion exercises are particularly important to prevent MP joint stiffness (B) and extensor tendon adhesion, especially for the index finger as its extensor tendon can be impeded by the pins in the second metacarpal.

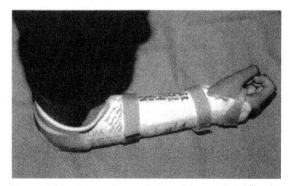

Figure 3.31 A sugar tong splint provides good stabilisation of the distal radioulnar joint (DRUJ). It prevents rotation and wrist motion, and only allows limited elbow flexion and extension. It may be necessary to hold the joint in full supination in order to maintain the DRUJ reduction.

Once stability of the DRUJ is achieved, gentle rotation exercises can be commenced. The elbow is flexed to 90 degrees and held by the side in order to prevent shoulder rotation and maximise forearm rotation. Wrist extension and flexion is also commenced at this time. Care should be taken with end range flexion exercises. Pushing into flexion may stretch out the healing soft tissues supporting the ulnar side of the wrist prematurely.

A grip strengthening programme done in various ranges of rotation (supination, neutral and pronation) aids in restoring stability. This aims to strengthen the deep head of pronator quadratus and the extrinsic tendon cage surrounding the wrist. The extensor carpi ulnaris (ECU) attaches indirectly through its tendon sheath to the ulnar wrist capsule. ECU exercises, both concentric and eccentric, may also help to stabilise the ulnar aspect of the wrist.

COMPLICATIONS

The incidence of complications has been reported in one study with varying methods of treatment as 22% of patients with major complications.[26]

A fracture of the distal radius often reduces the grip strength by 30% and reduces the range of motion of the wrist joint. Prolonged immobilisation causes stiffness from adhesions: these form in the tendons crossing the wrist as well as within the wrist joint and between ligaments. The fingers must be mobilised early so as to reduce stiffness within the MCP joints and decrease flexor tendon adhesions.

Extensor tendonitis may result from the tendons rubbing over the internal fixation due to their subcutaneous position. The EPL tendon may rupture in up to 1 in 300 Colles' fractures either from ischaemia within the tendon or from the roughened fracture edges.

Reflex sympathetic dystrophy (RSD or CRPS) can result in a very poor outcome. It usually presents or becomes apparent 1 or 2 weeks' post-fracture. The patient complains of severe pain out of proportion to the injury; the hand becomes warm, red and swollen (Fig. 3.32). A tight plaster may exacerbate or cause the symptoms. RSD needs

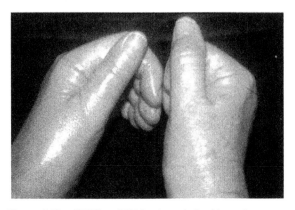

Figure 3.32 CRPS or RSD is characterised by redness, swelling, shiny skin and increased sweating in the early stages. There is pain out of proportion for the injury. Often symptoms don't become apparent until 3 weeks following the injury.

to be recognised early and appropriate changes in treatment implemented. The plaster needs to be removed and a new plaster or splint applied. Treatment should be directed at the RSD symptoms until they are under control. The stress loading programme or an active pain-free exercise programme, with pain control using TENS or other modalities, may be necessary.

Compression of the median nerve can occur from either the initial degree of displacement of the fracture or from subsequent swelling. In either situation this should be treated with open release. It has been reported in 13% of acute fractures.[26]

The ulnar nerve is less frequently compressed. The superficial radial nerve, however, may be irritated by the placement of percutaneous wires to secure the fracture from over the radial styloid or by insufficient protection when inserting external fixateur pins.

Any internal fixation can become infected and is often seen with external fixateurs. Vigilant pin site cleaning and monitoring is essential.

Malunion usually leads to a greater loss of range of motion, function and increased pain. Intra-articular involvement also increases the chance of developing early degenerative change, leading to arthritis. A corrective radial osteotomy must be considered – but can be a complex and difficult operation – to restore alignment at the radio-carpal joint.

REFERENCES

1. Bacorn RW, Kurtzke JF: Colles' fracture. A study of two thousand cases from the New York State Workmen's Compensation Board. J Bone Joint Surg 35A:643–58, 1953.
2. Paley D, Axelrod TS, Martin C, Rubenstein J, McMurty RY: Radiographic definition of the dorsal and palmar edges of the distal radius. J Hand Surg 14A:272–6, 1989.
3. Sanderson PL, Cameron IC, Holt GR, Stanley D: Ulnar variance and age. J Hand Surg 22B:21–4, 1997.
4. Ishii S, Palmer AK, Werner FW, Short WH, Fortino MD: An anatomic study of the ligamentous structure of the triangular fibrocartilage complex. J Hand Surg 23A:977–85, 1998.
5. Hollevoet N, Van Maele G, Van Seymortier P, Verdonk R: Comparison of palmar tilt, radial inclination and ulnar variance in left and right wrists. J Hand Surg 25B(5):431–3, 1999.
6. Lundy DW, Quisling SG, Lourie GM, Feiner CM, Lins RE: Tilted lateral radiographs in the evaluation of intra-articular distal radial fractures. J Hand Surg 24A:249–56, 1999.
7. Fernandez DL: Should anatomical reduction be pursued in distal radial fractures? J Hand Surg 25B(6):523–7, 1999.
8. Trumble TE, Schmitt SR, Vedder NB: Factors affecting functional outcome of displaced intra-articular distal radial fractures. J Hand Surg 19A:325–40, 1994.
9. Aro H, Koivunen T: Minor axial shortening of the radius affects outcome of Colles' fractures. J Hand Surg 16A:392–8, 1991.
10. Geissler WB, Fernandez DL, Lamey DM: Distal radioulnar joint injuries associated with fractures of the distal radius. Clin Orth Rel Res 327:135–46, 1996.
11. Roth JH, Miniaci A: Healing of extra-articular angulated apex volar fractures of the distal radius. Can J Surg 31:39–41, 1988.
12. Knirk JL, Jupiter JB: Intra-articular fractures of the distal end of the radius in young adults. J Bone Joint Surg 68A:647–59, 1986.
13. Baratz ME, Des Jardines JD, Anderson DA, Imbiglia JE: Displaced intra-articular fractures of the distal radius: the effect of fracture displacement on contact stresses in a cadaver model. J Hand Surg 21A:183–8, 1996.
14. Hannu AT, Korvunen T: Minor axial shortening of radius affects the outcome of Colles' fracture treatment. J Hand Surg 16A:392–8, 1991.
15. Palmer A, Werner FW, Murphy D, Glisson R: Functional wrist motion: a biomechanical study. J Hand Surg (Am) 10:39–46, 1985.
16. Ryu J, Cooney WP, Askew LJ, An K-N, Chao EYS: Functional ranges of motion and the wrist joint. J Hand Surg (Am) 15:409–19, 1991.
17. Laseter GF, Carter PR: Management of distal radius fractures. J Hand Ther 9:114–28, 1996.
18. Maitland GD: Peripheral manipulation, 2nd edn. London: Butterworths, 1977:152–87.
19. Kaltenborn F: Mobilization of the extremity joints. Universitetsgaten, Oslo: Olaf Norlis Bokhander, 1980:26–8.
20. Kay S, Haensel N, Stiller K: The effect of passive mobilisation following fractures involving the distal radius: a randomized study. Aust J Physio 46:93–101, 2000.
21. Campbell DA: Open reduction and internal fixation of intra articular and unstable fractures of the distal radius using the AO distal radius plate. J Hand Surg: 25B(6):528–34, 1999.
22. Geissler WB, Freeland AE, Savoie FH, McIntyre LW, Whipple TL: Intracarpal soft tissue lesions associated with an intra-articular fracture of the distal end of the radius. J Bone Joint Surg 78A:357–65, 1996.
23. Agee JM: External fixation. Technical advances based upon multiplanar ligamentotaxis. Orthop Clin N Am 24(2):265–74, 1993.
24. Gelberman RH, Szabo RM, Mortensen WW et al.: Carpal tunnel pressures and wrist position in patients with Colles' fracture. J Trauma 24:747–9, 1984.
25. Davenport WC, Miller G, Wright TW: Wrist ligament strain during external fixation: a cadaveric study. J Hand Surg 24A:102–7, 1999.
26. Cooney WP, Dobyns JH, Linschieid RL: Complications of Colles' fractures. J Bone Joint Surg 62A:613–19, 1980.

E.   CARPAL FRACTURES

Rosemary Prosser and Tim Herbert

The carpal bones have multiple surfaces which are covered in articular cartilage. Most carpal fractures are therefore intra-articular. Post-fracture stiffness caused by intra-articular adhesion formation can be countered by early motion, once the stability of the fracture is confirmed. Hand therapy plays an important role in restoring motion, strength and functional use of the hand and wrist following these fractures.

SCAPHOID FRACTURES

The most commonly fractured carpal bone is the scaphoid.[1,2] Botte and Gelberman[3] report the incidence as 60–70% of all carpal injuries.

The true incidence, however, is unknown as some are misdiagnosed as a sprain at the time of injury. A scaphoid fracture is not always immediately evident on plain X-ray.

The mechanism of injury has been postulated by Mayfield[4] and Weber and Chao,[5] as a high force applied to the radial half of the hand with the wrist in hyperextension. The proximal half of the scaphoid is stabilised between the radiocapitate and radioscaphoid ligaments and volar capsular ligaments. A bending load applied to the hand and distal half of the scaphoid causes a shear force at the waist of the scaphoid, resulting in a scaphoid waist fracture.

Fractures of the tubercle of the scaphoid appear to be caused by either compression or avulsion.[6] Similarly, small proximal pole scaphoid fractures may be caused by avulsion of the scapholunate ligament.

The primary source of vascularity of the scaphoid is its dorsal distally based artery. It supplies the scaphoid from its distal to proximal end. A fracture which disrupts the blood supply to the proximal fragment can cause avascular necrosis of this fragment.

Diagnosis and examination

History and clinical examination are just as important as radiographic findings. The history usually involves a high-velocity injury to the wrist in hyperextension. Minor injury may be sufficient to destabilise a fibrous non-union of a previously fractured scaphoid.

On examination, there is tenderness in the anatomical snuff box. There may also be tenderness over the scaphoid tubercle. Range of motion, particularly extension, is restricted. Grip strength may be reduced by more than 50%. The axial grind test may also be useful.

Established non-unions may produce pain at extremes of motion, particularly with forced extension. Radial and ulnar deviation may be reduced due to the deformation of the scaphoid. A painful block to radial deviation may indicate radiocarpal impingement. The prognosis is poor, if avascular necrosis is present.

Six standard X-ray views of the scaphoid are required to evaluate the scaphoid radiologically – posteroanterior (PA), lateral, deviation and oblique. Comparative examination of X-rays of the uninjured wrist usually gives the most valuable information with regard to the status of the injured scaphoid.[1,7] Other imaging techniques such as bone scans for acute fractures and avascular necrosis,[2] three-dimensional computer tomography (CT) scans along the plane of the scaphoid for conformation of fractures and union,[8] and magnetic resonance imaging (MRI) for acute fractures and avascular necrosis[9] have been reported to be useful in difficult cases.

Herbert's[1] classification of scaphoid fractures is widely accepted:

- type A – stable, acute fractures such as tubercle and incomplete waist fractures
- type B – unstable fractures such as distal oblique, complete waist, proximal pole, trans-scaphoid–perilunate dislocation
- type C – delayed union
- type D – established non-union.

Conservative management

Type A

Treatment of undisplaced fractures is generally accepted to be conservative. This involves cast immobilisation for at least 6 weeks. Many different types of cast immobilisation have been advocated, from long arm to short arm casts, with or without the thumb. Barton[7] studied 292 scaphoid fractures and found that including the thumb in a short arm cast did not improve the result. He recommends a short arm Colles'-type cast. Percutaneous fixation for undisplaced scaphoid waist fractures can enable early motion within the first week following fixation.

Therapy. For the first 6–8 weeks while the cast is on, therapy involves education of the patient with regard to reducing oedema with appropriate positioning, elevation and active digit exercises.

Following cast removal, therapy aims at reducing stiffness and strengthening the injured wrist and hand. At this time, residual oedema is in a subacute or chronic stage. Regular massage and a compression garment is more appropriate than ice and pressure pump therapy.

An exercise programme of both active and graded resistance for the wrist and hand is commenced immediately after cast removal. The initial exercise focus should be on grip and functional activities with wrist stability. Wrist stability with grip requires coordinated isometric control by the wrist muscles. Once this is achieved, treatment can be refocused on specific wrist exercises. Passive and active stretching, such as the contract relax technique[10] can be more beneficial when combined with heat.[11,12]

Passive joint mobilisations (PJMs) have in the past been a treatment of choice for intercarpal stiffness. Several studies[13,14] have shown that the Maitland[15] and Karltenborn[16] anteroposterior (AP) techniques do not necessarily change the final range achieved following Colles' fracture. The accessory movement of the carpals is complex and not strictly in an AP plane. For example, the scaphoid primarily rotates at a 45 degree angle to the radius. For this reason, we would recommend the physiological gliding, rocking and rotation described by McGee (see Chapter 3B). Clinically, the patients report that PJMs make it easier to move the stiff joint and that there is less discomfort with motion following the technique. It is our experience that radius–scaphoid gliding, radius–scapholunate gliding, lunate–capitate gliding and scaphoid rotation are the most useful mobilisations following scaphoid fractures. Scaphoid PJMs should not be commenced until radiologic union is adequate. PJMs are indicated if after appropriate massage, heat and muscle/soft tissue stretching techniques the joint(s) is assessed as still being stiff.

Joint mobilisation and strengthening should be balanced. Joint range achieved by stretching techniques including PJMs will not be maintained if strength is poor.

If joint range of motion is difficult to maintain between treatment sessions, serial night splinting may be helpful. The benefits of functional use of the hand and wrist in improving range of motion, and particularly strength, should not be underestimated. For this reason, splinting in the day is avoided and active use of the hand and wrist is encouraged.

Surgical management

Type B: acute fractures

We tend to favour open reduction with internal fixation (ORIF) for all acute fractures (tubercle fractures excepted), a policy favoured by our patients as it enables them to return to work within a few weeks of injury and is more predictable than casting. Whereas many surgeons continue to argue the case for conservative treatment, most would now agree that ORIF is indicated when X-rays show clear signs of instability (Fig. 3.33).

The principles of surgical management are adequate exposure of the fracture, stable anatomical reduction with accurate realignment of the articular surfaces, sound internal fixation, careful repair of the soft tissues and early postoperative mobilisation. The Herbert bone screw is a reliable method for providing stable fixation.

Therapy. Following ORIF of the scaphoid, postoperative therapy is seldom required. Satisfactory fixation enables joint motion to be commenced as soon as possible. Early motion encourages healing of the damaged articular cartilage and prevents intra-articular adhesions that may lead to joint stiffness.

The surgeon applies a firm compressive bandage of cast padding and crepe bandage with the wrist in extension immediately after the surgery. This remains in place until the stitches are

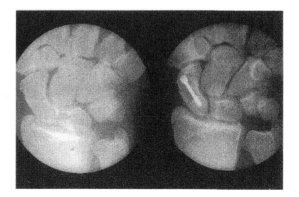

Figure 3.33 Open reduction with internal fixation (ORIF) with Herbert bone screw of a type B scaphoid fracture.

removed at 10–14 days post-surgery. At this time, the patient is instructed on wound and scar care, a home exercise programme and a gradual return to light to moderate activity. Heavy activity is not permitted until union is adequate on X-ray. A thermoplastic wrist extension splint is custom-made for those patients whose job or personality is such that they require more protection over the next 4–6 weeks.

Generally, only those patients who have very thick scar or excessive swelling following surgery require therapy.

Type D: non-unions

Non-union of the scaphoid remains a common problem, and if left untreated almost inevitably leads to progressive carpal collapse deformity and oesteoarthritis.[17–19] For this reason surgery to reconstruct the scaphoid is recommended, except in cases where significant degenerative changes throughout the wrist have become the primary problem.

Surgery includes reconstruction of the scaphoid with complete excision of the pseudoarthrosis and the use of an iliac crest bone graft to restore length and stability. Internal fixation is more reliable than plaster in maintaining the reduction. By avoiding postoperative plaster immobilisation, function is rapidly restored and early return to work is possible.

Therapy. Patients with non-unions who have been treated with immobilisation require preoperative therapy to reduce porosis and stiffness before surgery can be scheduled. The preoperative programme of approximately 2–3 weeks is aimed at increasing strength and mobility. This usually involves treatment with heat, active exercise, PJMs excluding the scaphoid and a grip strengthening regime within pain limits. A wrist support may be worn between exercise sessions.

Postoperative therapy is similar to acute fractures. If there is residual stiffness from the cast immobilisation, this is addressed with an exercise programme and PJMs. A grip strengthening and wrist strengthening programme is particularly important for those patients who have weakness due to prolonged immobilisation, particularly manual workers.

OTHER CARPAL FRACTURES

Fractures of the other carpal bones – e.g. hamate, trapezium, and capitate – are less common and can be treated along the same lines as scaphoid fractures. If the fracture is stable, cast immobilisation is recommended. This is followed by a period of therapy to mobilise the wrist and strengthen the wrist and hand. ORIF is the treatment of choice for unstable fractures. If the injury is a significant one with a high velocity or force, there will be considerable soft tissue injury and reaction. This must be carefully evaluated: the amount of soft tissue injury and reaction will determine how much therapy is needed.

TRIQUETRUM

Triquetral fractures are approximately 3–4% of all carpal fractures.[3] Clinically, they are the second most common fracture. They are often associated with perilunate dislocations or other carpal injuries. Dorsal avulsion fractures are associated with radiotriquetral or lunotriquetral ligament injuries. Palmar avulsion fractures can result from ligament avulsion occurring during perilunate dislocations. Body fractures usually result from impaction of the ulnar styloid into the triquetrum.[20,21]

Diagnosis and examination

Clinically, there is tenderness over the triquetrum; there may also be tenderness over the triquetrolunate joint and in the region of the triangular fibrocartilage complex (TFCC). In the case of small avulsion fractures there may be minimal swelling and stiffness; end range deviation and extension may cause discomfort. The diagnosis can be confirmed on X-ray; chip fractures can usually be seen dorsally in the lateral or oblique view.

Treatment

Fractures of the body require ORIF. Stable avulsion fractures usually only require protection in a splint or cast for comfort for approximately 3–4 weeks. Avulsion fractures associated with perilunate dislocations or triquetrolunate ligament rupture are serious high-energy injuries: they require surgical repair of the ligaments and prolonged therapy.

Therapy

Stable avulsion fractures associated with triquetrolunate ligament rupture need to be treated as a ligamentous injury. They require 6 weeks of protection against forces that may compromise healing or cause elongation of the healing ligament, which may lead to instability. This is followed by an appropriate exercise programme (see Chapter 3F).

Body fractures requiring ORIF may require protection in a splint or bandage for 4–6 weeks. The splint is removed three to four times a day for wrist range of motion exercises. Oedema can be managed with massage and a compression sleeve. Cryotherapy combined with compression, such as the Cryocuff, may be useful in the early stages if oedema is significant.

Once the fracture is united, usually 6 weeks following surgery, the exercise programme can be upgraded, and resisted exercise and activity commenced. Wrist stability with resisted grip is achieved first before a resisted wrist range of motion programme is commenced. Active resistive and passive stretching techniques can also be commenced at this time. Heat can enhance the effectiveness of the stretching techniques. PJMs must be directed at only those joints that are stiff. The triquetrum moves along a helicoid path on the hamate. Its motion is three-dimensional, involving a combination of anteroposterior, cephalic caudid and rotational motion. PJMs to the triquetrum should attempt to emulate this motion.

As mentioned previously, mobilisation should be balanced with strengthening. Objective reassessment of grip strength is very important. Grip strength may vary considerably. It is not unusual to see it 20–30% lower than the contralateral side after 6 weeks of cast immobilisation. Functional activities play a vital part in improving grip strength and wrist function, particularly stability.

LUNATE

Isolated lunate fractures include avulsion chip fractures, longitudinal compression fractures and transverse fractures. The incidence of lunate fractures is 2–7% of carpal injuries.[2,3] Palmar pole fractures may be the result of avulsion of the short radiolunate ligament. Dorsal pole fractures may result from either avulsion of the dorsal capsular attachment, or an impaction of the distal radius on the lunate following a wrist hyperextension injury. Dorsal avulsion fractures involving the scapholunate or lunotriquetral ligaments should be treated as ligamentous injuries of the wrist (see carpal instabilities) rather than lunate fractures. There is a possible association between lunate body fractures and the development of avascular necrosis, i.e. Kienböck's disease. Interosseous cysts of the lunate caused by either scapholunate ligament ganglion invasion or Kienböck's disease can also predispose the lunate to pathological fracture, usually transverse.

Treatment

Avulsion fractures do not require formal treatment; they usually heal spontaneously. Acute longitudinal and transverse fractures can be treated conservatively with cast immobilisation for 6 weeks. ORIF is warranted if the fracture is unstable.

Therapy

Once the fracture is united, the cast is removed; therapy is aimed at restoring motion, strength and functional use. The patient is assessed on an individual basis and the therapy programme constructed according to the findings. The basic programme has been discussed previously in the chapter under conservative management of scaphoid fractures. PJMs should be directed at the stiff joints and may include all joints associated with the lunate, particularly the lunocapitate and radiolunate joints.

TRAPEZIUM

Trapezium fractures are 1–5% of all carpal fractures.[3] There are two main types: a split fracture of the body or a ridge fracture.

A trapezium body fracture[21] can be the result of a direct blow or a fall on an hyperextended and radial deviated wrist in which the trapezium is compressed between the first metacarpal and the radial styloid.

Ridge fractures[21] are usually the result of a fall on the outstretched hand in which the transverse carpal ligament has caused an avulsion fracture.

Diagnosis and examination

A body fracture can be diagnosed on plain X-rays; a true anteroposterior (AP) and a lateral or oblique view may be required. Clinically, there is local tenderness and pain over the trapezium, and a weak pinch grip.

Ridge fractures are best diagnosed on carpal tunnel films. Clinically, there is point tenderness at the base of the thumb. Resisted wrist flexion may increase pain and there may be an associated carpal tunnel syndrome.

Treatment

Intra-articular or unstable fractures require open reduction and internal fixation.[3] Principles of fixation have been discussed in the scaphoid fracture section of this chapter.

Conservative treatment requires cast or circumferential splint immobilisation, including the metacarpophalangeal (MP) joint of the thumb, for 6 weeks or until there is clinical and radiographic union. Splint immobilisation is preferential when there is excessive swelling as it can be removed for massage and treatment using a pressure pump, Cryocuff or interferential. A compression sleeve can be applied underneath the splint. A firm fit can be maintained more readily in a splint as it can be remoulded as the oedema decreases.

Therapy

Following cast or splint application, the patient is instructed on active finger exercises to avoid finger stiffness. Wrist and thumb MP motion can be commenced at 6 weeks on cast/splint removal. Active and passive stretching techniques including PJMs can be utilised. A graded resisted exercise programme can also be commenced at 6 weeks: it

should be ungraded as necessary throughout the course of therapy.

If ORIF is necessary, a splint to protect the surgery is fitted and used for 4–6 weeks. Oedema control is commenced immediately postoperatively. Wound and scar care should be attended to as necessary. At 4–6 weeks, mobilisation and strengthening is commenced, as with conservative management.

TRAPEZOID

The incidence of trapezoid fracture is less than 1%.[3]

The mechanism of injury is usually the result of a high-velocity force pushing the index metacarpal into the trapezoid, causing fracture or dislocation of the trapezoid.

Diagnosis is made on the clinical findings of point tenderness, pain and oedema and on X-ray (AP and oblique views).

Treatment, both conservative and surgical, follows the same lines as that for trapezium fracture.

CAPITATE

The incidence of capitate fracture is also low, 1–2% of carpal fractures.[2,3,22]

Dorsal ligament avulsion injuries are the most common. The blood supply to the capitate enters dorsally on the distal two-thirds of the body and palmarly within the distal half. This pattern of blood supply may predispose the capitate to avascular necrosis following fracture.

The mechanism of injury may be direct trauma to the dorsum of the wrist in extension or to the heads of the second and third metacarpals with the wrist in flexion. Capitate fractures are usually seen in combination with other wrist injuries such as perilunar dislocation in major wrist trauma cases. In high-energy injuries, the proximal fragment may rotate 90 degrees.

Clinical presentation includes pain, swelling, local tenderness and loss of wrist motion. Diagnosis is confirmed on X-ray or CT scan.

Stable fractures can be treated conservatively with immobilisation in a short arm cast for 6 weeks, followed by a post-immobilisation therapy programme to restore motion, strength and function.

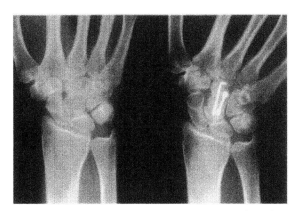

Figure 3.34 Open reduction with internal fixation (ORIF) using a K-wire and Herbert bone screw of a fractured capitate.

Unstable fractures require ORIF: postoperative therapy is similar to that following saphoid ORIF. Greater attention to mobilisation of the mid-carpal joint in particular may be necessary (Fig. 3.34).

HAMATE

Hamate fractures are also rare: 2–4% of carpal fractures.[2,3,22] There are two types – fractures of the hook and fractures of the body.

Fractures of the body often involve the joint surfaces and can be associated with fracture dislocations of the fourth and fifth carpometacarpal joints. These require percutaneous fixation or open reduction internal fixation.

Hook fractures are more common. They occur following a fall on the extended wrist, or are associated with abrupt impact following a forceful swing of a club or bat, such as the mistimed golf shot. The hook is fractured by the impact of the fall, causing avulsion of the transverse carpal and pisiohamate ligaments, or due to the force exerted through the handle of the golf club when the club comes to an abrupt halt as it hits the ground.

Hook fractures present with acute tenderness over the hook of the hamate. There is discomfort holding a racket, bat or club and there may be discomfort with resisted abduction or adduction of the little finger. Wrist motion is within normal limits. Grip strength may be reduced due to pain. Irritation of the ulnar nerve or flexor tendons may occur due to their close anatomical proximity to the hamate hook. Hook fractures can be seen on

carpal tunnel X-ray views and bone scans. CT scans can be useful for difficult cases.

Conservative treatment involves cast or splint immobilisation until the tenderness settles; an asymptomatic fibrous non-union usually results. If the fragment remains irritable, preventing grip on the golf club or bat, simple surgical excision is recommended. The irritable fragment can be removed without disturbing any of the major wrist ligaments. Surgical management is also necessary if there are any ulnar nerve or flexor tendon symptoms.

Therapy

No splintage is necessary following surgical excision of the hook of hamate. The two most common problems are a reactive hypersensitive scar over the hypothenar eminence and ulnar nerve irritability. Scar management involves massage, compression (wrap and/or pad) and ultrasound, particularly if the scar is hypersensitive. Ulnar nerve symptoms can be treated with desensitisation, TENS (transcutaneous electrical nerve stimulation) and brachial plexus mobilisations directed to the ulnar nerve.

PISIFORM

Pisiform fractures account for 1–3% of carpal fractures.[3] They are usually due to direct trauma to the volar aspect of the wrist or a chip avulsion caused by the pull of flexor carpi ulnaris (FCU) against a strong resistance.

Clinically, there is acute tenderness over the pisiform; there may be pain or tenderness on resisted FCU or abduction of the little finger. The diagnosis can be confirmed on an oblique X-ray.

Pisiform fractures can be treated conservatively by protection in a wrist splint for approximately 3 weeks. If symptoms do not settle the pisiform can be excised surgically.

Therapy

Therapy following pisiform fracture follows the same principles as mentioned previously. Appropriate protection may only be needed for 3–4 weeks; oedema control, mobilisation and graded strengthening exercises are employed as required.

PJM of the pisiform usually involves cephalic caudal gliding. Abductor digiti minimi (ADM) and FCU exercises will also aid in pisiform mobilisation: the pisiform acts as a sesamoid bone between the two tendons.

REFERENCES

1. Herbert TJ: The fractured scaphoid. St Louis: Quality Medical Publishing, 1990.
2. Taleisnik J: The wrist. New York: Churchill Livingstone, 1985:149–68.
3. Botte MJ, Gelberman RH: Fractures of the carpus, excluding the scaphoid. Hand Clin 3:149–61, 1987.
4. Mayfield JK: Mechanism of carpal injuries. Clin Orthop 149:45–54, 1980.
5. Weber ER, Chao EY: Experimental approach to the mechanism of scaphoid waist fracture. J Hand Surg 3:142–53, 1978.
6. Prosser AJ, Brenkel IJ, Irvine GB: Articular fracture of the distal scaphoid. J Hand Surg 19B:87, 1988.
7. Barton N: Diagnosis and management of acute scaphoid fractures. In: Nakamura R, Linscheid RL, Miura T (eds), Wrist disorders. Tokyo: Springer-Verlag, 1992:143–51.
8. Nakamura R, Horii E, Tanaka Y, Imaeda T, Hayakawa N: Three-dimensional CT imaging for wrist disorders. J Hand Surg 14B:53–8, 1989.
9. Imaeda T, Nakamurra R, Miura J, Makino N: Magnetic resonance imaging in scaphoid fractures. J Hand Surg 17B:20–7, 1992.
10. Vossa DE, Ionta MK, Myers BJ: Proprioceptive neuromuscular facilitation – patterns and techniques. 3rd edn. Philadelphia: Harper & Row, 1985.
11. McEntee P: Therapists' management of the stiff hand. In: Hunter JH, Schneider LH, Mackin EJ, Callahan AD (eds), Rehabilitation of the hand. St Louis: Mosby, 1990:328–41.
12. Sapega AA, Quedenfeld TC, Moyer RA, Butler RA: Biophysical factors in range of motion exercise. Phys Sports Med 9(12):57–65, 1981.
13. Taylor NF, Bennell KL: The effectiveness of passive joint mobilisation on return of active extension following Colles' fracture: a clinical trial. NZ J Physiother April:24–8, 1994.
14. Kay S, Haensel N, Stiller K: The effect of passive mobilisation following fracture involving the distal radius: a randomized study. Aust J Physio 46:93–101, 2000.
15. Maitland GD: Peripherial manipulation. London: Butterworths, 1977.
16. Kaltenborn FM: Mobilisation of the extremity joints. Oslo: Olaf Norlis Bokhandel Universitetsgaten, 1980.
17. Mack GR, Bosse MJ, Gelberman RH, Yu E: The natural history of scaphoid non-union. J Bone Joint Surg 66A:504–9, 1984.
18. Fernandez DL: Scaphoid non-union: current approach to management. In: Nakamura R, Linscheid RL, Miura T (eds), Wrist disorders. Tokyo: Springer-Verlag, 1992:153–64.
19. Shinya K, Herbert TJ: The natural history of 462 cases of scaphoid non-union: symptoms, degenerative change and the effect of plaster immobilisation [abstract]. J Hand Surg 19B (suppl 1):26–7, 1994.
20. Cooney WP: Isolated carpal fractures. In: Cooney WP, Linscheid RL, Dobyns JH (eds), The wrist – diagnosis and operative treatment. St Louis: Mosby, 1998:474–87.
21. Bauterbaugh GA, Palmer AK: Other carpal fractures. In: Barton N (ed.), Fractures of the hand and wrist. Edinburgh: Churchill Livingstone, 1988:236–50.
22. O'Brien ET: Acute fractures and dislocations of the carpus. In: Lichtman DM (ed.), The wrist and it's disorders. Philadelphia: WB Saunders, 1988:129–59.

F. MANAGEMENT OF CARPAL INSTABILITIES

Rosemary Prosser

DEFINITION

Stability of the wrist requires a compression force between the radius, ulna and carpus, and ligamentous tension between these structures. Carpal instabilities occur when there is a loss of normal articular contact or rhythm during a particular motion.[1] Garcia-Elias[2] defines carpal instability as carpal dysfunction which occurs when the wrist cannot maintain the normal balance between the articulating bones during the application of physiological loads.

PATHOLOGY

Instability can occur when there is a loss of static or dynamic intercarpal alignment, or axial alignment of the radius and ulnar. The instability can be due to the loss of integrity or laxity of the major retaining ligaments or a change in the bony configuration. Instability problems range from a wrist that gives way to the most severe state of dislocation. Dislocation can result from a progression of an instability caused by ligament injury or from direct high-energy injury which disrupts all the major retaining ligaments, resulting in dislocation.

TERMS AND CLASSIFICATIONS

There are many classifications and terms for wrist instabilities.[3] It is somewhat confusing when one is first reading the literature. They include:

- DISI (dorsal intercalated segment instability).
- VISI (volar intercalated segment instability). The dorsal and volar nomenclature refers to the position of the lunate on lateral X-ray.
- A SLAC (scapholunate advanced collapse) wrist is one that has a DISI and other associated X-ray findings such as post-traumatic osteoarthritis.
- CID (carpal instability dissociative) refers to instability that is within the carpal row, e.g. scapholunate ligament rupture.
- CIND (carpal instability non-dissociative) refers to instability between the carpal rows, e.g. a tear of the capsular ligaments or a midcarpal instability.
- Dynamic instability implies that the X-ray is normal; there may be signs of instability if force is applied, e.g. the clench fist view.
- Static instability implies that standard X-rays show signs of instability.

In 1991 Herbert described a classification (Table 3.10) that was simple, clinical and enabled all other terms of classifications to be encompassed in it.

Table 3.10 Classification of carpal instability (From Herbert[4])

Stage	Description
I	Giving way, normal clinically, normal X-ray
II	Provoked into an unstable position clinically, normal X-ray
III	Subluxed, malalignment on X-ray
IV	Fixed deformity, risk of osteoarthritis
V	Arthritic, arthritic changes on X-ray

Examination and treatment can be difficult if there is not a good understanding of the anatomy and biomechanics of the wrist and of the function required.

Important anatomical and biomechanical aspects to be considered are:

- The proximal carpal row is where the majority of carpal movement takes place, the intercalated segment of the wrist.
- The scaphoid rotates, the lunate glides in an arc and the triquetrum glides and rotates as it moves up and down on the helicoid surface of the hamate.
- By comparison there is very little movement between the bones of the distal row.
- The scaphoid has a biomechanical tendency to flex and the triquetrum a tendency to extend. The lunate lies between the scaphoid and triquetrum; the ligamentous attachments between these bones restrain the scaphoid and triquetrum.
- Loss of this fine balance causes instability at the proximal carpal level.

ASSESSMENT

Subjective history usually falls into two broad categories: injury or 'overuse'. Listen to the patient's complaint and history. Information about the mechanism of injury and any past injuries or problems relating to the wrist is helpful. Ask the patient what they can do to relieve the problem. What the patient does to relieve the pain is often a good indication of what will be helpful in treatment.

Predisposing factors may include:

- hypermobility
- ganglions
- repetitive twisting, radial and ulnar deviation, strong gripping and pushing at the end of range.

EXAMINATION

Examination should follow inspection, active movements, grip measurement, palpation, passive motion and tests that stress the wrist:

- Resting wrist posture, swelling and deformity are noted.
- The usual range of motion and grip strength measures are taken.
- Grip strength measures in supination and pronation may also be useful with ulnar side problems. In pronation the ulnar is in its long position. Grip in pronation which is painful and weak may indicate ulnar impingement or triangular fibrocartilage complex (TFCC) pathology.
- Palpation should include the carpals and radius and ulna and their associated structures.
- Scapholunate joint.
- Lunotriquetral joint.
- Lunocapitate joint.
- Triquetrohamate joint.
- Scaphocapitate joint.
- Scaphotrapezoid and trapezium joint.
- Distal radioulnar joint (DRUJ) – ulnar glide, compression.
- TFCC – stress/shear test (compression and shear).
- Extensor carpi ulnaris (ECU) – stability and strength.
- Flexor carpi radialis (FCR) – strength and tenderness.
- Overpressure at end ranges.
- Scaphoid shift test.
- Ulnar carpal critical test (see Fig. 3.38)/ ballottement tests.
- Piano key test.

X-ray and other imaging

Standard X-rays can be very useful. Both wrists need to be X-rayed so that subtle changes in carpal alignment can be evaluated. The standard views – anteroposterior (AP), radial deviation, ulnar deviation and lateral – are reviewed first. Dynamic instabilities will not often be seen on static views; stress views such as the clenched fist view may be useful. In our experience, even with stress views, a subtle dynamic instability may not be seen. Other authors[1,5–8] have advocated the benefits of bone scans, fluoradiographic views and magnetic resonance imaging (MRI).

MANAGEMENT

Conservative management – stages I and II

Conservative management is only recommended in stages I and II, where the instability is of a dynamic nature. Treatment involves patient education, splinting, activity modification and specific strengthening.

Surgical treatment – stages III, IV and V

Static instabilities in which there is subluxation or dislocation require surgical treatment.

ULNAR CARPAL INSTABILITY AND DRUJ INSTABILITY

The structures of the ulnar carpus include the articular surfaces of the ulna, lunate and triquetrum, plus the triangular fibrocartilage (TFC) and ulnocarpal ligaments (UCL). The TFC is stabilised by the volar radioulnar ligament and the dorsal radioulnar ligament: these are sometimes referred to as the volar and dorsal marginal ligaments or thickenings of the TFC. The TFC has also been referred to in the literature as the articular disc.[9] The UCL include the ulnotriquetral ligament and ulnolunate ligament volarly.[1] The TFC and UCL are generally known as the TFCC.[1,10] The dorsal ligaments, ECU and radiotriquetral ligament are the major dorsal stabilising structures; thus, the major retaining ligaments in the ulnar carpal region are the TFCC and the dorsal capsular structures, i.e. ulnar carpal instability encompasses distal radioulnar joint instability as well as ulnotriquetral instability.

The causes of ulnar carpal instability have been described as:

1. Major retaining ligament failure, in either the TFCC or dorsal capsular structures (Fig. 3.35).
2. Intra-articular surface defect in the radial sigmoid notch or ulnar head (Fig. 3.36).
3. A combination of 1 and 2.
4. Extra-articular defects with or without major retaining ligament defects. Angulation at a fracture site in the radius or ulnar can cause

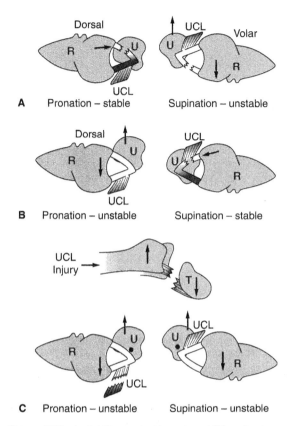

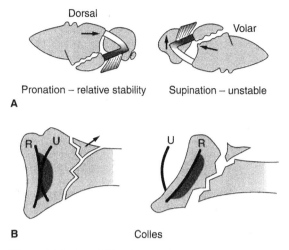

Figure 3.36 Instabilities that are the result of intra-articular fractures or defects of the sigmoid notch and their presentation in the rotation arc (A). The Colles' lesion produces both a dorsal radioulnar ligament defect and a significant ulnar positive variant (B). (Reproduced with permission from Bowers.[1])

Figure 3.35 Instability created by a dorsal (A) and volar (B) radioulnar ligament/TFC tear and from a UCL injury (C). Areas of remaining tension are in half tone. The thick arrow points to areas of remaining compressive load. (Reproduced with permission from Bowers.[1])

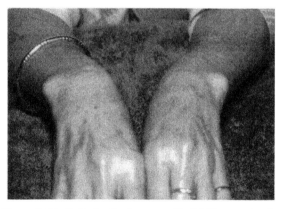

Figure 3.37 Patient with ulnar carpal instability, prominent ulnar head and supinated carpus (step down) can be seen.

intra-articular alignment changes. Length changes in the long bones can also cause alterations in ligamentous tension.

The mechanism of injury in ulnar instabilities caused by ligament failure is usually a twisting injury of the wrist under load, and may involve a fall. Signs and symptoms include ulnar-sided wrist pain, prominent ulna head, supinated carpus (Fig. 3.37), good range of motion, some weakness of grip and a positive relocation or critical test (Fig. 3.38). The relocation test is a combined movement of pronation and anterior to posterior glide of the carpus on the ulnar, which relocates the carpus into normal alignment. It is positive if the relocation of the carpus reduces pain. The TFCC stress/shear test may also be positive.

Where there is a significant ligamentous injury, a tendency toward a VISI position on X-ray may be seen.

Conservative management – stages I and II[11]

Support of the ulnar carpus takes the form of an ulnar carpal soft splint (Fig. 3.39). It is important to stabilise the ulnar head with the circumferential strap. The ulnar strap attempts to relocate the

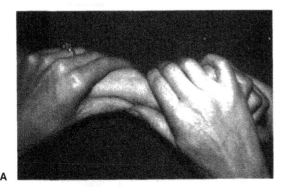

A

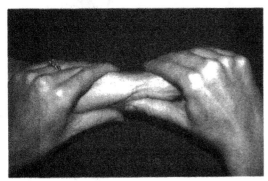

B

Figure 3.38 The ulnar carpal critical test is positive if there is excessive supination and volar translation on stressing the triquetrum on the ulna in this direction (A). Comparison to the contralateral side for each individual is essential. The relocation test is positive if realignment of the triquetrum on the ulna (B) improves pain and discomfort. The triquetrum is moved dorsally with some carpal pronation on the ulna.

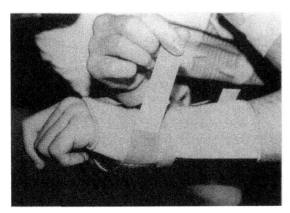

Figure 3.39 Ulnar carpal support. The circumferential strap provides some stability for the head of the distal ulnar, and the ulnar carpal strap, which is anchored volarly, provides a lift to the ulnar carpus. The elasticised piece in the middle of the ulnar strap is necessary to provide the lifting force and also serves to prevent compression of the TFCC.

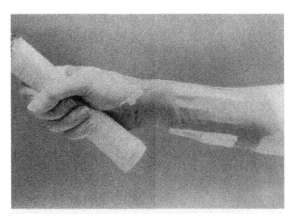

Figure 3.40 Ulnar carpal taping is an alternative for athletes who have high demands and low tolerance to bulk in the palm.

subluxed carpus, at least preventing further subluxation. It should be firm under the ulnar carpus (non-stretch) and more elastic at the lateral aspect of the wrist so that the tension is utilised to elevate the carpus and not compress it. Taping may also be utilised, especially for athletes (Fig. 3.40). Splinting or taping may be required for 4–6 months.

Activity modification usually involves avoiding ulnar deviation, loading the ulnar side of the wrist and rotational activity.

Grip strengthening is used to improve isometric wrist stabilisation while gripping. Grip strengthening is done in neutral, supination and pronation. It should be done within pain-free ranges of rotation. The deep head of the pronator quadratus[12] stabilises the distal radius and ulna; it is active primarily with strong gripping activity. The aim of the grip strengthening programme is to improve stabilisation of the DRUJ and control wrist stability during functional grip patterns. Eccentric ECU strengthening may also be indicated. Eccentric ECU action is particularly important in activities requiring slow rotational motion and lowering a weight.

Surgical treatment – stages III to V

Early attempts of capsulorraphy for the ulno-triquetral joint have been disappointing. In our experience the capsulorraphy attenuates at

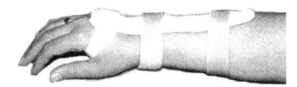

Figure 3.41 Ulnar gutter splint.

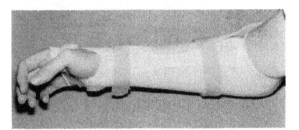

Figure 3.42 The sugar tong splint immobilises the forearm and prevents rotation.

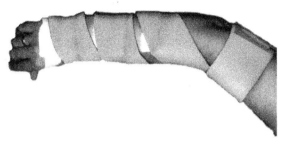

Figure 3.43 A neoprene rotation strap can be used with an ulnar gutter splint to provide a gentle dynamic rotation splint. The ulnar gutter splint ensures the force is applied to the forearm and not to the carpus.

approximately 6 months following the surgery. This has led to the development of ulnar shortening as the surgery of choice.[13] By shortening the ulna, the ulnar ligaments are tightened. Biomechanical studies (Hargreaves, pers. comm.) have shown that the oblique or step cut shortening osteotomy are much stronger than the transverse osteotomy. The osteotomy is fixed with a plate and screws. The ulna does not have as good vascularity as the radius. It has a relatively high delayed union rate due to this. Delayed union may delay postoperative therapy progress. The osteotomy plate is not normally removed until 1 year following the surgery.

Therapy

The step cut or oblique osteotomy has enough strength to allow immobilisation in an ulnar gutter wrist splint, which is two-thirds the length of the forearm (Fig. 3.41). If stability of the osteotomy is a concern, then a sugar tong splint (Fig. 3.42), limiting forearm rotation, may be used. The splint is used for 6 weeks, or until there is satisfactory healing on X-ray, then for 2 more weeks intermittently if necessary. An ulnar carpal support may be used for the following 2–4 weeks, until strength and mobility are restored.

In the first 4–6 weeks, small-range active wrist extension and flexion exercises are only necessary if there is a tendency toward wrist stiffness. The patient is allowed to do small range rotation about the midposition with the splint on. At 6 weeks, active exercise can be increased and assisted active exercises commenced if union on X-ray is sufficient. It is our experience that the ease of regaining full rotation is quite variable. In our series,[13] the type of radioulnar joint did not significantly impact on rotation range of motion. Gentle passive stretching techniques can be commenced at 8 weeks post-surgery. We have found the use of a neoprene rotation strap in conjunction with the ulnar gutter splint an effective gentle stretch splint for rotation (Fig. 3.43). At 12 weeks post-surgery, resistive activity can be commenced.

SCAPHOLUNATE INSTABILITY

The scaphoid plays a vital role in wrist biomechanics. Its ability to rotate and influence lunate and triquetrum motion facilitates flexion and extension and radial and ulnar deviation. Scaphoid rotation also allows midcarpal motion. When the carpus is subjected to a major deforming force in extension, the scaphoid link may fail by fracture or rupture of the proximal ligaments. When the scapholunate ligament fails, the scaphoid rotates into an anteverted or flexed position; with more extensive ligament damage, the lunate and triquetrum sublux dorsally, producing the classic DISI deformity. Blatt[14] reports that the three proximal ligaments (the interosseous scapholunate ligament, dorsal radioscapholunate ligament and volar radioscaphoid ligament) must be ruptured before complete scapholunate dissociation occurs. The scapholunate ligament has three parts: dorsal, volar and membranous. The dorsal part of the ligament is considered to be the most important for scapholunate stability.[15]

Structures requiring particular attention during assessment if scaphoid instability is suspected include the radiocarpal joint, the midcarpal joint, the motion of the scaphoid and lunate, and the scapholunate ligament.

The mechanism of injury varies from a fall on the outstretched hand to repetitive strong gripping, e.g. fitters and turners who are constantly using hand tools which require strong gripping. Patients with scaphoid instability report pain centrally or radially in the wrist: giving way of the wrist when it is loaded may be the functional complaint. They have a tender and sometimes minimally swollen scapholunate interval. Scapholunate interval swelling or ganglion are often seen more easily when the wrist is in the flexed position.

Range of motion is good, but often painful or tender at end range. Grip is often weak compared with the contralateral side. Stress applied to the midcarpal joint may provoke scaphoid subluxation. The scaphoid shift test (known also as the Watson test) is used to assess scapholunate ligament integrity (see Chapter 3A). It is positive if it reproduces the patient's pain in the scapholunate interval region. Proximal pole subluxation over the rim of the radius may be demonstrated with a clunk as the wrist is moved from full ulnar deviation to full radial deviation. The scaphoid shift test can also be used to assess the mobility of the scaphoid.

Comparative X-rays of the contralateral wrist may show subtle changes in scaphoid position and height. No X-ray changes may be apparent. Stress views in the form of the clenched fist view may not always indicate a ligament deficiency. Scaphoid anteversion (flexion) allows the triquetrum and lunate to extend, resulting in a DISI deformity (Fig. 3.44). A DISI present on X-ray indicates a complete dissociation of the scapholunate joint: this requires surgical treatment.

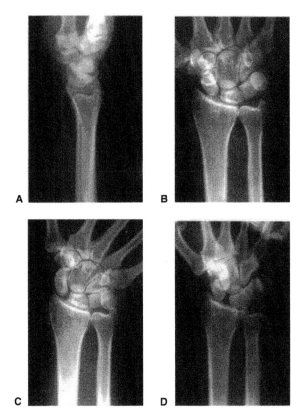

Figure 3.44 X-ray of scapholunate dissociation – instability late stage III. There is a DISI deformity on the lateral X-ray (A), a gap between the scaphoid and lunate is evident on the A–P (B), the scapholunate gap increases with ulnar deviation (C) and with the clenched fist view (D).

Conservative management – stages I and II

The scaphoid is under considerable force biomechanically from the other carpals. Splinting to block the scaphoid anteversion (flexion) is needed, which may be very difficult and often impossible. The splint or taping (Fig. 3.45) may simply serve as a reminder that the patient should limit his range of motion (radial deviation and end range extension). If conservative management is to be the treatment of choice, it should be done in an appropriate manner. An acute ligamentous tear requires 6 weeks to heal. Splinting or ligament protection must be instituted for this period of time. Inadequate protection will result in an attenuated ligament, poor carpal biomechanics and

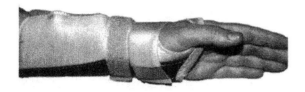

Figure 3.45 A wrist support that can be used for a scapholunate ligament injury.

a chronic instability. Chronic instabilities may only require protection with at-risk activities or activities causing pain, e.g. heavy lifting or gripping activities, or with repetitive deviation motion under load.

Restoration of range of motion is usually not a problem following acute minor tears or strains. Care must be taken with grip strengthening for scapholunate instabilities. The ligament is loaded with strong gripping. The grip 'strengthening' programme needs to be focused on functional needs. It may be done in the splint: endurance and not working into fatigue are more the focus rather than strength.

Activity modification is essential for those patients with stage I or II instabilities to prevent further progression of the instability. This usually involves avoidance of pressure or loading of the wrist in end range extension, e.g. instead of pushing on an extended wrist to get up out of a low chair the patient is advised to push up in a fist position on the proximal phalanges with the wrist in neutral. For some patients it is possible to teach them to activate the FCR isometrically before pushing on the wrist in extension. This attempts to reduce stress on the proximal carpal row, particularly the scaphoid. The patient can also learn to make greater use of the trunk and leg muscles to assist in standing rather than pushing on the wrist. Strong gripping and repetitive deviation, particularly under load, should also be avoided. Modification to hand tools may be necessary; using larger grip sizes, more adhesive grip surfaces and tools with longer lever arms may all help to reduce the force required to use a tool in a particular activity.

Scapholunate ganglions are usually an indication of a minor or minimal strain of the scapholunate ligament.[16] These patients usually need a period of rest and then assessment of their grip

and function. Patient education and activity modification may be all that is needed.

Surgical management – stages III and IV

Static dislocations require surgical treatment. Surgical options include scaphotrapezial trapezoid (STT) fusion,[17] wrist capsulodesis/capsulorraphy,[14,18] or, where possible, scapholunate ligament repair with or without capsulorraphy. Scapholunate ligament repair involves mobilisation of the scaphoid followed by direct repair of the ligament. The scaphoid may require arthrolysis if intra-articular adhesions are present. Following direct repair of the ligament, the repair is protected with K-wire fixation of the scapholunate joint. Further stabilisation of the distal end of the scaphoid can be achieved by insertion of another K-wire. A dorsal capsulorraphy[18] can also be used to protect and reinforce the scaphoid reduction.

Postoperative therapy

A plaster slab is applied in the operating theatre. In the first postoperative week an extension or limited motion splint (Fig. 3.46) is applied. Protective movement is commenced in a small range only if the wrist was stiff preoperatively. If the wrist was hypermobile preoperatively, then it is protected in a cast for 4–6 weeks.

Initially, movement is restricted to 30 degrees extension and flexion to prevent disruption or attenuation of the repair. Oedema control and wound care are instituted as required. Exercises, if appropriate in the first 6 weeks, are restricted to active movements only. After 6 weeks the K-wire(s) is removed and full extension and approximately 50% flexion is encouraged. This is the range aimed for by 3 months post-repair. Forced flexion, that is passive stretching techniques, are contraindicated. Overstretching into flexion will cause elongation of the repaired ligament and a recurrence of some degree of the instability. Gradually, with use, over time (usually 6–12 months), 60–75% of the preoperative flexion range is regained.

Passive stretching for extension and a graded resisted grip programme can be instigated at

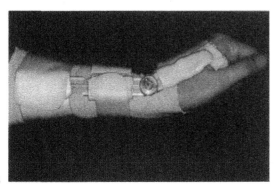 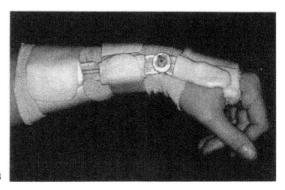

A   **B**

Figure 3.46 Limited motion splint: the hinge has a blocking rivet which is used to limit the motion. Extension (A) and flexion (B) permitted in the splint is shown.

6 weeks. Rarely are passive joint mobilisations (PJMs) necessary; however, if intercarpal stiffness persists, PJMs – excluding the scapholunate joint – may be used judiciously. Capsulorraphy is a general dorsal capsular tightening; PJMs which stress the healing dorsal capsule are not appropriate. Full resistance for the wrist and grip are not applied until 12 weeks postoperative.

Management – stage V

Arthritic scaphoid dislocations can be managed conservatively depending on the pain and activity level of the patient. Joint protection and activity modification is often helpful. An elastic or soft support with a thermoplastic or metal bar can provide symptomatic relief. A variety of surgical treatments are described in the literature. They include the SLAC procedure,[19] complete wrist fusion,[20] wrist denervation,[21] STT fusion and radial styloidectomy.[22] STT fusion is contraindicated in the presence of radioscaphoid arthritis.[23]

LUNOTRIQUETRAL INSTABILITY

Lunotriquetral instability is not seen as much as scapholunate instability. Instability may be due to a perilunar dislocation causing scapholunate ligament disruption, lunocapitate dissociation and then lunotriquetral ligament disruption or there may be an isolated lunotriquetral ligament tear. Bishop and Regan[8] report that the dorsal radiotriquetral ligament, dorsal scaphotriquetral ligament

and the lunotriquetral ligament must be divided for a VISI to be evident on X-ray. The ulnar half of the arcuate ligament may also be disrupted palmarly. The VISI is caused by the disruption in proximal row balance; once the influence of the triquetrum on the lunate is lost, the scaphoid moves into a flexed posture taking the lunate with it.

The proposed mechanism of injury of isolated lunotriquetral ligament ruptures is a fall on the wrist in extension and radial deviation; the impact is taken on the hypothenar eminence, causing a carpal hyperpronation. Weber[24] suggested that a dorsal force on the wrist in flexion or inflammatory arthritis could also result in a lunotriquetral ligament disruption.

Clinically, the patient presents with pain on the ulnar side of the wrist. Pain may be made worse with deviation or rotation of the wrist. The patient may report giving way of the wrist under load. Tenderness over the lunotriquetral joint can be elicited. Motion is usually only limited by pain; grip may be weak. Usually a painful clunk can be reproduced when the wrist moves from radial to ulnar deviation. Ulnar nerve paraesthesia may be present if there is a reasonable amount of inflammatory synovitis or oedema. Provocative tests include compression of the joint, ballottement and the shear test.[8] Ballottement and the shear test involve stabilisation of the lunate and stressing the lunotriquetral ligament by forcing the triquetrum in the volar or dorsal direction.

In stages III–V, a VISI on X-ray can be seen. In stages I and II, there may be minimal or no X-ray

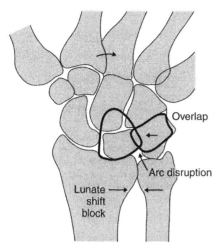

Figure 3.47 A lunotriquetral instability. Disruption of the smooth convexity of the proximal carpal row is more pronounced in ulnar deviation. There is also overlapping of the lunate and triquetrum. (Reproduced with permission from Alexander and Lichtman.[27])

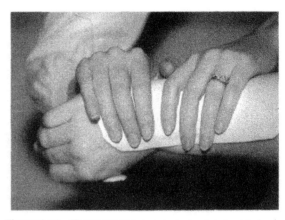

Figure 3.48 Thermoplastic ulnar carpal splint moulded in carpal pronation. Care must be taken to pad over the triquetrum so that the ulnar nerve is not compressed.

findings. Subtle X-ray changes include disruption of the smooth arc between the lunate and triquetrum (Gilula's line); occasionally an overlapping of the lunate and triquetrum or an ulnar lunate shift is seen (Fig. 3.47).

Conservative management

Acute minor tears can be managed in a cast or splint, which immobilises the wrist with some carpal pronation[8] (Fig. 3.48). Care must be taken when moulding into pronation not to compress the ulnar nerve volarly. If TFCC involvement is also diagnosed, the cast may include the elbow, or a sugar tong splint with carpal pronation moulding may be used. The wrist is immobilised for 6 weeks,[24] then intermittently for a further 2 weeks. Minor tears, stage I and early stage II instabilities may only require an ulnar carpal pronation support. A thermoplastic splint providing carpal pronation[25] may also be beneficial. Care must be taken in the application of the thermoplastic splint not to cause pressure areas over the ulnar head dorsally and pisiform volarly. Skirven recommends the use of silicone pads in these two areas.

At 6 weeks post-injury, active range of motion exercises are commenced. If there are concerns regarding stability, exercises may be delayed until 8 or even 10 weeks post-injury. Two to 3 weeks following the instigation of active exercises a graded resisted grip strengthening programme is commenced. Wrist strengthening exercises are not added until grip strength is at least 50–60% of the contralateral side. As with ulnar carpal instabilities, eccentric ECU exercises may need to be targeted. Strengthening and activity modification are similar to those for ulnar carpal instability, which have been discussed previously.

Surgical management

Acute complete tears should be repaired primarily. Surgical treatment for chronic lunotriquetral ligament deficits ranges from ligamentous repair or reconstruction to ulnar shortening, lunotriquetral or midcarpal arthrodesis, proximal row carpectomy (PRC) or total fusion.[8,26]

Lunotriquetral ligament repair requires suturing of the ligament, which is usually avulsed from the triquetrum. Dorsal augmentation by capsulodesis/capsulorrhaphy to tighten the dorsal radiotriquetral ligament has also been recommended.[8] Reconstruction with half of ECU is another option described.

Postoperative therapy

Cast immobilisation for 8 weeks is recommended by Bishop and Regan,[8] followed by a period of splintage of approximately 4 weeks. The wrist is mobilised once the cast is removed – firstly with active motion, then selective passive motion. PJMs to the lunotriquetral joint are contraindicated, as this may compromise the integrity of the repair. After dorsal capsulorraphy, passive flexion beyond 50% of flexion range would also be contraindicated for similar reasons. Graded resistive exercises are not commenced until 10–12 weeks: they should be carefully monitored; resistive exercise should be within the capability of the musculature so that the joint is not stressed unduly.

MIDCARPAL INSTABILITY

This is not as common as other types of instability. Midcarpal instability refers to an instability between the capitate and lunate.[26,27] The Mayo clinic group refer to this instability between the proximal and distal rows as CIND.[7] Lichtman and his associates[26–28] report it is more often intrinsic (volar), but may also be extrinsic (dorsal). Volar midcarpal instability is said[26–28] to be due to ligamentous laxity in the ulnar arm of the arcuate ligament complex (capitotriquetral ligament) and dorsal radiolunate-triquetral ligament, resulting in inadequate support of the proximal row and midcarpal joint. This causes a dynamic flexion deformity in the proximal row as the distal row is allowed to sublux volarly on the proximal row (Fig. 3.49). The clunk with ulnar deviation in pronation is thought to be due to an abrupt reduction of the distal row on the proximal row. Other authors[7] report that insufficiency in the radio-scaphocapitate ligament, dorsal wrist capsule and palmar capitotriquetral ligament may also be major causes of midcarpal instability.

Midcarpal instability may be primarily due to ligamentous laxity; there may be no history of trauma. Midcarpal instability may also develop following malunion of a distal radial fracture in which there is considerable dorsal angulation,

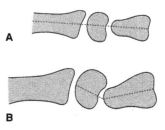

Figure 3.49 Normal lateral alignment of the radius and carpals (A). Altered lateral alignment in intrinsic (volar) midcarpal instability (B). The lunate is in a volar position, which may be seen on X-ray in the later stages of the instability. (Reproduced with permission from Brown and Lichtman.[29])

thereby causing a relative lengthening of the radiocarpal ligaments.

Clinically, there is a volar sag (carpal supination) on the ulnar side of the wrist, the ulnar head is prominent, and there is a clunk with ulnar deviation in pronation. A depression at the midcarpal joint may be seen when the wrist is in full flexion. There may be localised midcarpal synovitis and tenderness over the triquetrohamate joint. The clunk with ulnar deviation may become painful due to the synovitis, midcarpal articular wear or the gradual attenuation of the ligaments increasing the instability.[28] The midcarpal shift test involves the application of volar pressure to the dorsal aspect of the distal capitate. The wrist is then simultaneously axially loaded and ulnar deviated. The midcarpal shift test is positive if it produces a painful clunk. Wrist circumduction may also be used as a provocative test.

There may be a VISI on X-ray in severe cases of palmar midcarpal instability. Dorsal midcarpal instability, resulting in a DISI, has also been described, although this type of midcarpal instability is considered rare. Due to the dynamic nature of this instability, video fluoroscopy is considered the most helpful radiological examination.[28]

Management

Management is difficult. A simple wrist splint to rest in or wear when the wrist is stressed may be helpful. A dorsal thermoplastic wrist extension splint with moulding at the capitate dorsally and with a thermoplastic strap moulded palmarly over the lunate may help reduce a subluxation. Gaenslen and Lichtman[27] report that triquetral support reduces the clunk occurring with ulnar deviation. Skirven[25] has described a thermoplastic splint to provide triquetral support. The ulnar carpal support splint[11] may be adequate in stage I cases.

Activity modification and avoidance of ulnar deviation particularly may help reduce pain

levels. The need for grip strengthening should be evaluated carefully. Any exercise that causes pain should be avoided.

Surgical management

A wide variety of surgical options have been suggested in the literature,[28] including ligament tightening, partial fusion, ulnar shortening and correction of radial malunion.

REFERENCES

1. Bowers WH: Instability of the distal radioulnar joint. Problems of the distal radioulnar joint. Hand Clin 2:311–27, 1991.
2. Garcia-Elias M: The treatment of wrist instability. J Bone Joint Surg (Br) 79-B:684–90, 1997.
3. Dobyns JH, Cooney WP: Classification of carpal instability. In: Cooney WP, Linscheid RL, Dobyns JH (eds), The wrist – diagnosis and operative treatment. St Louis: Mosby, 1998: 490–500.
4. Herbert TJ: Carpal instability. Proceedings of the Sydney Hospital Hand Symposium. Update on the wrist joint. Sydney 1991:2–6.
5. Taleisnik J: The wrist. New York: Churchill Livingstone, 1985:149–68.
6. Nakamura R, Horii E, Tanaka Y, Imaeda T, Hayakawa N: Three dimensional CT imaging for wrist disorders. J Hand Surg 14B:53–8, 1989.
7. Wright TW, Dobyns JH: Carpal instability nondissociative. In: Cooney WP, Linscheid RL, Dobyns JH (eds), The wrist – diagnosis and operative treatment. St Louis: Mosby, 1998:550–68.
8. Bishop A, Regan D: Lunotriquetral strains. In: Cooney WP, Linscheid RL, Dobyns JH (eds), The wrist – diagnosis and operative treatment. St Louis: Mosby, 1998:527–49.
9. Kuhlmann J: Lunotriquetral dissociation. In: Buchler U (ed.), Wrist instability. London: Martin Dunitz, 1996:147–54.
10. Palmer AK, Werner FW: Biomechanics of the distal radioulnar joint. Clin Orthopaed Rel Res 187:26–35, 1984.
11. Prosser R: Conservative management of ulnar carpal instability. Austr J Physiother 41:41–6, 1995.
12. Stuart PR: Pronator quadratus revisited. J Hand Surg (Br), 21B(6):714–22, 1996.
13. Koppel M, Hargreaves IC, Herbert T: Ulnar shortening osteotomy for ulnar carpal instability and ulnar carpal impaction. J Hand Surg (Br) 22B(4):451–6, 1997.
14. Blatt G: Scapholunate instability. In: Lichtman DM (ed.), The wrist and its disorders. Philadelphia: WB Saunders, 1988:251–73.
15. Mayfield J: Pathogenesis of wrist ligament instability. In: Lichtman DM (ed.), The wrist and its disorders. Philadelphia: WB Saunders, 1988:53–73.

16. Watson HK, Rogers WD, Ashmead IV D: Reevaluation of the cause of the wrist ganglion. J Hand Surg 14A:812–17, 1989.
17. Kleinman W: Management of chronic rotary subluxation of the scaphoid by scaphoid-trapezio-trapezoid arthrodesis. Hand Clin 3:113–33, 1987.
18. Herbert TJ, Hargreaves IH, Clarke AM: A new surgical technique for treating rotary instability of the scaphoid. J Hand Surg 1:75–7, 1996.
19. Watson HK, Brenner LH: Degenerative disorders of the carpus. In: Lichtman DM (ed.), The wrist and its disorders. Philadelphia: WB Saunders, 1988:286–328.
20. Feldon P: Wrist fusions: intercarpal and radiocarpal. In: Lichtman DM (ed.), The wrist and its disorders. Philadelphia: WB Saunders, 1988:446–64.
21. Buck-Gramcko D: Denervation of the wrist joint. J Hand Surg 2:54, 1977.
22. Rogers WD, Watson HK: Radial styloid impingement after triscaphe arthrodesis. J Hand Surg 14A:297–301, 1989.
23. Herbert TJ: The fractured scaphoid. St Louis: Quality Medical Publishing, 1990.
24. Weber ER: Wrist mechanics and its association with ligamentous instability. In: Lichtman DM (ed.). The wrist and its disorders. Philadelphia: WB Saunders, 1988:41–52.
25. Skirven T: Splinting for midcarpal instability. In: Proceedings from Surgery and Rehabilitation of the Hand – '99 with emphasis on the wrist. Philadelphia: WB Saunders, 1999:124–5.
26. Alexander C, Lichtman D: Triquetrolunate and midcarpal instability. In: Lichtman DM (ed.), The wrist and its disorders. Philadelphia: WB Saunders, 1988:274–85.
27. Gaenslen E, Lichtman D: Midcarpal instability: description, classification and treatment. In: Buchler U (ed.), Wrist instability. London: Martin Dunitz, 1996:163–9.
28. Brown DE, Lichtman DM: Midcarpal instability. In: Management of wrist problems. Hand Clin 3(1):136, 1987.

G. SALVAGE PROCEDURES FOR THE WRIST

Bryce M Meads and Rosemary Prosser

Late presentation of a wrist injury or a poor result from attempts at reconstructive surgery can lead to early degenerative changes within the wrist.

A predictable pattern of arthritis develops within the wrist for scapholunate instability and has been termed scapholunate advanced collapse or a SLAC wrist. Similar patterns of degenerative change also develop in non-unions of scaphoid fractures.

Changes initially develop at the tip of the radial styloid. Subsequently, degeneration progresses to the radioscaphoid joint and then the capitolunate joint. Involvement of the radiolunate joint was far less common and occurred typically after the previously mentioned stages, as determined by Watson and Ballet.[1]

Pain and degenerative changes occur with fragmentation of an avascular lunate in Kienböck's disease.

A range of salvage procedures have been developed to deal with such patterns of progression of degenerative changes. They act only to preserve some function in a compromised wrist rather than restore function to normal.

INDICATIONS

The failure to stop the pattern of degenerative change at the wrist, whatever the initial pathology, leads to the three primary indications for salvage procedures:

- pain
- stiffness
- loss of function.

MANAGEMENT OPTIONS

The pathology may vary significantly and will need to be taken into account when deciding upon procedures. Involvement of the lunate fossa in Kienböck's disease may occur earlier than the pattern seen in a SLAC wrist.

DENERVATION OF THE WRIST

Denervation can range from excising the articular branch of the posterior interosseous nerve to a full denervation procedure. A full denervation is selected occasionally for troublesome chronic wrist pain that is not responsive to simple anti-inflammatories or analgesics or to restorative wrist procedures. This procedure attempts to manage the symptoms rather than treat the primary disorder.

For these reasons, a detailed clinical and radiological work-up must be performed prior to recommending this procedure. A diagnostic block of local anaesthetic can be performed on the posterior interosseous nerve (PIN). If function improves with the block then a partial denervation procedure is thought to be helpful.

Dellon[2] found greater than 90% of patients had subjective and objective improvement in hand function after a PIN resection. Fukomoto et al.[3] describe a more extensive denervation procedure with 95% good results. The deep articular branches of the ulnar nerve are unable to be divided and thus ensure that a Charcot joint does not occur. However, progression of the original pathology may occur, causing further deformity and pain, as with a SLAC wrist.[2]

MOTION PRESERVING

An arthroscopy is often required before deciding the most appropriate treatment method, either motion preserving or not. The arthroscopy can better determine the extent of radiocarpal and midcarpal joint cartilaginous damage, as this is not well visualised with conventional imaging. Thus, salvage procedures can be selected more appropriately.

Radial styloidectomy

The presentation of arthritis at the radial styloid or of the radioscaphoid joint is an indication to consider a radial styloidectomy. It is also an adjunct to other wrist salvage procedures for non-union of the scaphoid and SLAC wrists, particularly with STT (scaphotrapezial trapezoid) joint fusions to improve radial deviation.

This procedure does not compromise the pre-operative range of wrist movement. However, instability may occur, causing increased radial ulnar and palmar displacement of the carpus if more than 4 mm of the styloid is removed.[4] This is due to the disruption of the origin of the radial collateral and the palmar radioscaphocapitate ligament. A short oblique osteotomy removing 2 mm of bone was found to preserve the radioscaphocapitate ligament in 91% of cases.[5]

Proximal row carpectomy

This procedure involves the resection of the scaphoid, lunate and triquetral bones. It is essential to ensure that the articular surfaces of the corresponding lunate fossa and the proximal pole of the capitate are undamaged, as this may compromise the outcome. The indications are Kienböck's disease, scapholunate dissociation and scaphoid non-union with periscaphoid arthritis, as well as chronic perilunate dislocations or a dislocated lunate.

The radius of curvature of the capitate is only 60% of the lunate fossa in the lateral view, although adaptive changes are thought to occur. The axis of movement at the new articulation of the wrist becomes a combination of translation and rotation, which acts to dissipate the load on the wrist and may account for some of the success of the procedure.[6]

A proximal row carpectomy will preserve or slightly improve the range of motion of the wrist from preoperative values, achieving an arc of 115 degrees or 64% of the opposite normal wrist: grip strength achieved values of 70–94% of the opposite side.[6,7] A return to work was achieved in 91% of patients within 5 months, including 9 out of 13 heavy labourers.[8]

Longer-term results have noted only a small incidence of progressive radiocarpal arthritis in 13% of patients at 6 years.

Therapy

The primary aim of therapy is to obtain a stable pain-free wrist with some motion. The configuration of the joint surface of the capitate in the

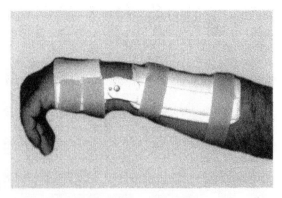

A

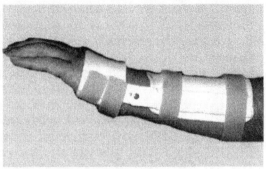

B

Figure 3.50 A limited motion wrist splint can be fabricated with a set range of motion. Wrist hinges are expensive. Cost-effective hinges can be fabricated from thermoplastic material. It is relatively easy to limit the motion of the hinge to the range desired by cutting a 'V' at the appropriate angle and using a rivet as a stopper. Range of extension (A) and flexion (B) permitted by the splint is shown.

lunate fossa of the radius is not very stable immediately after surgery, particularly with deviation. The surgeon applies a plaster volar slab in slight wrist extension (20 degrees) on completion of the procedure. This is removed for removal of sutures at 10–14 days postoperatively. At this time, the surgeon will assess the stability of the wrist. The patient is then fitted with a limited motion splint that allows 20–30 degrees of extension and flexion of the wrist but no deviation (Fig. 3.50). A compressive sleeve is fitted beneath the splint to control oedema around the wrist. If the wrist is very unstable at the time of suture removal, a cast is applied for 2 or more weeks before limited motion is allowed.

Full range of motion is encouraged for all proximal joints. Forearm rotation is practised within the confines of the splint. Full range of motion of the digits is also practised. The patient is encouraged to use the hand for light activities with the splint on.

Specific instructions are given for wrist exercises. Wrist extension is done with finger flexion and wrist flexion with finger extension within the splint. This is essential if independent wrist extension is to be achieved. The splint is only removed in therapy for massage and limited extension and flexion exercises. If the wrist range is less than 20 degrees in either direction at 4 weeks, active exercises with a 10-second hold at the end of range and active assisted exercises are commenced.

Six weeks following proximal row carpectomy, if the wrist is stable, the limited motion splint is exchanged for an elasticised support with or without a metal or thermoplastic bar, depending on wrist stability and strength and the demands of the patient. Wrist exercises are increased to maximise extension and flexion. A light graded resisted grip strengthening programme is commenced. Resisted wrist exercises are not commenced until grip strength is at least 50% of the unoperated hand. Grip strengthening provides indirect isometric exercise for the wrist in a functional position.

Strong resisted activity is not allowed before 12 weeks post-surgery at the earliest. It may be delayed longer if grip is still weak. It is advisable to use a wrist support for heavy lifting and activities for at least 6 months following surgery. At 8–10 weeks post-surgery, deviation range is assessed. If deviation range is lagging behind wrist extension/flexion range, gentle deviation exercises can be commenced. Care should be taken and the exercises done cautiously to avoid the wrist becoming unstable. A stable stiffer wrist is much more useful than an unstable one (Fig. 3.51).

Partial wrist fusion

There are a number of partial wrist fusions performed for varying pathologies. The most common indications are, according to Minami et al.:[9]

1. painful radiocarpal arthritis or intercarpal arthritis
2. established carpal collapse

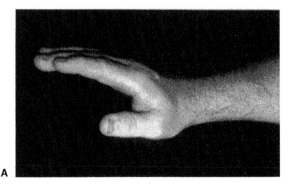

A

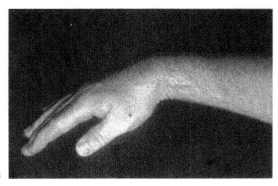

B

Figure 3.51 A good range of motion is achieved by this patient following proximal row carpectomy: extension (A) and flexion (B). The range achieved enabled him to carry out all functional daily activities.

3. Kienböck's disease
4. failed ligamentous repair or reconstructions
5. bone tumours with limited carpal involvement.

STT fusion

Fusion of the scaphoid, trapezium and trapezoid joint prevents rotation of the scaphoid, with the fusion mass crossing the radial side of the midcarpal joint.

Indications are rotatory subluxation of the scaphoid, stage IIIA or IIIB Kienböck's disease.[9]

A radial styloidectomy is usually performed at the same time, due to impingement with radial deviation that is more common with those patients with a fixed DISI deformity.[10] The scaphoid must be fused at 45 degrees of flexion to the longitudinal axis of the radius. If it is not reduced, it will have an incongruent articulation at the radioscaphoid joint, which may lead to early degenerative changes at this joint:[11] 80% of patients reported no pain or aching after activity at 5 years of follow-up.[10]

Postoperative range of motion showed wrist flexion, extension and ulnar deviation around 75% of the opposite side, leaving the patient with a useful arc of 100 degrees of wrist motion. Mean grip strength was greater than 80% of the unoperated side;[12] however, a troublesome non-union rate of 4–10% has been found, with immobilisation averaging 6–7 weeks.

Eighty-six per cent of patients returned to their original employment at 14.8 weeks.[12] Rogers et al.[10] has reported that there was no evidence of further degenerative changes at 5 years.

Radioscapholunate fusion

Fusion of the scaphoid and lunate to the distal radius is used in SLAC wrists or in degenerative changes due to distal radial fractures where the midcarpal joint has been well preserved (Fig. 3.52).

Movement of the wrist occurs at the midcarpal joint while eliminating radiocarpal motion. Final range of motion reported was 18 degrees flexion, 32 degrees extension and 25 degrees ulna deviation. Radial deviation was limited to an average of 3 degrees.

Long-term follow-up demonstrated a failure rate of 33% with subsequent total fusion of the wrist, with good results reported in 46%.[13] A recent modification of excising the distal pole of the scaphoid can improve the range of radial deviation.

Progressive degenerative change of the midcarpal joint occurred in 27% of those patients with a radioscapholunate fusion at an average follow-up of 8 years. The contact area within a normally articulating midcarpal joint is less than 40%. The load distribution across the midcarpal joint is relatively evenly distributed, with the STT 23%, scaphocapitate 28%, lunatocapitate 29% and triquetrohamate in 20%.[14] It is unknown how fusing the scaphoid and lunate to the radius affects this, but it presumably increases the biomechanical stress across the joint, leading to degenerative changes.

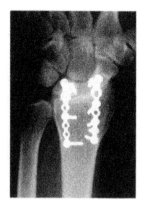

Figure 3.52 Radioscapholunate arthrodesis. (X-ray with permission from Dr D Wheen.)

Four-corner fusion

Four-corner fusions involve fusing the capitate, lunate, hamate and triquetral bones with excision of the scaphoid. Resection of part or all of the scaphoid can be performed at the same time. The midcarpal joint is usually degenerative but the radiolunate joint should be preserved for this procedure to be indicated. Thus it is used for the middle phase of a SLAC wrist and scaphoid non-union.[12] Combined with excision of the scaphoid, it can be referred to as a SLAC wrist procedure.

It is important to correct carpal malalignment at the time of this procedure. In a DISI wrist, it is critical to reduce the dorsal rotation of the lunate on the capitate prior to fusion: 91% of patients reported improvement in pain with a similar satisfaction level.[12] The wrist motion preserved is approximately 50% of the opposite side and the grip strength 80%.[7,12]

There is a 3–17% non-union rate reported with this procedure.[7,12] The length of immobilisation is around 6–7 weeks. Fusion with a Herbert screw may improve the quality of fixation and reduce the non-union rate. Eighty per cent of patients returned to their original employment at an average of 14 weeks.

Therapy following partial wrist arthrodesis

A partial wrist arthrodesis requires a period of at least 6 weeks immobilisation. The cast is removed when bony union is confirmed on X-ray. During the time in the cast full range of motion of all unimmobilised joints is maintained. Excessive oedema is controlled with cold packs, elevation and gentle compressive wraps. Forearm rotation exercises to maintain some motion at the distal radioulnar joint (DRUJ) are done within the cast.

Once the cast is removed, range of motion exercises for the wrist are commenced. The exercise programme may include assisted active, active, gentle passive and active stretching techniques such as hold relax. The patient is instructed in independent wrist extension with finger flexion and vice versa. A light graded grip strengthening programme is also commenced at this time. The functional position of wrist extension during grip activity is reinforced in the grip strengthening programme. Forearm rotation exercises are continued and, once a good pattern of wrist extension/flexion is developed, further assessment of wrist deviation range is made and addressed.

Passive joint mobilisations (PJMs) are contraindicated for the arthrodesed joints. Great care and caution should be exercised in adjacent joints so that the arthrodesed joints are not stressed. Given recent results in the literature[15] indicating that PJMs made no difference in the final outcome following distal radial fracture, and the risk of stressing the new arthrodesis PJMs for the carpals may be considered as a contraindication.

Arthroplasty

Various prostheses have been tried over time. Initially, a silicone rubber prosthesis was used. Results[16] at an average of 6 years showed only 48% with good results. Breakage of the implant in 52% and silicone synovitis in 30% have been troublesome complications, resulting in a 30% revision rate.

A biaxial unconstrained metallic arthroplasty with a polyethylene spacer on the radial component has been in use since 1983 (Fig. 3.53). Components can be cemented or uncemented with no significant difference in survival. Seventy-five per cent of patients reported no pain in the wrist at 5 years, with a 92% subjective improvement in symptoms.[17]

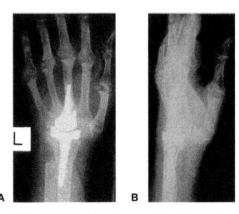

Figure 3.53 Biaxial wrist replacement. A: Anteroposterior view. B: Lateral view. (X-ray with permission from Professor WB Conolly.)

Short-term 5-year follow-up results had an 83% survivorship. Failure was mostly due to loosening and then subsidence of greater than 3 mm of the distal component. Correct alignment of the prosthesis and soft tissue balancing is important so as to avoid early failure. At an average of 6 years of follow-up, 81% of patients reported no pain. A flexion–extension arc of 65 degrees and radioulnar deviation of 30 degrees was found in patients at 5 years. Grip strength improved from 4.1 to 5.9 kg.[17]

Rheumatoid patients also had satisfactory pain relief, stability and a functional range of motion in 50% of cases with a cemented distal component and an uncemented radial component,[18] although these authors performed this unilaterally on the dominant hand. However, failure of this prosthesis results in a more difficult salvage, with revision to either a custom-designed prosthesis[17] or a wrist arthrodesis. The loss of bone stock from loosening and removal of the implant compromise both procedures.

Therapy

Generally, arthroplasty is reserved for patients with rheumatoid arthritis. Wrist implants generally do not stand up to heavy use. The biaxial implants have gained favour recently due to the problems of implant fracture and synovitis of the silicone spacer implants. The biaxial implants are not as stable as the silicone spacers immediately postoperatively; consequently, they generally require a longer period of immobilisation.

The period of immobilisation following biaxial implant arthroplasty will vary depending on the fit of the prosthesis at the time of surgery and the stability of the wrist at 2 weeks post-surgery when sutures are removed. Beckenbaugh[19] recommends a long arm cast for 2 weeks.

If the prosthesis was a tight fit and the range of wrist motion at 2 weeks is 20 degrees or less (10 degrees or less for both flexion and extension), then a thermoplastic wrist splint is used for a further 6 weeks.[19] The patient is commenced on isometric and active wrist exercises. Deviation and passive or assisted active exercises are contraindicated due to the risk of destabilising the arthroplasty. Light gripping activities with the splint on are encouraged. The aim of the therapy programme is to provide the patient with a stable pain-free wrist with some motion. The therapist should aim for a range no greater than 30 degrees of both flexion and extension. Ranges greater than this may produce instability. Use of the hand for gripping activities without the splint is not recommended until there is adequate wrist strength to maintain wrist stability in extension with grip. From 8 weeks a light graded resisted grip programme may be commenced. The patient should be able to use the hand for daily activities without the splint by 3 months.

If the prosthesis is a tight fit and the range at 2 weeks is greater than 20 degrees, a cast is applied for a further 2 weeks. At 4 weeks, the thermoplastic splint is applied and the postoperative exercise programme commenced.[19]

If the wrist can be partially distracted after insertion of the prosthesis (medium fit), the long arm cast is recommended for 6 weeks followed by 6 weeks of splinting.[19] Exercises are also started at 6 weeks.

If the fit of the prosthesis is loose, the long arm cast is recommended for 8 weeks. At 8 weeks, if motion is 20 degrees or less, a splint is applied for a further 4 weeks and exercises commenced. If motion is greater than 20 degrees, the splint is applied but no exercises are commenced for a further 4 weeks.[19] Light graded resisted grip may

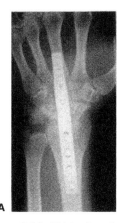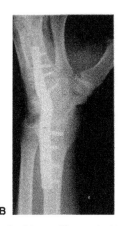

Figure 3.54 Total wrist arthrodesis. (X-ray with permission from Dr D Wheen.)

not be commenced for a further 6–8 weeks in this case.

The exercise programme should be tailored for the individual. The stability of the wrist joint should be continually assessed during therapy and the exercise and splinting requirements adjusted accordingly.

MOTION SACRIFICING

Arthrodesis

Total wrist fusion is a reliable procedure and the end point for many painful wrists (Fig. 3.54). It eliminates movement at the wrist, except for pronation and supination at the distal radioulnar joint.

The use of a premoulded wrist fusion plate in 10 degrees of extension has simplified the procedure. The radiocarpal, midcarpal and often the second and third carpometacarpal joints are decorticated. The plate is placed dorsally from the third metacarpal to the distal radius with bone graft packed between the decorticated surfaces of the carpal bones. Avascular bone must be replaced with a block of iliac crest bone to restore carpal height and reduce the chance of ulnar impingement, as in Kienböck's disease.

Improvement in wrist pain relief is usually around 90% with no or mild pain.[20] Many patients after experiencing the pain relief that a fusion provided indicated they would have liked the procedure performed earlier.[21]

Grip strength is maximal in 30 degrees of wrist extension whilst the fusion is usually in 10 degrees extension. Grip strength of fusion improved by 50%, returning to approximately 65–75% of the strength of the uninjured side.[20,21]

Pronation and supination of the forearm is usually not affected, with an average of 72 degrees of each seen preoperatively and postoperatively.[22]

Patients are usually restricted in a removable wrist splint or plaster for 6 weeks. After union has occurred, usually at 3 months, the patient is cleared for unrestricted lifting. Extensor tendonitis may occur, with irritation over the dorsum of the plate, which may then require removal. Flexion of the MCP joints can also be restricted by the same mechanism and patients are encouraged to mobilise the fingers with flexion–extension exercises at the MCP joints.

Carpal tunnel syndrome can complicate the early postoperative period and has been reported in 25% of cases.[21]

Therapy

Following arthrodesis, the patient is immobilised in a cast or splint for a period of 6 weeks, depending on the demands of the patient. During this time, range of motion exercises for the digits and proximal joints are instigated. Particular attention to MP flexion and full combined finger flexion is necessary in order to avoid MP joint stiffness and long extensor tightness and adhesion. Forearm rotation exercises are done within the confines of the splint or cast to maintain DRUJ motion.

At 6 weeks, the splint or cast is exchanged for a wrist support, which is used for approximately 4 weeks. Low-demand patients may not require

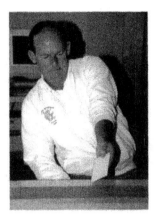

Figure 3.55 One of the difficulties following fusion reported by the patient was difficulty with supination with the hand positioned across the body due to the lack of ulnar deviation at the wrist; the shoulder works to compensate for the wrist. Forearm rotation with the arm by the side was unimpeded.

any further support. A compression sleeve such as tubigrip gives some circulative and psychological support immediately following cast removal.

A resistive grip and functional strengthening programme is commenced at 6 weeks. Functionally, the most difficult activities following total wrist fusion[21] (Fig. 3.55) are poor inner range grip strength and motion of the digits and an inability to do rotational activities with the hand positioned across the body.

Specific tips

Poor inner range motion and strength is best addressed with early range of motion and stretching exercises for both the joints and long extensors. Passive stretching techniques in the form of splinting and manual stretching techniques can be started at 2–3 weeks post-surgery if active motion is tardy.

REFERENCES

1. Watson HK, Ballet FL: The SLAC wrist: scapholunate advanced collapse pattern of degenerative arthritis. J Hand Surg 9A:358–65, 1984.
2. Dellon AL: Partial dorsal wrist denervation: Resection of the distal posterior interosseous nerve. J Hand Surg 10A:527–33, 1985.
3. Fukumoto K, Kojima T, Kinoshita Y, Koda M: An anatomic study of the innervation of the wrist joint and Wilhelm's technique for denervation. J Hand Surg 18A:484–9, 1993.
4. Nakamura T, Cooney WP, Lui W et al: Radial styloidectomy: a biomechanical study on stability of the wrist joint. J Hand Surg 26A:85–93, 2001.
5. Siegel DB, Gelberman RH: Radial styloidectomy: an anatomical study with special reference to radiocarpal intracapsular ligamentous morphology. J Hand Surg 16A:40–4, 1991.

6. Imbriglia JE, Broudy AS, Hagberg WC, McKernan D: Proximal row carpectomy: clinical evaluation. J Hand Surg 15A:426–30, 1990.
7. Wyrick JD, Stern PJ, Kiefhaber TR: Motion-preserving procedures in the treatment of scapholunate advanced collapse wrist: proximal row carpectomy versus four-corner arthrodesis. J Hand Surg 20A:965–70, 1995.
8. Tomaino MM, Delsignore J, Burton RI: Long term results following proximal row carpectomy. J Hand Surg 19A:694–703, 1994.
9. Minami A, Kimura T, Suzuki K: Long-term results of Kienböck's disease treated by triscaphe arthrodesis and excisional arthroplasty with a coiled palmaris longus tendon. J Hand Surg 19A: 219–28, 1994.
10. Rogers WD, Watson HK: Radial styloid impingement after triscaphe arthrodesis. J Hand Surg 14A: 297–301, 1989.
11. Minami A, Kato H, Iwasaki N, Minami M: Limited wrist fusions: comparison of results 22 and 89 months after surgery. J Hand Surg 24A:133–7, 1999.
12. Watson HK, Weizenweig J, Guidera PM, Zeppieri J, Ashmead D: One thousand intercarpal arthrodeses. J Hand Surg 24B:307–15, 1999.
13. Nagy L, Buchler U: Long term results of radioscapholunate fusion following fractures of the distal radius. J Hand Surg 22B:705–10, 1997.
14. Viegas SF, Patterson RM, Todd PD, McCarty P: Load mechanics of the midcarpal joint. J Hand Surg 18A:14–18, 1993.
15. Kay S, Haensel N, Stiller K: The effect of passive mobilisation following fractures involving the distal radius: a randomized study. Aust J Phys 46:93–101, 2000.
16. Jolly SL, Ferlic DC, Clayton ML, Dennis DA, Stringer DA: Swanson silicone arthroplasty of the wrist in rheumatoid arthritis: a long term follow-up. J Hand Surg 17A:142–9, 1992.
17. Cobb TK, Beckenbaugh RD: Biaxial total-wrist arthroplasty. J Hand Surg 21A:1011–21, 1996.
18. Courtman NH, Sochart DH, Trail IA, Stanley JK: Biaxial wrist replacement. Initial results in a rheumatoid patient. J Hand Surg 24B:32–4, 1999.
19. Beckenbaugh RD: Total wrist arthroplasty. In: Gelberman RH (ed.), The wrist. New York: Raven Press, 1994:253–78.
20. O'Bierne J, Boyer MI, Axelrod TS: Wrist arthrodesis using a dynamic compression plate. J Bone Joint Surg 77B:700–4, 1995.
21. Field J, Herbert TJ, Prosser R: Total wrist fusion. A functional assessment. J Hand Surg 21B:429–33, 1996.
22. Weiss APC, Hastings H: Wrist arthrodesis for traumatic conditions: a study of plate and local bone graft application. J Hand Surg 20A:50–6, 1995.

H.   THE STIFF WRIST

Rosemary Prosser

Wrist stiffness is usually a consequence of:

1. Severe extensive trauma of the wrist or forearm, such as that caused by a high-velocity injury such as severely comminuted fractures of the distal radius or perilunate trans-scaphoid dislocation.
2. Following prolonged immobilisation, particularly in flexion: e.g. after a Colles' fracture, which is usually cast in flexion, and ulnar deviation.

Undoubtedly the best treatment for wrist stiffness is prevention. Protected wrist motion should be commenced as soon as fractures, dislocations or soft tissue injuries are stable.

Stiffness in the wrist can be classified as:

1. intrinsic, involving joint ligaments and capsule
2. extrinsic, involving the tendons, fascial connective tissue, subcutaneous tissue and skin.

ASSESSMENT

A thorough evaluation of the joints and soft tissues of the wrist and distal radioulnar joint (DRUJ) is essential to determine which structures are limiting function and require treatment.

Every case requires evaluation of:

1. skin and subcutaneous tissue for scarring and oedema
2. strength, length and mobility of the extensor tendons to digits and wrist
3. strength, length and mobility of flexor tendons to digits and wrist
4. wrist range of motion (ROM), including DRUJ
5. wrist accessory glides, including DRUJ (Fig. 3.56)
6. strength of both grip and wrist motors
7. hand function and wrist stability

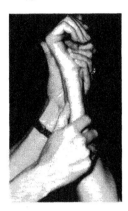

Figure 3.56 Wrist accessory glides for the distal radioulnar joint; volar glide of ulna on radius.

8. other structures affecting hand function, e.g. intrinsic muscles.

Thick woody oedema will invariably lead to stiffness of all the soft tissues. Oedema at the wrist level involves all carpal joints. A scaphoid fracture treated by cast immobilisation will produce stiffness in other joints in the carpus, e.g. C-L (capitolunate) and L-T (lunotriquetral) joints. Judicious use of physiological accessory glide testing will locate these joints.

When assessing forearm rotation, attention and differentiation between the DRUJ and carpal rotation must be made.

Wrist stability should be assessed in conjunction with grip strength. Good grip strength cannot be gained with poor wrist extension. Inadequate wrist extension will have a great impact on activities requiring cylindrical or power grip.

Extensor tendons are particularly susceptible to becoming bound down in adhesions due to their location and anatomy. They are broad flat tendons lying immediately adjacent to the joints and bones of the wrist and hand with thin overlying soft tissue.

TREATMENT TECHNIQUES

The following treatment techniques are considered below:

- massage
- heat
- stretching – active and passive
- exercise
- passive joint mobilisations (PJMs)
- continuous passive motion (CPM)
- splinting
- functional activity.

Massage

Massage is probably the oldest form of therapy: its benefit in terms of softening scar tissue and mobilising the skin and subcutaneous tissues are well recognised. Massage should be firm but not overvigorous in order to avoid inflammation, and it should be performed about four times a day.

Heat

All the usual indications and precautions should be followed. Heat applied before stretching techniques will enhance the stretch.

Stretching

Passive stretching[1] should be applied slowly and gently over time, approximately 10 seconds. The stretch should be pain-free to avoid causing microtrauma to the tight structures. Inflamed tissues will not tolerate as much stretch as those that are not inflamed. Both flexors and extensors may require stretching.

Active stretching techniques involve an active maximal contraction of the tight muscle in its lengthened position. This is followed by a maximal relaxation; the result should be a gain in musculotendinous length. Proprioceptive neuromuscular facilitation (PNF) techniques such as hold relax or contract relax are effective active stretch techniques. It is less likely that there will be overstretching or microtrauma of the tight tissues with these techniques.

Exercise

The role of exercise cannot be underestimated. Only active and resisted exercises can provide the tendon with appropriate proximal tendon glide. They also provide the muscle with the stimulus to strengthen and lengthen its passive component and strengthen its active component. Exercises should include both wrist and digit ROM and strengthening.

When working on wrist extension, the finger extensors should be relaxed. Finger extension with wrist extension is not functional. If the EDC (extensor digitorum communis) are activated to aid wrist extension as soon as functional gripping is required, wrist extension power and thus wrist stability is lost. Resisted grip exercises ensuring that wrist extension is maintained is vital in increasing wrist stability with grip. It provides isometric wrist strengthening and coordinated action of both flexors and extensors of the digits.

Wrist stability with grip is more important than achieving full wrist ROM. Several authors[2,3] have shown that a range of 30/30 extension/flexion is adequate for activities of daily living. Conversely, a larger range of rotation, i.e. 50/50 supination/pronation, is necessary for everyday activities.

Rotation exercises for the DRUJ should not be neglected. They should be commenced as soon as possible. It is more difficult to compensate for loss of supination than pronation. Loss of forearm rotation will place extra stress on the shoulder rotators, which attempt to compensate for the lack of forearm rotation.

PJMs

PJMs provide a stretch force to the ligaments and capsule of the carpus. Strict adherence to the convex/concave rule is essential so that joint surfaces are not damaged. Much has been reported regarding PJMs in the treatment of joint stiffness. Several studies[4,5] have shown that they do not provide significant long-term benefits. They are very effective in determining joint mobility and thus aid in treatment planning and implementation.[6] Clinically, there are some patients who appear to benefit from joint mobilisations.

There are two well-known PJM techniques – Maitland[7] and Kaltenborn.[8] Both provide gliding techniques for the intercarpal joints. Careful assessment of the specific joints that are stiff and consideration of the biomechanics and kinematics of wrist motion is essential before embarking on any PJM technique. It is important to include the physiological rotation that occurs at the scaphoid and triquetrum when carrying out intercarpal joint mobilisation. The most beneficial glides are:

1. For extension:
   - scaphoid and lunate on radius (SL-R) posteroanteriors (P-As)
   - capitate on lunate (C-L) P-As
   - scaphoid rotation into the upright position (Fig. 3.57)

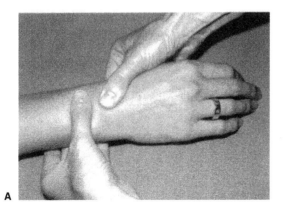
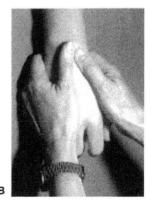

Figure 3.57 Passive joint glides for the scaphoid. A: Rotation of the scaphoid on the radius. B: Rotation of the scaphoid on the lunate.

- triquetral proximal rotation and glide on the hamate.
2. For flexion:
   - SL-R anteroposteriors (A-Ps)
   - C-L, A-Ps
   - scaphoid rotation into flexion
   - triquetral distal rotation and glide on the hamate.
3. For deviation:
   - scapholunotriquetral (SLT) lateral gliding on radius
   - C-L lateral gliding
   - scaphoid rotation
   - triquetral rotation and glide on hamate.
4. For supination:
   - radius on ulna (R-U) A-Ps
5. For pronation:
   - R-U, P-As.

CPM

CPM is only beneficial in the early stages. If the oedematous tissue is fibrotic and organised, the patient will gain more benefit from stretch/mobilisation splinting. CPM is helpful when the end range position is not tolerated for long periods, or if the joint is inflamed and will only tolerate a very gentle stretch. Salter and his associates[9–11] report that it improves articular cartilage healing and clearance of haemarthrosis from synovial joints. It is an important part of treatment following arthrolysis.[12] It can be adjusted to maintain maximum passive range of movement (Fig. 3.58) while the patient and therapist concentrate on active range of movement and regaining glide and strength.

Salter[10] reports that CPM should be applied for 24 hours/day for up to 3 weeks. Clinically, experience[13] has shown that for CPM to be effective it has to be applied in a pain-free manner for at least 8 hours/day for a minimum period of 2 weeks. At this time, the patient's wrist is reassessed, and other options such as mobilisation splinting are considered.

Splinting

Splinting for the stiff wrist usually aims to either stabilise the wrist in a functional position to maximise use of the hand or to improve wrist range of motion. It can be either static or dynamic.

Static splinting

Static splinting to mobilise the wrist usually involves a serial splinting regime. The thermoplastic material used needs to be remoulded, often many times. Thermoplastics which stretch out, become thin and lose their strength are not the material of choice. Thermoplastics with memory are more suited to the task. For a very stiff wrist it is often difficult biomechanically to apply appropriately directed torque to the joint with a dorsal or volar splint. In this circumstance, it is more appropriate to apply a serial cylindrical splint or plaster cast.

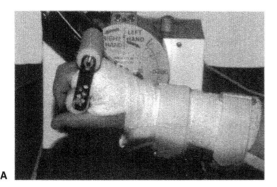
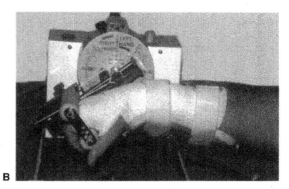

A   B

Figure 3.58   The CPM machine can be adjusted to provide maximal comfortable wrist extension (A) and flexion (B).

Generally, serial static splinting is used primarily to regain extension: rarely is it necessary to regain flexion. However, following capsulorraphy for scapholunate ligament repair, where flexion may be limited initially to protect the surgery, stiffness into flexion may become a problem and require serial static splinting. Diligent monitoring of median nerve function is required as the wrist is being held in a position which may cause median nerve compression.

Dynamic splinting

Dynamic splinting can be utilised to regain extension, flexion, supination or pronation. The design and construction, fit and wearing time of these splints should follow basic splinting principles[13] and be dictated by the individual patient's needs. A dynamic wrist splint needs to apply an appropriate torque to the joint given the size and complex structure of the wrist joint and the weight of the hand.

Flexion/extension splints

A dynamic flexion/extension splint may be the splint of choice if the patient has a wrist with a stiff end-feel and very limited motion, i.e. 25 degrees or less of flexion (Fig. 3.59) or extension (Fig. 3.60). Clinically, it appears that a dynamic splint can provide a better torque to the joint, due to the leverage and better moment arm provided by the outrigger at these angles. Migration of flexion/extension splints can be addressed by ensuring the forearm base is a good fit and extends circumferentially around the arm to the midline. Padded flares that hug the styloid processes may also be helpful.

Supination/pronation splints

There are many different dynamic splint designs[14–17] that address rotational stiffness. Low-profile outrigger splints use various materials to provide the power force, including rubber bands (Colello–Abraham or cradle design)[14,15] (Fig. 3.61), rubber tubing (Roylan)[14,15] (Fig. 3.62), static progressive devices such as the MERiT,[15]

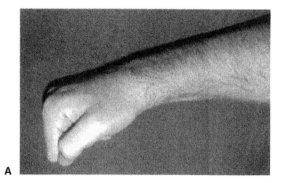

A

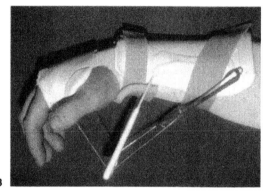

B

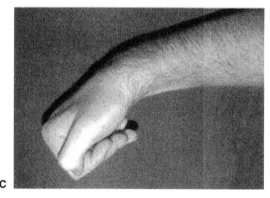

C

Figure 3.59 Dynamic wrist splintage to gain flexion. A: Wrist flexion before the splint is fabricated and fitted. B: Dynamic wrist flexion splint. C: Wrist flexion after splinting.

elastic Velcro[16] and neoprene. The splint utilised will depend on the patient's status with regard to joint stiffness and irritability, tolerance and availability of time and components for the therapist.

The two designs the author prefers are the low-profile rotation splint using elastic Velcro and the

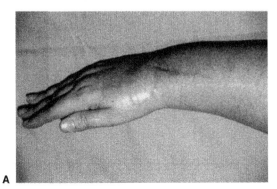

A

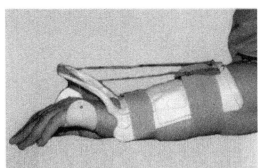

B

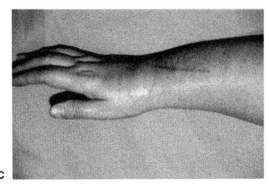

C

Figure 3.60 Poor wrist extension following distal radius fracture. The X-ray showed no bony impingement. Even after arthrolysis, extension range did not achieve neutral (A). A dynamic wrist extension splint was custom-made and fitted. The patient had a tapering forearm, which predisposed the splint to migrate distally. Extra attention to moulding and padding condyles were used to help alleviate this (B). Extension range after splinting (C). The wrist achieved 30 degrees extension after 6 months of splinting.

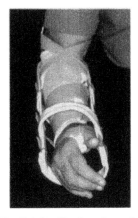

Figure 3.61 The Colello–Abraham type of rotation splint was used here to improve pronation.

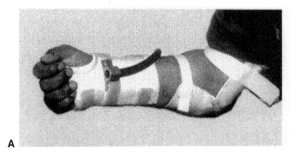

A

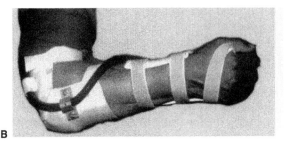

B

Figure 3.62 The Roylan rotation splint used for supination is shown. A: Volar view. B: Dorsal view.

neoprene rotational strap splint (Fig. 3.63). The elastic Velcro splint is low profile, easy to construct in a reasonable time and inexpensive. It is easy to adjust and not as cumbersome as the other low-profile splints. The Roylan splint components are very expensive and the cradle splint, while being very effective, takes a long time to construct.

The neoprene rotational strap splint can be used with and without an elbow piece. Without the elbow piece it is very comfortable. Clinically, I have found it is the only rotational splint that

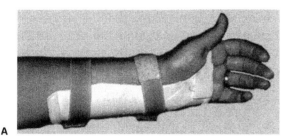

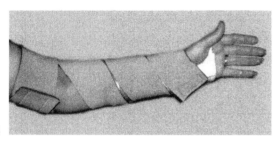

Figure 3.63 A neoprene rotation strap splint used for supination following DRUJ surgery is shown here. An ulnar gutter splint or wrist extension splint is fitted to control carpal rotation and disperse pressure evenly along the splint. The neoprene strap is fixed with Velcro to the forearm splint; tension is applied in the direction of the motion required. The neoprene strap is fixed on to itself at the elbow. The tension of the rotational force will change with changes in elbow flexion: more flexion reduces the tension. To maintain the tension constant, an elbow splint can be fitted in 90 degrees of flexion. Night-splinting is particularly difficult for patients with DRUJ problems, as most splints are quite cumbersome. Clinically, it appears that tolerance and wearing time for the neoprene rotation strap splint (with the forearm splint only) is better than the other splints mentioned.

is well tolerated at night. When worn at night it should be applied with the elbow in at least 90 degrees of flexion, as the elbow is flexed more the force applied by the neoprene strap is decreased. It is an extremely good splint, as it provides a very gentle force for those patients who have an irritable joint or for patients post-surgery where there is concern regarding the force that the tissues can tolerate.

Functional activity

It is important that the patient has some period of the day without a splint in which he is using the hand. Use of the hand and wrist provides functional strengthening for both grip and wrist muscles in terms of strength and stability. It focuses on completion or achievement of an activity rather than exercising a particular muscle. Goal-oriented strengthening may be seen by the patient as more rewarding and interesting than a formal structured exercise programme. Both types of strengthening are necessary. Formal exercises can provide specific strengthening for weak muscles; functional activity programmes help to translate this to everyday activity and use of the hand.

Wrist stability is just as important as wrist strength, for without wrist stability in slight extension, grip strength cannot be maximised. The patient is encouraged to maintain slight wrist extension while using the hand. If the wrist is too weak a light semi-flexible wrist splint may be necessary until the wrist stability improves. Emphasis on wrist isometric exercises is indicated in this circumstance.

ARTHROLYSIS

Indications

Arthrolysis of the wrist is not a very common surgical procedure for two reasons: first, most functional activities only require 35–40% of extension and flexion and 60–65% of rotation; secondly, a stiff pain-free wrist is more functional than a mobile painful one.

Arthrolysis is indicated for those patients who have a stiff pain-free wrist and can demonstrate a need for greater range of motion. Past injury and treatment and X-rays need to be reviewed regarding possible early arthritis or any potential instability that may result from arthrolysis.

The most common wrist arthrolysis seen by the author is that following scaphoid fracture treated by cast immobilisation or following open reduction with internal fixation (ORIF) of complicated wrist fractures.

Contraindications and precautions

Arthrolysis is contraindicated if there is arthritis, already good functional use and a potential for wrist instability. It is worth repeating that a pain-free stiff wrist is much more functional than a painful one with better range. A painful or unstable wrist does not provide enough stability for many functional grip tasks, especially those which require strong gripping or lifting.

Postoperative therapy

Day 1

Oedema control, digit ROM exercises, gentle assisted active and active wrist extension/flexion and supination/pronation.

Days 1–3

CPM in a relatively pain-free range for extension/flexion and rotation is applied. CPM is utilised for at least 8 hours/day or longer if tolerated. A wrist splint in approximately 30 degrees of extension is used as a resting splint when the CPM is not being used. Manual passive motion is also commenced. The amount of passive motion necessary will depend on the status of the joint and if CPM is being used. Light functional tasks are encouraged.

Day 14

Removal of sutures, wound and skin care in the form of lux baths, massage, silicone and compression. Passive and resisted exercises are commenced (earlier if stability and pain allow). CPM may be continued for another 4 weeks or serial static or dynamic splinting initiated.

Week 3

All forms of exercise are continued. Serial static or dynamic splinting may prove more helpful in gaining range than CPM at this time. Increased use of the hand is permitted within pain limits.

Weeks 4–12

A strengthening programme is commenced. Return to work is allowed for office workers at 2 weeks; for manual workers this may not be possible because of job demands until 6–12 weeks, depending on the patient's progress, stability and strength. Night-splinting may be necessary for several months postoperatively.

REFERENCES

1. Kottke F, Pauley D, Ptak R: The rationale for prolonged stretching for correction of shortening of connective tissue. Ach Phys Med Rehab 47:345–52, 1966.
2. Palmer A, Werner FW, Murphy D, Glisson R: Functional wrist motion: a biomechanical study. J Hand Surg (Am) 10:39–46, 1985.
3. Ryu J, Cooney WP, Askew LJ, An K-N, Chao EYS: Functional ranges of motion and the wrist joint. J Hand Surg (Am) 15:409–19, 1991.
4. Taylor NF, Bennell KL: The effectiveness of passive joint mobilisation on the return of active wrist extension following Colles' fracture: a clinical trial. NZ J Physiother April:24–8, 1994.
5. Kay S, Haensel N, Stiller K: The effect of passive mobilisation following fractures involving the distal radius: a randomized study. Aust J Phys 46:93–101, 2000.
6. Reiss B: Therapists management of distal radial fractures. In: Hunter JM, Mackin EJ, Callahan AD (eds),

Rehabilitation of the hand: surgery and therapy, 4th edn. St Louis: Mosby, 1995:337–51.
7. Maitland GD: Peripheral manipulation, 2nd edn. London: Butterworths, 1977:152–87.
8. Kaltenborn F: Mobilization of the extremity joints. Universitetsgaten, Oslo: Olaf Norlis Bokhander, 1980:26–8.
9. Salter RB: The physiologic basis of continuous passive motion for articular cartilage healing and regeneration. Hand Clin 10:211–19, 1994.
10. Salter RB: History of rest and motion and the scientific basis for early continuous passive motion. Hand Clin 12:1–11, 1996.
11. O'Driscoll SW, Kumar A, Salter RB: The effect of continuous passive motion on the clearance of a haemarthrosis from a synovial joint. Clin Orthopaed Rel Res 176:305–11, 1983.
12. Breen TF, Gelbermann RH, Ackerman GN: Elbow flexion contractures: treatment by anterior release and continuous passive motion. J Hand Surg 13B:286–7, 1988.

13. Prosser R: The effectiveness of CPM for treatment of isolated joint stiffness following hand injury. Proceedings IFSHT 1st International Congress, Tel Aviv, Israel, 1987:31–4.
14. Fess E, Phillips C: Hand splinting, 2nd edn. St. Louis: Mosby, 1987.
15. Laseter GE, Carter PR: Management of distal radius fractures. J Hand Ther 9:114–28, 1996.
16. Schultz-Johnson K: Splinting the wrist: mobilisation and protection. J Hand Ther 9:165–77, 1996.
17. Wilton JC: Hand splinting. London: WB Saunders, 1997:67–113.

4

Hand and wrist arthritis

A.   OSTEOARTHRITIS

W Bruce Conolly and Anne Wajon

TYPES OF ARTHRITIS AFFECTING THE HAND, WRIST AND UPPER LIMB

Osteoarthritis

Degenerative osteoarthritis may be primary, or secondary to injury, infection, abnormal anatomical configuration or metabolic disease. Arthritis is primary when no predisposing factor can be identified. Classic radiological findings include joint space narrowing, subchondral sclerosis, subchondral sclerotic cysts, marginal osteophytes and ossicles and alteration of articular surfaces.[1]

Clinical presentation of osteoarthritis includes pain, localised joint swelling, limitation of motion and deformity.[2] The joints in the hand most frequently involved are the distal interphalangeal (DIP) joints of the fingers and the trapeziometacarpal joint of the thumb. The proximal interphalangeal (PIP) and metacarpophalangeal (MP) joints of the digits may also be involved.

Rheumatoid arthritis – including Still's disease (juvenile RA)

Rheumatoid arthritis is a chronic, systemic, inflammatory condition with chronic proliferative synovitis. It presents initially in the joints, secondarily involving the articular cartilage, underlying bone and associated muscle tendon units. There may be extra-articular manifestations such as rheumatoid nodules. Rheumatoid arthritis, although mostly affecting the wrist and MP joints, can also involve the PIP and DIP joints.

Crystalline arthropathy

Gout

In gout, uric acid crystals are deposited in the soft tissues of the joints. The great toe is most commonly affected but gout can involve any of the joints of the hand. Classically, there are well-demarcated punched out para-articular areas. Gout may present as an acute infection.

Pseudogout

In pseudogout there are deposits of calcium pyrophosphate crystals. Clinical presentation is often as an acute arthritis with carpal tunnel syndrome. Chondrocalcinosis and tenosynovitis may be present.

Seronegative spondyloarthropathies

- Reiter's syndrome
- Psoriatic arthropathy
- Enteropathic arthritis
- Post-infective arthritis
- Ankylosing spondylitis.

Miscellaneous

- Haemophilic arthropathy
- Neuropathic arthropathy
- Hypertrophic osteoarthropathy.

CONSERVATIVE MANAGEMENT OF OSTEOARTHRITIS IN THE HAND

Conservative management of osteoarthritis includes consultation with a rheumatologist and referral to hand therapy. Therapy includes splintage, exercise, pain control and joint protection.[3]

Joint protection includes patient education, with analysis of activity and modification of use.

Initial assessment may include an activities of daily living (ADL) checklist, with description of the mechanism of injury (where applicable) and description of any aggravating activities. A general history should also be obtained, including the use of medication and involvement of other joints. X-rays assist in staging the arthritis,[4] and will be helpful when discussing the disease process with the patient (Fig. 4.1).

Objective assessment should include palpation, measurement of active and passive range of motion and specific provocative tests such as the grind test at the trapeziometacarpal joint. Grip and pinch strength provides an indication of overall hand function, and is tested using commercially available devices. Isolated muscles are tested when appropriate. Details of these assessment and measurement techniques are covered in detail elsewhere in the book.

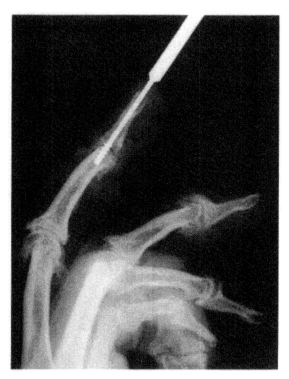

Figure 4.1 X-ray of osteoarthritis at the DIP joint. The index finger DIP joint is being treated by arthrodesis. (Reproduced with permission from Conolly.[5])

Splintage

Splinting should address pain control, joint protection and prevention of deformity, while improving independence with ADL. The splint should meet the needs of the individual patient's requirements, with the materials used in its fabrication dependent on the severity of the disease. Generally, the larger and more rigid the splint, the more support and restriction of motion it will provide.

Thermoplastic splinting material provides rigid support, and may be used to immobilise an inflamed joint. Alternative materials include neoprene and lycra, which do not restrict motion yet still provide a firm, comforting support. Some patients like a variety of splints, which they wear as required. For example, a patient with PIP joint osteoarthritis may wear a dorsal finger splint at night and a neoprene or lycra stall during the day (Figs 4.2 and 4.3).

Patient education

It is essential to outline to the patient the nature of the disease process. Frequently, they are able to identify an activity that increases their pain. They should understand that it is the joint's posture and movement during performance of that activity that aggravates pain.

Advice in joint protection may simply involve avoiding the specific aggravating activity, such as turning taps. If this is not desirable or possible, then the patient may need to wear a protective splint (such as a neoprene stall), use assistive devices (such as tap turners), or change their technique (use two hands). Such adaptations will allow the patient to control their symptoms, possibly delaying the need for surgery.

Pain-relieving techniques are also important, as the chronicity of the condition makes it unrealistic for the patient to attend hand therapy every time they have an aggravation of symptoms. Self-treatment techniques include frequent warm soaks, massage, anti-inflammatory creams, self-traction of the affected joint and the use of splints and supports as appropriate.

Therapy

As well as providing appropriate splintage and advice regarding joint protection, therapy is able to offer symptomatic relief. Techniques include the use of ice or heat, massage, ultrasound and/or traction when the pain is acute and the joint inflamed. Once the acute episode has settled, it may be appropriate to gradually increase functional activities and begin strengthening exercises. Strengthening programmes should be carefully monitored, as repetitive resisted exercises may aggravate symptoms and worsen deformity if not appropriate to the patient's condition. Similarly, stretches of tight structures must be taught with consideration to preventing further joint deformity.

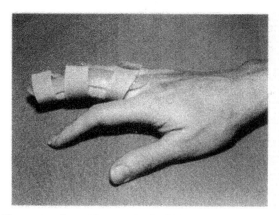

Figure 4.2 Dorsal finger splint for PIP joint.

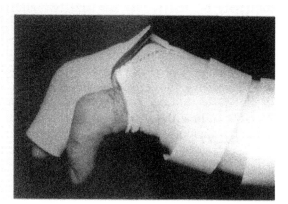

Figure 4.3 Neoprene stall for PIP joint.

Drug treatment

Corticosteroid injections may be both diagnostic and therapeutic, and relief of pain may last from 2 to 6 months, or longer. Nonsteroidal anti-inflammatory drugs (NSAIDs) may provide some symptomatic relief of pain and inflammation, with other specific medicines being appropriate for the affected arthritis, e.g. anti-immune drugs for RA, methotrexate, gold, etc.

SURGICAL PROCEDURES FOR OSTEOARTHRITIS IN THE HAND

Indications for surgery

The main indication for surgery is persistent pain that has not responded to conservative measures.[5] Specifically, guidelines for surgical treatment may include pain that interferes with daily function, or is refractory to splinting, muscle strengthening or NSAIDs.[6] Similarly, gross instability or deformity may interfere with function to such an extent that surgery is the desired course of treatment. Surgical options include resection arthroplasty or arthrodesis. In the case of an unstable and painful index finger DIP joint, prohibiting normal hand writing, an arthrodesis would both relieve pain and restore stability to permit normal function.

DIP JOINT

Surgical techniques

Arthrodesis

Arthrodesis by the K-wire cerclage technique (Fig. 4.4A) or Herbert screw (Fig. 4.4B) should result in a painless and stable distal digit. The DIP joints are fused in varying degrees of flexion based on individual functional requirements. From a cosmetic perspective, the digit looks better with the DIP joint in near full extension, whereas it may be preferable to fuse the IP joint of the thumb in enough flexion to allow it to oppose the digits.

Postoperative care

For the first 10–14 days the operated digit may be supported in a volar plaster slab. Following

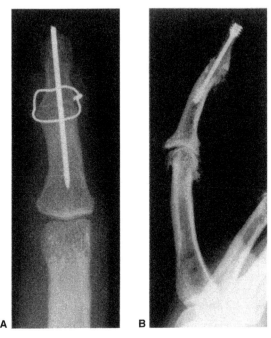

Figure 4.4 A: DIP arthrodesis with K-wire cerclage technique. B: Herbert screw arthrodesis of the DIP joint.

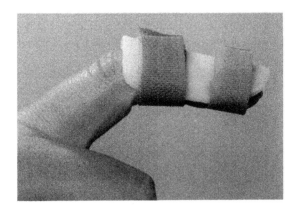

Figure 4.5 Dorsal DIP joint resting splint.

removal of sutures, a light dorsal thermoplastic splint (Fig. 4.5) should be used for protection until there is clinical and radiological union, which may take 8–10 weeks. Light activities may be performed during this time. Coban or a lycra finger stall may be used to control swelling, and early motion at the PIP joint should be encouraged to minimise the risk of PIP joint stiffness.

Complications

Non-union can occur in up to 5–10% of procedures, depending on the surgical technique and the nature of the bone.

Other surgical techniques

Osteophytes and bone spurs can be removed to improve the appearance of the digit but some motion may be lost.

PIP JOINT

Surgical techniques

Arthrodesis

Arthrodesis is preferred for the index and middle fingers and is usually performed by the tension band technique (Fig. 4.6A). This provides inherent stability, enabling early motion of the MP and DIP joints and requiring little postoperative care. Arthrodesis will eliminate pain, but the stiffened joint and resultant finger deformity might prove a significant disability if the patient needs to work with the hand in confined spaces. In these instances, a silicone implant arthroplasty or amputation through the PIP joint would be preferable.

Silicone interposition arthroplasty

Flexible silicone interposition arthroplasty (Fig. 4.6B) of the ulnar two or three digits can give satisfactory pain relief and a 40–60 degree range of motion. Patients must be informed prior to surgery of the need for intensive and prolonged postoperative therapy to maximise the return of function.

Postoperative therapy following interposition arthroplasty

The primary goal of therapy is to protect the involved joint from any lateral stress while encouraging motion into flexion and extension. It is

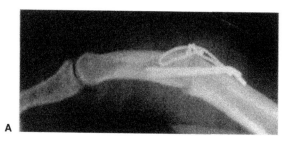

A

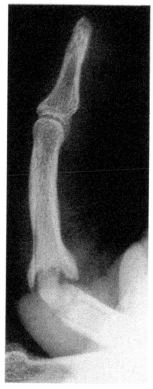

B

Figure 4.6 A: Arthrodesis of the PIP joint using the tension band technique. B: Implant arthroplasty at the PIP joint.

essential to protect the healing collateral ligaments and joint capsule during the early postoperative phase, and advise the patient to avoid any strong lateral pinch against the operated digit during functional activities.

It is common to have difficulties in regaining passive flexion, and so the digit is splinted in a dynamic PIP flexion splint at approximately day 3 (Fig. 4.7). Depending on extension range, it may also be necessary to incorporate a dorsal component to the splint to allow the digit to be held

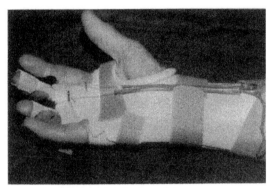

Figure 4.7 Dynamic PIP flexion splint.

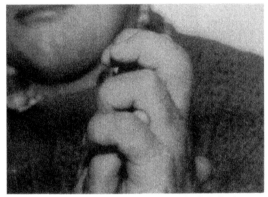

Figure 4.8 Isolated blocking exercises for PIP flexion.

passively in extension at night. Isolated blocking exercises for PIP extension are begun early to maximise active PIP extension and tendon glide. Similarly, blocked flexion exercises assist in regaining flexion for gripping (Fig. 4.8).

Oedema control with the use of coban begins in the first postoperative week, and wound care with lux baths, lanoline massage and compression pads begin once the sutures are removed.

The splint is worn at all times for the first 4 weeks. After this time, it may be removed for light functional activities, with the use of buddy straps, while in therapy. There must be no lateral stress to the PIP joint. The splint is worn between exercise sessions until 6 weeks.

At 6 weeks, the splint is removed for light functional activities at home, with splintage maintained at night as needed. Light resisted gripping

activities are gradually progressed in resistance and frequency over the subsequent 6 weeks, maintaining the buddy straps until the patient is able to return to full function, usually by 3 months following surgery.

MP JOINTS

Indications for surgery

Painful arthritis of the MP joint of the thumb is far more common than for the MP joints of the fingers. In the thumb, arthrodesis is the treatment of choice, as implant arthroplasty does not provide enough stability to resist lateral forces in pinch grip. The MP joints of the fingers are better managed by silicone interposition arthroplasty.

Surgical techniques

Arthrodesis

The tension band technique gives a painless stable joint and allows early motion of uninvolved joints.

Silicone interposition arthroplasty

This procedure reliably eliminates pain and permits both passive and active motion. Postoperative care is the same as for the rheumatoid MP joint replacements.

Long-term problems may include stiffness into flexion, or fatigue and fracture of the prosthesis. It may be necessary to incorporate night flexion splintage to counteract the loss of flexion range.

TRAPEZIOMETACARPAL (CMC) JOINT

Conservative management of trapeziometacarpal osteoarthritis

Most patients with trapeziometacarpal (TM) or pan-trapezial arthritis present initially to their therapist reporting pain at the base of the thumb which is made worse by activities requiring fine manipulation with pinch. Turning keys, opening jars and handcrafts are frequently the aggravating activities in the predominantly postmenopausal female population. Patients frequently report an acute localised pain at the base of the thumb during a specific activity, and subsequently complain of a persistent ache which may last for some hours.

Objective assessment should include the following measures:

1. Active range of motion:
   - IP extension/flexion
   - MP hyperextension/flexion
   - TM palmar/radial abduction, opposition to the base of the little finger, retropulsion and the ability to place the hand flat
2. Passive tests
   - grind test and compression during pinch
3. Strength
   - grip, pinch (tip, three-point chuck, lateral), APL grade (abductor pollicis longus strength – grade 0–5).

Examination will reveal localised thickening at the TM joint. In the advanced stages of disease, the thumb will posture in a typical collapse deformity with dorsoradial subluxation of the base of the first metacarpal, adduction contracture, MP hyperextension and IP flexion.

This joint is subject to compression forces much greater than those at the IP and MP joints. Cooney and Chao[7] report that compression forces of up to 120 kg at the TM joint may occur in strong grasp. Attenuation of the ligaments and capsule in degenerative arthritis, in combination with large rotational movements associated with pinch, may result in instability, weakness and pain. A vicious cycle of the disease process and mechanical factors may ultimately lead to deformity.

It is necessary to differentiate TM arthritis pain from De Quervain's disease and carpal tunnel syndrome using Finkelstein's manoeuvre and Phalen's test, respectively. A positive grind test and negative Finkelstein's manoeuvre and Phalen's test will help localise the problem to the trapeziometacarpal joint. X-rays should be viewed to exclude pantrapezial arthritis (scaphotrapezial trapezoid osteoarthritis).

The neoprene thumb support can provide some relief in the early stages of the disease or when the patient reports a generalised ache at the base of the thumb. It encloses the first ray, leaving the IP free, and is attached with a Velcro strap around

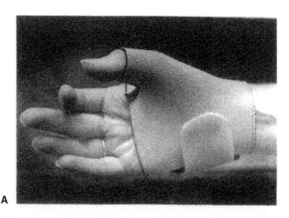

A

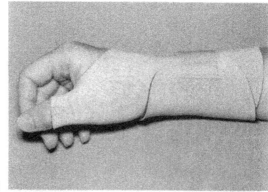

B

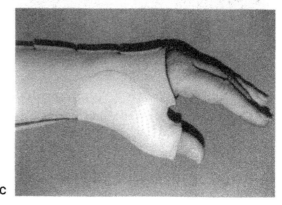

C

Figure 4.9 A: Neoprene thumb support. B: Neoprene thumb and wrist support. C: Neoprene support with added thermoplastic component.

the ulnar border of the hand (Fig. 4.9A). A longer support may be used if the scaphotrapezial joint is involved (Fig. 4.9B), while a thermoplastic piece may be adhered to the neoprene if extra support and control of the trapezimetacarpal (TMC) and MP joints is required (Fig. 4.9C).

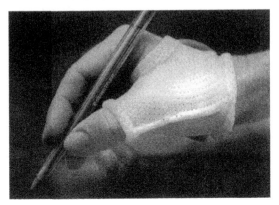

Figure 4.10 Thermoplastic short opponens thumb splint.

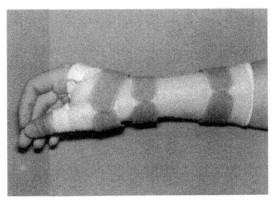

Figure 4.11 Long opponens splint.

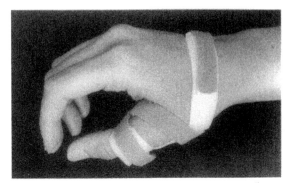

Figure 4.12 Trapeziometacarpal three-point strap splint.

A thermoplastic 'short opponens' thumb post (Fig. 4.10) similarly covers the first metacarpal and proximal phalanx, fixing the MP joint in some degree of flexion and permitting opposition to the index and middle fingers. This splint has been used with some clinical success for the TM joint. Alternatively, a 'long opponens' splint (Fig. 4.11) is described by Swigart et al.[8] as being 'well-tolerated and an effective conservative treatment to diminish, but not completely eliminate, the symptoms of carpometacarpal joint arthritis and inflammation' (p. 86).

The three-point strap splint[9] was designed to enhance stability at the TM joint. It is moulded with the MP joint in flexion, and uses a system of straps to restrict dorsoradial subluxation of the base of the first metacarpal, maintain metacarpal abduction and prevent MP hyperextension (Fig. 4.12). This positioning prevents dynamic collapse of the first ray under load, reducing stress to the affected joint, and permitting the patient to perform previously aggravating activities without pain.

Indications for surgery include failure of conservative measures with persisting pain, increasing deformity or an increase in thumb web contracture.

Surgery for isolated TM arthritis includes arthrodesis, first metacarpal osteotomy or resection arthroplasty. Pantrapezial arthritis should be treated by trapeziectomy with ligament reconstruction and tendon interposition.

Surgical technique

Arthrodesis (for TM OA)

Arthrodesis can be performed using a small buttress plate (Fig. 4.13) or by the tension band technique. The thumb is positioned with the first metacarpal in about 40 degrees each of radial and palmar abduction. The patient is still able to oppose the thumb against the other fingertips and flex the thumb across the palm but will lack the ability to place the hand flat on a surface. This makes it an undesirable technique for golfers, who will not be able to adduct their thumb.

Trapeziectomy, ligament reconstruction and tendon interposition (for pantrapezial OA)

The trapezium is removed through a dorsoradial approach, protecting the superficial branches of

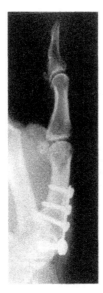

Figure 4.13 Buttress plate arthrodesis of the trapeziometacarpal joint.

the radial nerve and preserving the capsule. Proximal first metacarpal migration is prevented by reconstruction of the ulnar ligament of the base of the thumb. A slip of flexor carpi radialis (FCR) or abductor pollicis longus (APL) kept attached distally is threaded through the base of the first metacarpal and so sutured to maintain the scaphometacarpal space, which is then filled with the remainder of that tendon as an 'anchovy'. The capsule is then repaired (Fig. 4.14).

MP joint of the thumb

For advanced arthritis the procedure of choice is arthrodesis in about 10–15 degrees of flexion, usually by the tension band technique, preserving IP joint movement. Where there is secondary hyperextension of the MP joint in association with arthritis at the base of the thumb, some form of volar capsulodesis or sesamoid arthrodesis should prevent the hyperextension and still allow flexion.

Implants

Implants have been designed for this joint after trapeziectomy. For years, silicone implants

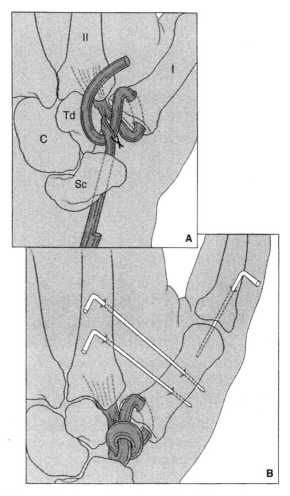

Figure 4.14 Suspension arthroplasty with ligament reconstruction and tendon interposition using flexor carpi radialis (FCR) (A); the free end of FCR is used as an 'anchovy' to fill the space left by the removal of the trapezium. The first metacarpal is held in abduction by K-wires and the MP joint held in slight flexion by another K-wire (B). I = metacarpal I, II = metacarpal II, C = capitate, Sc = scaphoid, Td = trapezoid.

(Fig. 4.15) were used at the base of the thumb. More recently, titanium implants have been developed.

Postoperative care

Patients require 6 weeks in a position of safe immobilisation for the thumb following interposition arthroplasty. This position holds the wrist

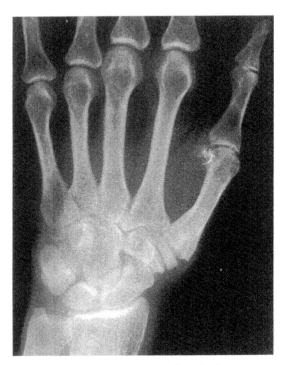

Figure 4.15 Silicone implant arthroplasty for the trapeziometacarpal joint.

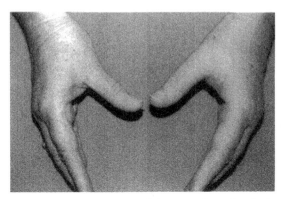

Figure 4.16 Eight weeks post left suspension arthroplasty compared with nonoperative side.

at 20–30 degrees of extension, the trapeziometacarpal joint in palmar abduction with the MP in slight flexion to control any tendency to hyperextension (see Fig. 4.11). The position should allow opposition to the index and middle fingers to allow for ADL and writing. The thumb IP joint and all digits should be left free.

The splint is generally fabricated in the first postoperative week and the patient instructed to wear it at all times. The usual warnings regarding pressure areas and circulatory disturbances are discussed.

Once the sutures are removed at 2 weeks, warm lux soaks and lanoline massage are begun. The massage is continued four to six times per day, for up to 3 months, to minimise scar sensitivity and adherence. The patient is instructed to move the IP joint through its full range of pain-free motion from the first week. This may be performed with the splint on.

At 4 weeks, gentle active pain-free exercises begin, including MP flexion/extension, opposition, palmar and radial abduction. The patient is instructed to wear the splint between exercise sessions.

At 6 weeks, the splint may be removed for light functional activities such as stacking cones or grasping foam pieces. It is essential to avoid any activity that causes pain. The patient may require a light neoprene thumb support, or a short opponens thumb post splint, to assist them in weaning from the postoperative splint.

Light resistive pinch and grip exercises begin between 6 and 8 weeks postoperatively. Exercises with sponges, pegs or soft putty are appropriate: these should be progressed in resistance and repetition very slowly, being careful not to cause any aggravation of the patient's symptoms.

Eighty per cent of patients will report good pain relief, reasonable motion (Fig. 4.16) and adequate stability. Return to full activities, including sport, may take 3–6 months. The main complication following this surgery is radial neuritis.

Tomaino et al.[10] reviewed patients at 2, 6 and 9 years post ligament reconstruction–tendon interposition arthroplasty. They found function of the thumb continued to improve for as long as 6 years following surgery, with excellent relief of pain and significant improvement in strength.

Therapy following arthrodesis aims to achieve a mobile scar, with no loss of range at either the MP or IP joints. The patient needs to keep the thumb protected until union has occurred, and begin resistance strengthening as tolerated. A strong and pain-free thumb usually results with little loss of function, other than being unable to place the hand flat on a table.

SPECIFIC TIPS

MP hyperextension

It is essential to control the MP joint when splinting the trapeziometacarpal joint. If the MP joint is allowed to hyperextend with activity, it will increase the tendency of the thumb to collapse into dorsoradial subluxation of the base of the first metacarpal with subsequent loss of web space.

Patient education

Patients must be made aware of their role in aggravation of symptoms. They are frequently able to modify their activities or use assistive devices to avoid causing pain.

Exercises

Care must be taken when prescribing exercise programmes for patients with osteoarthritis, as repetitive activities, especially against resistance, can aggravate their symptoms. The exercise programme should avoid any increase in joint deformity, with careful instructions regarding repetitions and frequency. In the hand, the home programme must not cause any increase in pain, with the patient instructed to reduce the frequency and/or repetitions of their exercises to ensure they do not aggravate their symptoms.

Splintage

Splintage may be necessary for long periods to help control pain with certain activities.

REFERENCES

1. Dray GJ, Jablon M: Clinical and radiologic features of primary osteoarthritis of the hand. Hand Clin 3:351–67, 1987.
2. Bora FW, Miller G: Joint physiology, cartilage metabolism, and the etiology of osteoarthritis. Hand Clin 3:325–36, 1987.
3. Poole UP, Pellegrini VD: Arthritis of the thumb basal joint complex. J Hand Ther 13:91–107, 2000.
4. North ER, Eaton RG: Degenerative joint disease of the trapezium: a comparative radiographic and anatomic study. J Hand Surg 8:160–7, 1983.
5. Conolly W (ed.): Atlas of hand surgery. New York: Churchill Livingstone, 1997.
6. Pellegrini VD: Osteoarthritis of the trapeziometacarpal joint: the pathophysiology of articular cartilage

degeneration. I. Anatomy of the aging joint. J Hand Surg 16:967–74, 1991.
7. Cooney WP, Chao EYS: Biomechanical analysis of static forces in the thumb during hand function. J Bone Joint Surg 59A:27–36, 1977.
8. Swigart C, Eaton R, Glicket S, Johnson C: Splinting in the treatment of arthritis of the first carpometacarpal joint. J Hand Surg 24A:86–91, 1999.
9. Wajon A: The thumb 'strap splint' for dynamic instability of the trapeziometacarpal joint. J Hand Ther 13:236–7, 2000.
10. Tomaino MM, Pellegrini VD, Burton RI: Arthroplasty of the basal joint of the thumb. J Bone Joint Surg 77A:346–55, 1995.

B.   RHEUMATOID ARTHRITIS

Rosemary Prosser and W Bruce Conolly

DEFINITION AND PATHOLOGY

Rheumatoid disease, the most common of the connective tissue disorders is a systemic disease manifesting mostly as a chronic inflammation of the synovial membranes of the joints and tendons (Fig. 4.17). The joint synovitis stretches the joint capsule, ligaments and the extensor apparatus, displaces and dislocates the tendons and infiltrates and erodes the bone. The tendon synovitis causes tendon nodules and can infiltrate the tendon, causing ischaemia and restricted glide, which may lead to rupture. Tendon rupture may also occur by attrition from friction of the tendon over bony spicules.

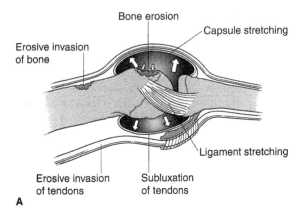

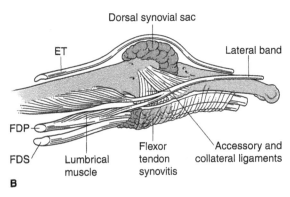

Figure 4.17 A: Pathological anatomy of the rheumatoid process at the MCP joint. Note the distension of the capsule by the proliferative synovitis, the secondary bone erosion, the stretching of the ligaments, the extension into the volar pouch and the potential invasion of the flexor tendon system. B: Disturbance to the balance of the intrinsic and extrinsic tendon forces. ET = extensor tendon, FDP = flexor digitorum profundus, FDS = flexor digitorum superficialis.

Synovitis in closed compartments can cause secondary nerve and tendon compression e.g. carpal tunnel syndrome, trigger finger.

Rheumatoid disease can be associated with skin nodules, vasculitis, purpura, myositis, peripheral neuropathy and intrinsic muscle fibrosis.

PHASES OF RHEUMATOID DISEASE

Rheumatoid arthritis can be classified into three clinical phases:

1. Inflammatory phase. Inflammatory synovitis of the joint and tendon mechanism manifests as pain and stiffness.

2. The destructive phase. The synovium invades local tissues, causing destructive changes. Joint instability may progress to deviation deformities, dislocation or subluxation due to ligament attenuation and destruction of cartilage and bone. Tendons may dislocate or rupture. Changes in joint and tendon alignment and stability cause altered biomechanical forces that can precipitate further deformity.

3. The healing or remission phase. This may lead to fibrosis and ankylosis of the joints and tendon adhesion.

PATTERNS OF DEFORMITY

As the joint capsule and ligaments stretch and weaken, the intrinsic and extrinsic muscle tendon forces cause zigzag deformities of the skeletal system of intercalated joints. In the sagittal plane one sees flexion collapse of the wrist, flexion deformity of the MP joints and either swan-neck or buttonhole deformity to the PIP joints with secondary deformity to the DIP joint.

In the coronal plane there may be radial deviation of the carpus associated with carpal translocation and ulnar drift of the MP joints.

The wrist

The synovitis usually predominates on the ulnar side, leading to radial deviation of the wrist. Weakening of the dorsal capsule and proximal intercarpal ligaments causes carpal translocation, ulnar carpal supination, volar subluxation of the proximal carpal row and ultimately carpal collapse.

As the wrist is the key to hand function, deformities of the wrist will lead to deformities at the more distal CMC, MP and IP joints.

The MP joints

As the wrist proceeds to radial deviation, the MP joints will tend to ulnar deviate to maintain some form of functional alignment of the hand as a whole. Other factors contributing to this ulnar drift include:

1. attenuation of the radial sagittal extensor hood at the MP joint, allowing ulnar subluxation of the extensor tendons

2. attenuation of the A1 pulley, allowing the flexor tendons to pull more ulnarly
3. differential contracture of the ulnar side intrinsics.

As with the wrist joint, where the flexors are more powerful than the extensors, there will be a tendency with the wrist and the MP joints to volar subluxation. Laxity of the radial lateral ligaments also contributes to ulnar drift at the MP joints.

The PIP joints – Swan-neck deformity (Fig. 4.18B)

Swan-neck deformity can be caused by tight intrinsics, weakening or rupture of the FDS tendon or attenuation of the palmar plate. Swan-neck deformities often occur secondary to MP volar subluxation due to joint disease, or may be secondary to DIP mallet deformity due to overaction of the extensor acting on the PIP joint.

The PIP joints – Buttonhole deformity (Fig. 4.18C)

Buttonhole deformity occurs when proliferative synovitis erodes the central slip; the lateral bands migrate volarwards, causing PIP flexion and secondary hyperextension of the distal interphalangeal joints.

The distal interphalangeal joints

The commonest deformity is the 'mallet' finger, which is usually secondary to hyperextension deformities of the PIP joint.

The thumb (Fig. 4.19A)

Nalebuff[1] described classic deformities of the thumb:

- type I – buttonhole deformity, flexion of the MP joint with secondary IP hyperextension (Fig. 4.19B)
- type II – type I together with adduction of the metacarpal (Fig. 4.19C)
- type III – where the CMC joint is involved with adduction of the first metacarpal and compensatory hyperextension of the MP joint

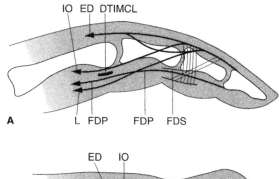

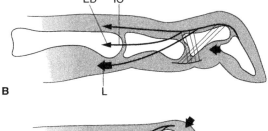

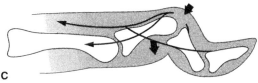

Figure 4.18 A: The normal relation between the extrinsic extensor tendon and the intrinsic interosseous (IO) and the lumbrical (L) tendons, acting on the three joint system connecting four small finger bones. B: Swan-neck deformity. Attenuation of the volar plate and loss of stability over the volar part of the PIP joint with hyperextension of the PIP and flexion of the DIP joint. C: Buttonhole deformity. PIP synovitis with attenuation of the dorsal capsule and the central slip, causing volar subluxation of the lateral bands, flexion of the PIP joint and hyperextension of the DIP joint from shortening of the oblique reticular ligament (ORL). There is also hyperextension of the MCP joint. DTIMCL = deep transverse intermetacarpal ligament, ED = extensor digitorum, FDP = flexor digitorum profundus, FDS = flexor digitorum superficialis.

and flexion of the interphalangeal joint – this is analogous to swan-neck deformity of the finger (Fig. 4.19D)
- type IV – subluxation of the first CMC joint with metacarpal adduction and rupture of the ulnar lateral ligament of the MP joint.

ASSESSMENT AND CONSERVATIVE THERAPY MANAGEMENT

Despite severe deformity, hand function in rheumatoid patients can be reasonably good, depending on the patient's needs and lifestyle.

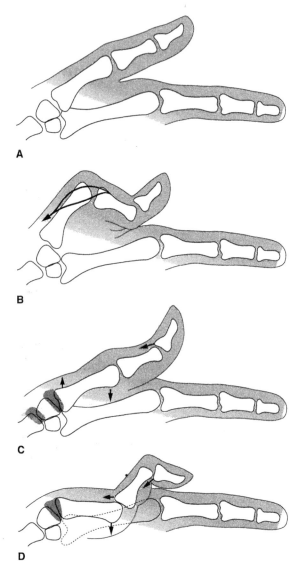

Figure 4.19 Types of thumb deformity in rheumatoid arthritis (after Nalebuff[1]). A: Normal thumb. B: Type I deformity, buttonhole (reverse swan-neck). Synovitis of the MCP joint distends the capsule, stretches the EPB, and dislocates EPL to the ulnar side, causing hyperextension of the interphalangeal joint. C: Type II deformity. There is CMC joint subluxation with thumb web contracture from an adducted first metacarpal. D: Type III deformity, swan-neck. Synovitis of the CMC joint causes destruction and dislocation of that joint with adduction of the first metacarpal. In this deformity, there is secondary volar plate attenuation with swan-neck deformity of the MCP joint and a secondary flexion deformity of the interphalangeal joint. The prime pathology at the CMC joint is probably best solved by trapeziectomy with ligament reconstruction. The swan-neck deformity of the MCP joint is treated by soft tissue volar plate tenodesis, sesamoid arthrodesis or MCP joint fusion.

Close questioning regarding individual requirements and pain levels is essential. Activity and function is subjectively assessed in the areas of morning stiffness, self-care, domestic tasks, work and leisure activities.

Examination includes assessment of:

- The soft tissues (synovitis, tendon integrity or attenuation and nodules).
- Joint range of motion and deformities.
- Muscle length and strength, including grip and pinch strength.
- Functional testing, which may include specific tests such as the Jebson[2] or Sollerman[3] functional tests. However, analysis of simulated aggravating activities may prove more beneficial in assessing the functional needs of the individual.

Joints and tendons with synovitis are recorded on an upper limb or hand chart. Deformities, ROM and strength are also charted.

Conservative management

Conservative management is focused on maximising functional use of the hand while avoiding deforming forces and postures. Range of motion and strengthening exercises, and improving activity endurance are encouraged within pain and strain limits. Exercise sessions are short, at regular intervals. Exercise and activity needs to be balanced with rest, depending on the status of the arthritis. Rest may be relative and confined to one or two joints using functional splints. Work simplification or modification may assist in energy conservation, e.g. sitting to prepare vegetables – peeling or chopping for 2–3 min at a time.

Patient education with regard to the effects of the disease and appropriate management strategies are essential to maximise independence. Philips[4] reports that clinical experience finds that most activities of daily living (ADLs) require a grip strength of 9 kg and a pinch grip strength of 2–3 kg. Patients with grip strength less than this will require to modify their grip or the activity: e.g. by using two hands to lift rather than one. Joint protection[5] to avoid deformity and loss of functional use is emphasised. Larger joints are

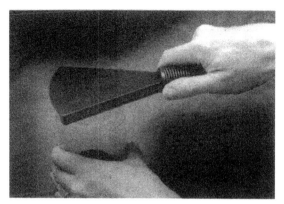

Figure 4.20 This jar and bottle opener provides a gripping action combined with extra leverage, allowing opening of the jar by a much reduced grip strength.

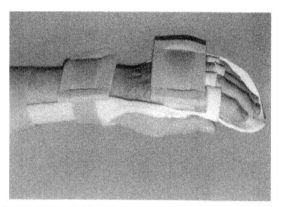

Figure 4.21 Night resting splint; the MP joints are held in comfortable extension and the PIP joints in slight flexion. Finger ulnar deviation can be managed with individual finger straps.

used when possible, as they are able to tolerate greater loads than smaller joints: e.g. closing drawers with the hip rather than the hands. The use of adaptive devices to increase leverage and decrease joint strain is encouraged: e.g. bottle/jar openers, electric knives and can openers, tap turners, lever taps, spring-loaded scissors and adaptive large handles for cooking and eating utensils (Fig. 4.20).

Management of the three phases

1. Inflammatory phase

'Appropriate' rest in this phase is essential. All painful activity should be avoided if possible. Night resting splints in a comfortable position are beneficial (wrist 20 degrees extension, MPs in a comfortable extension, IPs in 20–30 degrees flexion and thumb in abduction and opposition to the index finger; Fig. 4.21). The ultimate position decided will depend on the individual's condition; i.e. which joints are involved and the degree of inflammation and deformity. Wrist splints stabilising the wrist to allow more pain-free hand use during the day may also be helpful (Fig. 4.22).

A formal exercise programme at this stage may not be appropriate. Exercises are restricted to activities only within pain limits. Warm red inflamed joints often respond favourably to cold packs or cool water baths. Medication to

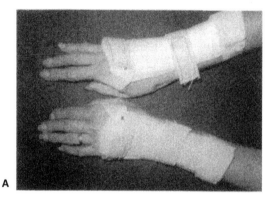

A

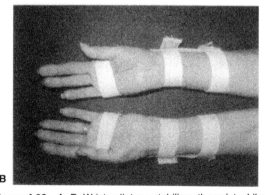

B

Figure 4.22 A, B: Wrist splintage stabilises the wrist while facilitating a better functional grip of the digits.

control the acute inflammatory phase is essential. Any therapy intervention including splinting should not aggravate the patient's condition in any way.

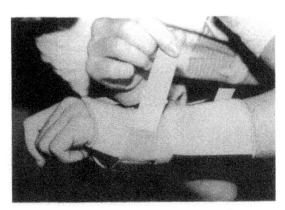

Figure 4.23 The ulnar carpal pronation wrist splint supports the ulnar carpus and attempts to try and control ulnar carpal subluxation and supination.

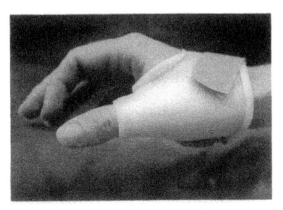

Figure 4.24 A thermoplastic hand-based splint can control stability of the MP joint with minimal interference with functional use.

2. The destructive phase

Following the acute phase, joint and tendon structures may be damaged and attenuated. It is important in this phase to protect these structures to prevent further deformity. Some of the structures requiring support may include the thumb MP joint ulnar collateral ligament (UCL), finger MP joints from ulnar deviation forces and PIP joints from flexion or hyperextension.

Gentle heat, e.g. wax, hot packs, warm water and ultrasound, may help relieve pain. Gentle exercises, actively or with minimal resistance such as sponge squeezing in warm water, are encouraged. Hydrotherapy may be particularly helpful for patients with elbow, shoulder, spine and lower limb involvement.

Specific attention in the hand should be given to:

1. Wrist balance to prevent radial deviation: an ulnar carpal pronation wrist splint (Fig. 4.23) may be of benefit if the ulnar carpus is supinated.

2. MP joint alignment: MP ulnar deviation is usually primarily due to MP joint subluxation. A working splint or resting splint supporting these joints may be beneficial. Improving radial intrinsic strength may help combat the ulnar deviation tendency at the MP joints before subluxation occurs.

3. Finger intrinsic muscle length: intrinsic muscle contracture secondary to MP joint subluxation may develop. Intrinsic tightness may also add to or cause swan-neck deformity. Very gentle IP flexion stretching with the MP joints supported in extension stretches the intrinsic muscles.

4. Integrity of the thumb MP joint UCL: good UCL function is required for a functional stable pinch. A small thermoplastic hand-based thumb splint (Fig. 4.24) can be used during pinch activities to support the UCL.

5. Swan-neck and buttonhole deformities are difficult to manage conservatively in the late stages. Early in the development of the deformity, swan-neck deformities can be managed by FDS exercises and prevention of PIP hyperextension using a digit-based PIP extension block splint[6] or a ring splint. The beauty of this splint is that it is small, functional, does not interfere with motion or function and is very cosmetically acceptable (Fig. 4.25). MP joint motion and stability should be monitored if the splint is worn full time. Protection of the PIP joint may transfer more force to the MP joint and cause a progression of MP joint deformity. Buttonhole deformities are more difficult to control, as splintage to prevent PIP flexion contracture may prevent PIP motion and interfere with hand function.

If the extensor mechanism or flexor tendons are attenuated or subluxed by the rheumatoid process at any joint in the digit, the biomechanics of the finger are altered and all one can hope to do is to prevent the deformity progressing.

3. The healing or remission phase

Joint range of motion and muscle strength can be maximised. Pain levels are lower in this phase, allowing gentle passive joint stretching when

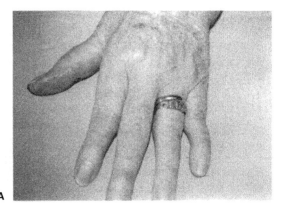
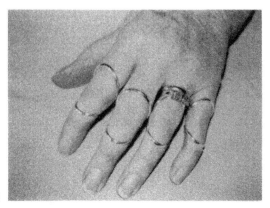

A

B

Figure 4.25 A, B: Ring splints offer an extremely good cosmetic splint that can control PIP hyperextension and swan-neck deformity progression. MP joint stability should be carefully monitored; extra stress on the MP joint may expose it to deforming forces.

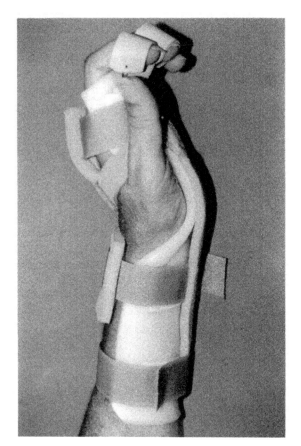

Figure 4.26 A night intrinsic stretch splint can be coordinated with an MP joint extension splint. The stretching force should be very gentle and well tolerated by the patient.

indicated and muscle and grip strengthening in the form of a graded resistance programme. Altered joint and tendon biomechanics resulting from the inflammatory and destructive phases should be respected. Further strain on attenuated structures should be avoided.

Night-splinting to prevent further progression of deformity may help maintain range and function. Splinting for the MP joints, finger deformities and thumb has already been mentioned. Tight intrinsics can be gently stretched at night in a forearm-based splint which also supports the MP joints and wrist (Fig. 4.26).

SURGICAL TREATMENT OF THE RHEUMATOID HAND

General principles

Patients presenting for surgery should be under the overall care of a physician or rheumatologist. Before any surgical procedure, the patient should be assessed by a hand therapist.

Patients present with multiple joint problems, often in both upper and lower limbs. In general, hand procedures should follow other limb procedures: e.g. shoulder and elbow and lower limb procedures should be carried out before hand procedures. MP implant arthroplasty and other hand reconstructive measures will not stand up to weight-bearing forces required when using crutches.

The surgical management may be divided into preventive or reconstructive procedures. The surgery may be for the joints or soft tissues.

In general, wrist deformities should be corrected before MP and PIP joint surgery. Where there is the need for multiple reconstructive procedures, Souter[7] advises proceeding from simple to more complex operations. He advises the following sequence:

1. dorsal wrist surgery, including extensor tendon synovectomy and excision of the head of the ulna, with wrist stabilisation as necessary
2. flexor tendon surgery
3. metacarpophalangeal joint surgery
4. PIP joint surgery and correction of finger deformities
5. realignment of the thumb in the most useful position relative to the reconstructed fingers.

Indications for surgery include:

1. to relieve pain
2. to improve function
3. to arrest the progression of deformity
4. to improve appearance.

In general, the types of surgery for rheumatoid arthritis include:

1. Joint:
   - synovectomy
   - soft tissue reconstruction
   - arthroplasty
   - arthrodesis.

2. Soft tissue:
   - tenosynovectomy and release of tendon entrapment
   - tendon reconstruction
   - removal of soft tissue nodules
   - decompression of nerves.

Hand therapy principles

The aim of hand therapy following surgery is to maximise the gains made from the surgery. Consideration of the patient's medications and tissue status (fragile tissues require more gentle handling) is necessary. Removal of sutures may be delayed if the patient is taking corticosteroids. Arthritis in other joints may also affect the treatment programme: e.g. shoulder and elbow function will directly affect hand function. Shoulder and elbow exercises following hand surgery are necessary to maintain ranges at these joints.

RHEUMATOID HAND SURGERY AND THERAPY

Extensor procedures for the hand, wrist and finger MP joints

Extensor tenosynovectomy

Through a midline dorsal approach the extensor tenosynovium is removed, together with rheumatoid nodules from the tendons in each of the six extensor compartments, though the first and second compartments are less frequently involved. Frayed tendon ends may be trimmed, and tendons with incipient ruptures sutured or reconstructed. Rough bony spikes are removed from the extensor aspect of the distal ulna and radius.

Hand therapy. Early mobilisation of the MP and IP joints is vital to maximise tendon glide following tenosynovectomy. A frayed or fragile tendon will not tolerate as much exercise as a healthy one. Patients with fragile tissues or in difficult circumstances may need splintage during the day for 3 weeks to help rest the hand and protect the tendons when engaged in moderate to heavy activity.

Active exercises and light activity is encouraged immediately (2–3 days postoperatively) following the surgery. The exercises include EDC through range, intrinsic extension and global extension of the digits. The amount and vigour of the exercises will depend on the condition of the tendons at the time of surgery. For tendons in good condition, exercises are done second hourly for 5–10 min.

For healthy tendons, resisted activity and exercise can be commenced at 3 weeks post-surgery. This may be delayed until 4–6 weeks post-surgery if the tendons are frayed.

A repaired or reconstructed tendon will need full-time protection in a splint for 6 weeks and an exercise programme suitable for the surgery (see extensor tendon repairs).

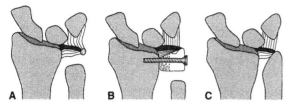

Figure 4.27 Procedures for the DRUJ. A: Darrach excision of the ulnar head. B: Sauve–Kapandji procedure involves fusion of the DRUJ and creation of a pseudojoint proximally. C: Bowers' partial resection of the distal ulnar head, leaving the DRUJ ligamentous complex intact. Darrach excision of the ulnar head is the most common procedure performed for the DRUJ.

Excision of the ulnar head and other procedures for the distal radioulnar joint (DRUJ)

In the Darrach procedure (Fig. 4.27), about 2 cm of the distal ulna is removed subperiostially, maintaining where possible the TFCC and other ligaments in the area. The distal ulnar stump is protected by an ulnar basal flap of extensor retinaculum.

In the Sauve–Kapandji[8] procedure a pseudo-arthrodesis is created just proximal to the fused DRUJ. This operation maintains the ulnar side of the wrist.

In the Bowers'[9] procedure the articular surface of the distal ulna is resected but the ulna length and its ligaments are maintained, preserving integrity of the TFC.

Ulnar head replacement with a ceramic and titanium prosthesis, e.g. the Herbert ulnar head, is still at the experimental stage: it is only considered if the patient is young, requires both motion and strength at the joint and has good inherent tissue quality (Herbert, pers. comm.).

Hand therapy. Stability of the distal ulna and preservation of maximum forearm rotation (particularly supination) are the two most important aims for the postoperative therapy programme. Splintage following surgery may vary, depending on whether a soft tissue procedure was used to stabilise the distal ulna and the final stability assessed at the end of surgery. Splints that could be used include the 'sugar tong' splint (Fig. 4.28), an ulnar gutter, wrist splint in 20 degrees of extension or a simple forearm strap. Generally, a splint is worn full time for 4–6 weeks and then intermittently for a further 3 weeks.

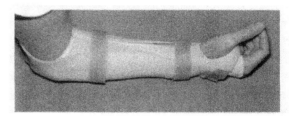

Figure 4.28 A sugar tong splint can be used very effectively to control forearm rotation after DRUJ procedures.

Forearm rotation exercises are commenced as soon as the acute inflammation has settled and there is reasonable clinical stability. This may vary from 1 to 4 weeks. Clicking in the area of surgery, prominence of the distal ulna head dorsally or full rotation with pain are all indications that further relative rest in a sugar tong- or forearm-based wrist splint is necessary. Patients with thin fragile tissues may require full-time splintage for up to 6 weeks.

The Sauve–Kapandji procedure, Bowers' procedure and ulnar head replacement require a similar postoperative programme to the Darrach procedure.

Extensor tendon reconstruction

Extensor tendon reconstruction for rupture of the extensor tendons usually involves the little and ring fingers (see Chapter 2E). There may be:

1. direct repair, which is seldom possible because of retraction of the unhealthy proximal tendon stumps
2. side junction of the distal stump of the ruptured tendon to the extensor tendon to the adjacent normal one
3. tendon transfers, using EI, EDM or FDS, if unaffected by the disease
4. tendon grafting.

Hand therapy. The postoperative therapy programme is the same as that following extensor tendon repair or tendon transfer (see relevant chapters).

Wrist synovectomy and stabilisation

Persisting painful synovitis of the radiocarpal joint can be treated by synovectomy of the radiocarpal and the intercarpal joints. The wrist can be stabilised temporarily by Kirschner wires. Occasionally, a thick reinforced silicone sheet is used as interposition between the radius and the proximal carpal bones. At the end of this procedure, the dorsal radial carpal capsule and ligaments are repaired to the distal end of the radius.

In all these procedures the distal half of the extensor retinaculum is placed deep to the extensor tendons to prevent friction on the underlying rheumatoid joint, and the other half is replaced as the extensor retinaculum to support and prevent bowstringing of the tendons.

Hand therapy. An unstable wrist decreases hand function and grip strength. Splintage needs to be balanced with the exercise programme. The ability to maintain wrist extension with grip is the most important functional postoperative goal. Maintainence of forearm rotation is also important functionally.

The wrist is splinted in 20 degrees of extension for 4–6 weeks following surgery. Digit exercises are commenced immediately following surgery.

Wrist motion is assessed at 2 weeks, at the time of suture removal. If the wrist is stiff, i.e. has less than 50% of the preoperative range, wrist exercises are started. If wrist motion is 75–80% of the preoperative range, the wrist is rested for a further 2 weeks. If wrist motion is between 50% and 75% of the preoperative range, limited small-range exercises are advocated.

Resisted grip activity without a supportive splint is not recommended until the wrist is stable. Resisted wrist exercises are not commenced before 6 weeks following the surgery.

Limited wrist fusion

Where arthritis is limited to the radiocarpal joint and where there is reasonable preservation of the midcarpal joints, a radiolunate[10] (Fig. 4.29) or radioscapholunate arthrodesis is a useful procedure which may prevent progressive ulnar translocation of the carpus. This fusion may be internally fixed by screws (e.g. Herbert screw), K-wires or staples.

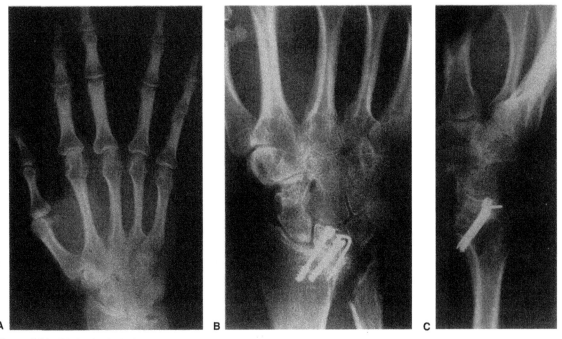

Figure 4.29 Limited wrist fusion. A: Preoperative X-ray. B: Radiolunate fusion using a Herbert screw, a Whipple screw and K-wire. C: Lateral view.

Hand therapy. The wrist needs sufficient splintage, usually in the form of a wrist extension splint, to protect the fusion and a protected and controlled exercise programme to maximise the residual range of motion at the midcarpal joint.

Young male patients may need cast immobilisation as their everyday activities will stress the wrist. A simple wrist extension splint is enough protection for elderly patients with sedentary lifestyles. Finger exercises are commenced within a few days following surgery.

Gentle active wrist ROM exercises to preserve range of the midcarpal joint may be commenced between 2 and 4 weeks post-surgery, depending on the type of internal fixation, patient compliance, lifestyle and quality of bone stock. Resisted activity should not be commenced before confirmation of bony union at 6 or more weeks post-surgery.

Wrist arthrodesis

Persisting painful instability of the wrist, if relieved by wearing a wrist splint, can be treated highly successfully by arthrodesis (Fig. 4.30). Intramedullary rods or pins are passed from the metacarpus to the radius. Alternatively, a standard wrist fusion technique can be carried out using a plate and screws, with or without bone graft.

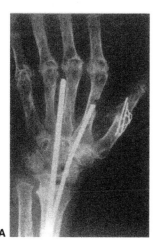 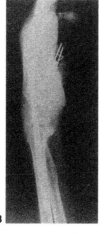

A   **B**

Figure 4.30 A, B: Wrist fusion for severe rheumatoid arthritis with intramedullary fixation. There has also been tension band arthrodesis of the thumb MP joint.

Hand therapy. The fusion needs to be protected either by a wrist extension splint or a lightweight fibreglass cast until the fusion is solid. This may vary from 6 to 10 weeks. Finger exercises should be commenced early, so that tendon glide is maintained, particularly the extensor tendons, which are retracted at the time of surgery and more prone – due to their anatomical position – to becoming stuck down in adhesions.

Wrist arthroplasty

Wrist implant arthroplasty is indicated when some wrist motion needs to be maintained, such as painful wrist destruction in association with stiffness of the fingers. The wrist joint can be excised and an implant (e.g. Swansonn or biaxial) used. The dorsal capsule is preserved and repaired after inserting the prosthesis.

Hand therapy. Range of motion following wrist arthroplasty is quite limited. The expected ROM is approximately 20–30 degrees. Therapy should aim to maximise this range in a functional position, i.e. around the neutral axis with slightly more extension than flexion. Lateral stability is also important; the arthroplasty should be protected from lateral forces using a wrist extension splint or a limited motion splint for at least 6 weeks.

Exercises for the wrist are usually commenced at 1–2 weeks post-surgery. The wrist extension goal is 20 degrees by 4 weeks.

The primary concern is wrist stability in a functional position to maximise grip strength and functional use. If wrist extension is poor (less than 20 degrees) at 6 weeks, night wrist extension assist splintage is indicated. Static, progressive static or dynamic splinting may be used, depending on the patient's compliance and tissue tolerance.

MP joint synovectomy and correction of ulnar drift

Synovectomy is only indicated if there is synovitis without joint changes or joint subluxation. After MP synovectomy if significant ulnar drift remains, the ulnar-side intrinsics of the index, middle and ring fingers can be transferred to the intrinsics on the radial side of the MP joint of the middle, ring and little fingers. In the index finger the extensor indicis is transferred to the radial side of the extensor hood.

Hand therapy. Early motion within a few days of surgery is essential if ROM is to be restored. Pain should be respected. The joint(s) may need to be protected and supported with a splint initially: i.e. the first 2 weeks.

Rest and exercise are balanced. IP motion should be restored to preoperative measures by 2 weeks post-surgery. Reasonable MP range (15/60) is expected by 3–4 weeks. This may vary, depending on the preoperative condition of the patient. MP joint flexion is emphasised with isolated MP joint flexion with concurrent IP extension (intrinsic flexion) and FDS fist exercises.

Patients with a combination of MP synovectomy and crossed intrinsic transfer should be rested in a static dorsal protective splint in the intrinsic plus position (MP flexion of 40–60 degrees and IP extension) for 6 weeks. Lateral straps position the digits in extension and prevent recurrence of MP ulnar deviation.

Gentle MP flexion exercises are practised within the confines of the splint in the first week. Gentle active IP flexion and extension is also practised within pain limits. Early assisted active radial deviation exercises are also advocated.

Strict maintainence of the correction of the ulnar deviation deformity is necessary for at least 8–12 weeks. If necessary, a corrective splint to maintain lateral alignment and allow motion of the MP joints can be made and fitted at 6 weeks.

Graded resisted exercise and activity are commenced with light activity at 6 weeks.

MP joint implant arthroplasty

Where there is gross deformity of the MP joints and the patient is unable to open the hand, has loss of pinch and a severe cosmetic disfigurement, implant arthroplasty, either using the Swansonn, the Sutter or Avanta implant joints, can give good results (Fig. 4.31).

Either through a transverse incision or through separate longitude ulnar incisions the head of the metacarpal is resected, the proximal phalanx and metacarpal shafts are reamed, the implant placed

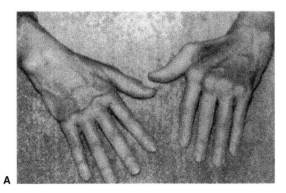

A

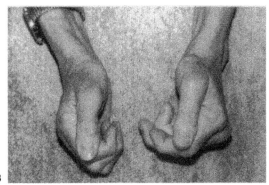

B

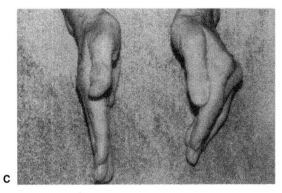

C

Figure 4.31 MCP joint silicone implant arthroplasty of the right hand (A), flexion achieved (B) and extension (C).

and the extensor apparatus repaired, centralising the extensor tendon (Fig. 4.32).

Often the radial lateral ligament of the index finger is repaired to minimise ulnar drift at that finger and the ulnar-side intrinsics for the little finger are divided.

Hand therapy. Preoperative assessment of the patient's condition is helpful for setting appropriate realistic postoperative goals. It also enables

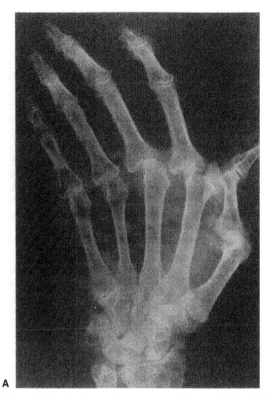
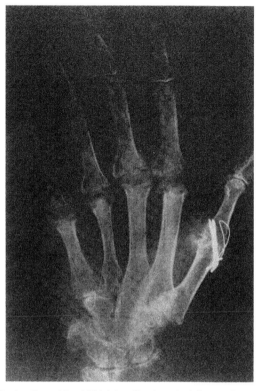

A B

Figure 4.32 Radiographs of a case of rheumatoid arthritis. Destruction of the MP joints with ulnar deviation and flexion deformity can be seen (A). The postoperative view (B) shows resection of all four MP joints with silicone implant arthroplasty together with MP arthrodesis of the thumb (tension band technique).

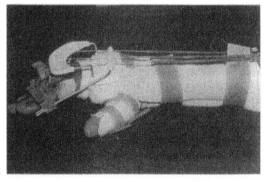
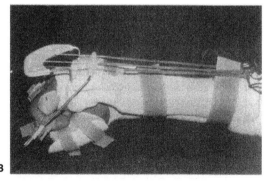

A B

Figure 4.33 A, B: A dynamic extension splint following MP arthroplasty supports the joints in the corrected position; the rotation bar controls deviation, while still allowing flexion and extension motion to be achieved in the splint. This patient also had a thumb MP joint arthrodesis. The thumb static digit-based splint is used to protect the arthrodesis.

the hand therapist to tailor the postoperative programme to the patient's needs.

The postoperative programme following this procedure is protracted. The patient will require an extended period of splintage and exercise.

A minimum of 3 months of full-time (day and night) splintage is usually required. A dynamic extension splint with an ulnar deviation correction bar (Fig. 4.33) is worn for the first 6 weeks, followed by another 6 weeks of a hand-based

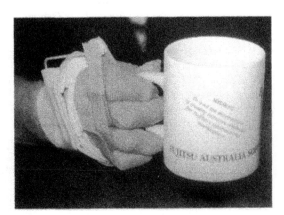

Figure 4.34 A hand-based ulnar deviation correction splint is maintained for several months after MP arthroplasty. It prevents recurrence of ulnar drift by supporting the joint against ulnar deviation forces encountered in functional activity until the intrinsics are strong enough to take over this role.

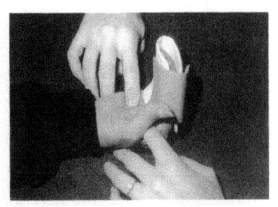

Figure 4.35 An IP extension splint can be used to isolate and facilitate MP flexion motion after MP arthroplasty.

ulnar deviation correction splint. When the forearm is in mid-rotation, any hand activity involving lifting or manipulating objects transmits an ulnar deviation force to the MP joints. For this reason, a hand-based ulnar deviation correction splint is recommended. The splint allows MP motion but prevents ulnar deviation (Fig. 4.34).

From 6 weeks to 4–6 months night-splintage, maintaining MP extension and/or ulnar deviation correction is often required.

The exercise programme is commenced in the first postoperative week. Good IP motion needs to be maintained. IP and MP exercises are commenced within a few days of surgery. Initially, active and assisted active MP exercises only are instituted. Passive exercises are added at approximately 2–3 weeks, depending on the range of motion that is achieved; resisted exercise is commenced at 6 weeks. Isolated active MP flexion with IP extension is emphasised. An IP extension splint (Fig. 4.35) facilitates MP flexion in the presence of poor intrinsic function. Functional use of the hand in the splint for light activities is encouraged from 4 weeks after surgery.

Often the intrinsics are tight and weak due to them being in the shortened position for years. Re-education of intrinsic action is one of the most challenging aspects of MP arthroplasty rehabilitation. MP intrinsic flexion with IP extension and

radial deviation exercises are focused on from the first postoperative week. Intrinsic strengthening is commenced as soon as the intrinsic muscles are strong enough to cope with resistance. Functional electrical stimulation may also be beneficial.

The expected MP range is 20/50–70 degrees with flexion to the palm if IP range is not limited. The implants do not stand up well to heavy use. Long-term heavy activity such as repeated lifting and carrying, some heavy gardening activities and scrubbing may cause failure or fracture of the implants. Heavy activity requirements may be a contraindication to MP implant arthroplasty.

Extensor procedures for the fingers: The PIP and DIP joints

PIP joint synovectomy

Persistent painful synovitis in joints with a potential range of movement and function without bone or joint change on X-ray can be treated by synovectomy. The synovectomy may be done through a dorsal, lateral or volar approach. If either the lateral ligaments or the central slip needs division for the synovectomy, these structures are repaired before wound closure.

Hand therapy. Following synovectomy, the digit is rested in a digit-based extension splint for 2–4 weeks. Wound and scar care and oedema control are attended to as required. PIP exercises are started a few days following the synovectomy. Graded activity is commenced as soon as the patient is able to tolerate light resistance. This may be as early as 3–4 weeks.

If the collateral ligament has required repair, care is taken to prevent lateral forces at the joint. Buddy taping is utilised for 6 weeks for this purpose.

The therapy programme following central slip repair will follow a similar programme to that described under extensor tendon repair. The short arc active programme may be preferred if the patient has a tendency to have stiffer arthritic joints.

Buttonhole deformity (BHD)

- Stage I: where there is PIP synovitis and mild deformity, synovectomy with relocation of the lateral bands and terminal tendon tenotomy may be performed.
- Stage II: where there is 30–40 degree flexion deformity in a flexible joint with preservation of joint space on X-ray, surgical synovectomy with central slip reconstruction and lateral band relocation is practised (Fig. 4.36).
- Stage III: where there is fixed deformity with joint stiffness not correctable passively, arthroplasty or arthrodesis will be necessary.

Hand therapy. Therapy following surgery needs to be carefully managed so that the joint structures and tendons are protected while they are gaining strength and the flexion and extension motion is balanced in such a way that the most functional range is achieved for each patient. Some type of PIP extension splintage is usually required for 6 weeks during the day and 3 months at night. The patient is usually required to work just as hard to restore DIP flexion. This may also need some type of flexion splintage.

Stage I. Following PIP synovectomy and distal tendon tenotomy, the PIP and DIP joints are splinted in extension for 6 weeks. DIP gentle active flexion is started in the first postoperative week. DIP motion should be monitored closely. If a DIP extension lag develops, flexion exercises may need to be discontinued in the short term. PIP exercises are commenced at 3 weeks once the

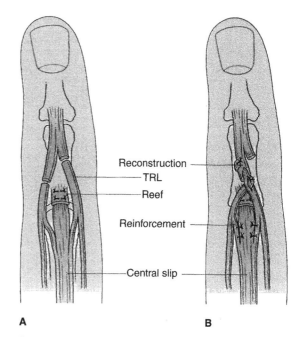

A   **B**

Figure 4.36   A: Surgical correction of buttonhole deformity. After synovectomy of the PIP joint, release the volar subluxing lateral bands by cutting the transverse retinacular ligament (TRL). Reconstruct the central slip mechanism by reefing what remains of the central slip. B: To enhance PIP extension, the lateral bands are divided distal to the PIP joint at different levels, and the central slip reinforced proximal to the joint using the lateral bands, and so a central slip is reconstructed just distal to the PIP joint by suturing the lateral bands together.

DIP is under control and the dorsal extensor structures start to have some strength. Resisted exercises are not commenced before 6 weeks postoperation.

Stage II. Both PIP and DIP joints are splinted in extension for 6 weeks. The exercise programme is similar to stage I. At 6 weeks gentle resisted grip activities are commenced. Night-time extension splinting may be necessary for a further 6 weeks. If there is a tendency for PIP extensor lag in the day, a neoprene sleeve provides a gentle extension force while still allowing flexion. The force of the neoprene sleeve can be altered by using different thicknesses of neoprene: at our clinic we use 1 mm, 2 mm and 3 mm neoprene, depending on the individual's requirements.

Stage III. PIP arthroplasty is discussed in detail following swan-neck deformities. PIP arthrodesis requires splintage of the PIP joint for protection for 6 weeks until the fusion is united. MP and DIP exercises should be commenced within the first postoperative week to ensure that range is maintained at these joints. Once the fusion is united, resisted hand activity can be commenced.

Swan-neck deformity

- Type I: if the PIP joint is flexible in all positions, DIP joint fusion may suffice.
- Type II: where there is MP joint deformity with secondary intrinsic tightness causing limited PIP flexion, intrinsic release should correct the MP joint deformity and the swan-neck deformity.
- Type III: where the PIP joint flexion is limited in all positions and the joint is preserved on X-ray, the PIP joint can be stabilised by FDS tenodesis or lateral band transfer (Fig. 4.37).
- Type IV: where the PIP joint is stiff and X-ray shows joint destruction, arthrodesis for the index and middle fingers or arthroplasty for the ring and little finger PIP joints is considered.

Hand therapy. Primarily, the aim following this surgery is to prevent PIP hyperextension and

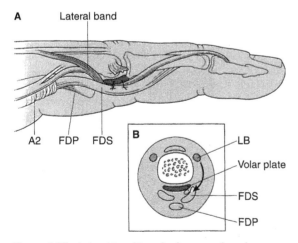

Figure 4.37 Lateral band transfer for correction of swan-neck deformity. A: Radiolateral view. B: Cross-section showing the radial lateral band transposed and held by the sling between the volar plate and the FDS tendon. A2 = A2 pulley, LB = lateral band, FDP = flexor digitorum profundus, FDS = flexor digitorum superficialis.

maintain flexion and regain DIP movement. A simple digit-based PIP blocking splint is usually adequate to control the hyperextension. FDS flexion exercises are emphasised with the aim of increasing PIP joint stability post-surgery.

Type I. DIP fusion is protected in a static digit-based splint for 6 weeks. PIP joint exercises are commenced approximately 1 week following surgery. If there is a tendency for PIP hyperextension following surgery, the PIP is included in the splint in 30 degrees of flexion. FDS exercises are emphasised to increase volar PIP joint strength.

Type II. Following intrinsic release the patient is splinted in the intrinsic stretch position for 6 weeks in the day and 3–6 months or more at night. IP exercises are commenced within the first postoperative week. MP joint motion is monitored. If stiffness into flexion is developing, MP flexion exercises are initiated before 6 weeks. At 6 weeks, MP joint motion and gross extension and flexion exercises are commenced along with light resisted activity.

If there is concurrent MP pathology, this must be addressed at the time of intrinsic release. MP joint subluxation is a contributing factor to intrinsic tightness. If uncorrected, intrinsic tightness will recur over time.

Type III. FDS tenodesis or lateral band transfer requires a dorsal blocking splint with MP flexion (approximately 50 degrees), PIP flexion (30 degrees) and DIP extension. After a few days, the surgical wounds have settled and DIP and PIP exercises are commenced within the dorsal blocking splint. The splint is worn for 6 weeks and then a further 6 weeks at night. A digit-based ring or figure of eight splint can be worn in the day from 6 weeks if protection from strong extension forces is necessary for patients engaged in manual activity.

DIP joint

For the DIP joint there may be:

1. synovectomy – rarely practised or
2. arthrodesis by the Herbert screw or K-wire or cerclage technique.

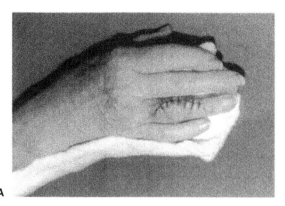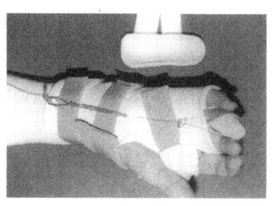

Figure 4.38 PIP arthroplasty 2 days after surgery (A). A dynamic flexion splint is the splint of choice following PIP arthroplasty for joints stiff in extension prior to surgery. This can be alternated with some type of extension splintage, such as a simple static digit-based splint (B).

PIP silicone implant arthroplasty

This procedure can be performed either through a dorsal, palmar, lateral or volar approach. The principle is to resect the head of the proximal phalanx and ream the middle and proximal phalangeal shafts: an implant where the width of the hinge is the same as the width of the skeleton is chosen and then the extensor apparatus repaired.

Hand therapy. Splintage following this surgery is very individual. If the patient has difficulty with flexion pre-surgery (swan-neck deformity), then this will be the emphasis post-surgery, and vice versa (buttonhole deformity). Flexion and extension splintage may need to be balanced, depending on the progress in ROM. Dynamic outrigger splintage allows motion while maintaining a gentle corrective torque at the joint. The dynamic splint is usually worn for 6 weeks. Dynamic flexion splintage (Fig. 4.38) with intermittent static extension splintage may be utilised following arthroplasty for swan-neck deformity. Buttonhole deformities require more extension splintage, which may be dynamic or static and combined with intermittent flexion splintage during the day.

Joint range is monitored: if there is stiffness into flexion, the dynamic flexion splint may be used intermittently in the day after the first 6 weeks for 6 more weeks. For stiffness into extension, a neoprene sleeve provides adequate extension force while allowing flexion. It can also be combined easily with buddy straps.

As with MP arthroplasty, restoration of lateral stability is vital in order to produce a functional digit. The PIP joint needs to be protected from lateral forces using buddy strapping or a hinged splint device acting at the PIP joint (Fig. 4.39); this is usually applied at 6 weeks when the dynamic splint is discontinued. Protection from lateral forces may be necessary for 3–6 months.

It is interesting to note that in patients with a tendency to stiff arthritic joints, in the long term the arthroplasty gets stiffer in extension rather than flexion. Some patients may require some type of night flexion splint one to two nights per week for years in order to maintain their flexion. The patients who require this protracted course usually manage it very well themselves if the functional benefits are apparent. Not all patients are prepared to undergo such a programme.

An exercise programme is commenced in the first postoperative week. Initially, active and assisted active exercise only are instigated. Passive exercises may be commenced in the second week if the joint is stiff. At 6 weeks, gentle resisted grip activity is begun.

Flexor procedures for the wrist and fingers

Flexor tenosynovectomy at the wrist

Where there is restricted flexor tendon glide, or secondary compression of the median nerve

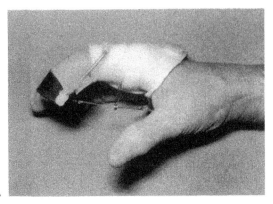 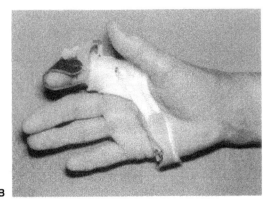

A   B

Figure 4.39 A, B: A rotation bar can also be used to control deviation at the PIP joint level after arthroplasty. This is essential if there is a preoperative deviation deformity.

manifesting as carpal tunnel syndrome, a flexor tenosynovectomy is indicated.

The approach is as for a carpal tunnel release with an extended interthenar approach protecting the median nerve. Hypertrophic synovium is systematically removed from each of the flexor tendons and, as with extensor tenosynovectomy, nodules may need to be removed from the tendons and frayed tendons repaired and ruptured tendons reconstructed.

Flexor tenosynovectomy in the digits

This procedure is performed through a volar zigzag approach from the mid-palm to the DIP joint. The A1, A2 and A4 pulley systems are dissected and preserved to prevent bowstringing of the tendons after operation.

Occasionally, one-half of the FDS is removed to make more space beneath the A1 and A2 pulleys.

Hand therapy for tenosynovectomy. Early active and passive motion is vital if flexor tendon glide is to be restored. It is important for the surgeon to convey to the therapist the state of the tendons at the time of surgery. Greater care with the exercise programme needs to be taken if the tendons are frayed. The exercise programme includes passive and active motion. Resistance is added at 4–6 weeks or earlier if the tendons are in good condition. Isolated FDS and FDP exercises as well as tendon gliding exercises are necessary.

The digital pulley status also alters the therapy programme. If the pulleys are attenuated or frayed, they must be supported during exercises. Pulley supports include simple taping, manual pressure, ring splints made of various materials and jewellery rings. Pulley support may be necessary for several months. The flexor retinaculum is the pulley at the wrist level. Following carpal tunnel release, strong gripping in wrist flexion should be avoided, as this places undue stress on the healing retinaculum and may cause volar displacement of the flexor tendon at this level.

Surgery for the thumb in rheumatoid arthritis

Thumb stability is essential for good thumb function. There are numerous splints that address thumb instability and deformities, including the hand-based thumb splint made of thermoplastic or fabric such as neoprene, three-point stabilising splints and splints that are forearm based. Splinting plays a major part in improving stability following surgery.

Synovectomy

Synovectomy can be carried out with respect to the interphalangeal or metacarpophalangeal joint of the thumb along the same principles as for the MP and PIP joint of the fingers.

Hand therapy. MP joint stability is extremely important for effective pinch grip. Following synovectomy, joint stability with some joint motion is the goal of therapy. Full-time splintage for 6 weeks may be necessary. Active exercises may not be commenced until 4 weeks post-surgery if motion is reasonable (30–40 degrees) at 2 weeks when the sutures are removed.

The MP joint

Type I – Flexion deformity of the MP joint. Where the flexion deformity is reversible and the joint surfaces intact, an MP joint capsulodesis and extensor hood reconstruction is carried out (Fig. 4.40). Splinting following MP joint capsulodesis and . extensor hood reconstruction for buttonhole deformity requires the MP joint to be maintained in extension. Attention to early IP joint flexion in terms of both active and passive exercise is necessary.

Type II and Type IV deformities. These deformities are due to disease at the CMC joint and adduction of the metacarpal. Treatment needs to be at the CMC joint level.

Type III – swan-neck deformity. Thumb swan-neck deformity is treated by volar plate tenodesis, sesamoid arthrodesis or MP joint arthrodesis. Splinting following MP volar plate tenodesis or sesamoidesis requires flexion of approximately 25 degrees. Restoration of IP motion is usually not difficult.

Occasionally, MP joint arthroplasty is needed where there is severe disease of the CMC joint. The largest silicone implant is used to fit the joint space, aiming at stability rather than movement.

The TMC (CMC) joint of the thumb

Because of the potential associated disease and deformity and destruction of the MP and IP joints, arthrodesis of the TMC joint is rarely feasible. Therefore, one is left with trapeziectomy and ligament reconstruction or implant arthroplasty (see TMC joint in osteoarthritis).

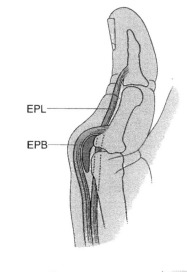

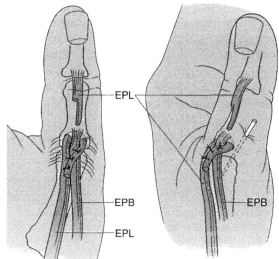

Figure 4.40 Capsulodesis and extensor hood reconstruction for type I deformity. EPB = extensor pollicis brevis, EPL = extensor pollicis longus.

MISCELLANEOUS PROCEDURES FOR THE RHEUMATOID HAND

Peripheral nerve decompression

The three major nerves of the hand and upper limb – the median, ulnar and radial nerves – are more liable to compression in their various tunnel situations where there is associated joint and tendon synovitis (see Chapter 7C). When surgical decompression is indicated, the tunnel is decompressed and the synovial bulk is removed from the associated joint and tendon.

Tendon decompression

Trigger finger, trigger thumb and de Quervain's condition are more common in patients with rheumatoid synovitis. Decompression of these tendons is often indicated (see Chapter 2F).

Rheumatoid nodules and bursae

Rheumatoid nodules and bursae can be large and multiple, functionally disabling and cosmetically unacceptable. They can be removed surgically. *Dorsal nodules* usually occur in the loose skin over the digital joints and are readily removed. *Palmar nodules* can be intimately related to the digital neurovascular bundles in the finger and in the distal pulp. Dissection can be difficult. Damage to the neurovascular structures is a risk. *Rheumatoid bursae* can occur over any joint. The olecranon is a common site. To prevent

recurrence, all the synovia of the bursae must be removed.

Gentle handling of the skin, drainage of the wound and an occlusive compression dressing for 7–10 days is necessary to avoid fluid collection, seroma, haematoma and wound problems. Immobilise the elbow for at least 10 days. Nodules and bursae can recur after resection.

Juvenile arthritis (Still's disease)

The disease itself causes growth arrest. It is important that drug management and surgery do not add to that arrest of growth. Non-operative splintage and rest of inflamed joints and tendons should alternate with gentle mobilising exercises of joints and tendons (see conservative management in this chapter).

Before epiphyseal closure, surgery may be necessary in the form of resection of tendon nodules and tenosynovectomy and, occasionally, joint synovectomy. After the epiphyses are closed, the standard rheumatoid procedures, e.g. joint fusion and replacement, may be indicated.

REFERENCES

1. Nalebuff EA: Diagnosis, classification and management of rheumatoid thumb deformities. Bull Hosp Joint Dis 29:119, 1968.
2. Jebson R, Taylor N, Trieschmann R et al: An objective and standardized test of hand function. Arch Phys Med Rehab 50:311, 1969.
3. Jacobson-Sollerman C, Sperling L: Grip function of the healthy hand in a standardized hand function test. Scan J Rehab Med 9:123–9, 1977.
4. Philips C: Therapists management of patients with rheumatoid arthritis. In: Hunter J, Mackin E, Callahan A (eds), Rehabilitation of the hand: surgery and therapy. St Louis: Mosby, 1995:1345–50.
5. Leonard J: Joint protection for inflammatory disorders. In: Hunter J, Mackin E, Callahan A (eds), Rehabilitation

of the hand: surgery and therapy. St Louis: Mosby, 1995: 1377–83.
6. Colditz J: Arthritis. In: Malick M, Kash M (eds), Manual on management of specific hand problems. Pittsburgh: AREN, 1984.
7. Souter WA: Planning treatment of the rheumatoid hand. Hand 11:3, 1979.
8. Kapandji IA: The Kapandji–Sauve procedure. J Hand Surg 17B:125–6, 1992.
9. Bowers WH: Arthroplasty of the distal radioulnar joint. Curr Conc Clin Orthop 275:104–9, 1992.
10. Chamay A, Della Santa D, Vilaseca A: Radiolunate arthrodesis, factor of stability for the rheumatoid wrist. Ann Chir Main 2:5, 1983.

5

The elbow

A. FUNCTIONAL ANATOMY AND CLINICAL ASSESSMENT

Jeff Hughes and Maureen Williams

INTRODUCTION

The elbow is part of an upper limb complex of articulations, the function of which is to place the hand in space. These articulations include the humeroulnar, radiocapitellar, proximal and distal radioulnar joints, and the middle radioulnar union (interosseous membrane and oblique cord).

The humeroulnar joint is a modified hinge allowing flexion/extension and a small degree of internal and external rotation. The axis of rotation of the elbow approximates a line from the anterior inferior aspect of the medial epicondyle through to the lateral epicondyle. The normal elbow extends straight to 0 degrees and flexes to 140 degrees (±10 degrees). Normal supination is 85 degrees and pronation is 75 degrees. Studies of normal elbow movement demonstrate that the functional range is between 30 and 130 degrees of flexion, and between 50 degrees of pronation and 50 degrees of supination.[1]

STABILITY

Stability of the elbow joint is provided by the congruent bony articulation, ligament complexes and the compressive forces provided by the triceps, forearm flexor and extensor muscles, brachialis

Table 5.1 Percentage contribution of stabilising structure

Elbow position	Stabiliser	Varus force	Valgus force
Extension	MCL	–	31
	LCL	14	–
	Capsule	32	38
	Articulation	55	31
Flexion (90°)	MCL	–	54
	LCL	9	–
	Capsule	13	10
	Articulation	75	33

LCL = lateral collateral ligament, MCL = medial collateral ligament.

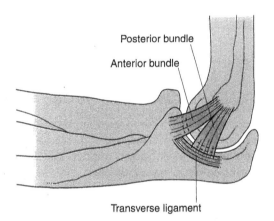

Figure 5.1 The medial collateral ligament complex is made up of the anterior, posterior bundles and the transverse ligament. The main valgus stabiliser of the elbow is the anterior bundle.

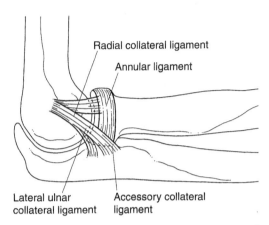

Figure 5.2 The lateral collateral ligament is made up of the radial collateral ligament, the annular ligament and the accessory collateral ligament.

and biceps. The various contributions these structures provide in various degrees of flexion/extension has been determined.[2]

The medial collateral ligament (MCL) complex (Fig. 5.1) has an anterior and posterior bundle (joined by a transverse ligament); both arise on the humerus posterior to the axis of rotation of the elbow and thus the tension varies with elbow flexion. The anterior bundle inserts into the medial coronoid process. The *anterior bundle is the primary valgus stabiliser of the elbow* and the radial head is a secondary stabiliser.

The lateral collateral ligament (LCL) complex (Fig. 5.2) is made up of the radial collateral ligament (RCL), the lateral ulnar collateral ligament (LUCL) and the annular ligament. The RCL and

LUCL arise from the lateral epicondyle (axis of rotation). The RCL inserts into the annular ligament. The *LUCL* inserts into the tubercle of the supinator crest, distal to the annular ligament and is *the primary lateral stabiliser of the humeroulnar joint* and, if deficient, results in posterolateral rotatory instability of the elbow.[3]

Radial head stability

The annular ligament is attached at the anterior and posterior margins of the radial notch and, in combination, encircles the radial head and stabilises the head against the ulna. It has no attachment to the radial head. It provides no stability to proximal migration of the radius.

Longitudinal stability

The position of the elbow and forearm and muscle action determines the extent of longitudinal load that is transferred through the radial head. In elbow extension, static compression results in the radial head transmitting approximately 60% of the axial load. If the radial head is excised, then the central band of the interosseous membrane (IOM) transmits 70–85% of the axial load from the radius to the ulna.[4] Thus, in the absence of a radial head, the IOM is the main longitudinal stabiliser of the forearm preventing acute longitudinal radio-ulnar dissociation (ALRUD or Essex–Lopresti lesion).

CLINICAL ASSESSMENT

Clinical examination of the elbow should be systematic. As the joint is subcutaneous to a large extent, it lends itself to inspection and palpation. The anterior and lateral aspects are easily inspected for bony and soft tissue landmarks, including the lateral epicondyle, common extensor origin, radial head, lateral collateral ligament, radial tunnel, triceps, olecranon, olecranon fossa, ulna nerve, medial epicondyle and common flexor origin. The posterior and medial aspects are examined with the patient lying supine and the arm fully elevated overhead. In addition, instability and stress manoeuvres can also be performed in this position. The clinical assessment of entrapment and tendonopathies are covered in other sections.

Clinical examination should include assessment of range of movement, deformity, joint swelling, joint congruency or crepitus, joint and skeletal stability, neurological deficit and musculotendinous integrity.

Range of movement

Range of movement can be measured in a highly reproducible manner, with a goniometer. With both forearms supinated the extremes of active and passive flexion and extension are demonstrated. The normal elbow extends straight to 0 degrees and flexes to 140 degrees ($\pm$10 degrees). Hyperextension is recorded as a negative integer. If hyperextension is greater than 10 degrees, it suggests hypermobility or periarticular deformity. A loss of full extension is often the earliest sign of an intra-articular elbow problem. Both sides should be compared. Even subtle unilateral loss of range is significant.

Forearm rotation is demonstrated by flexing both elbows to 90 degrees, while adducting the arms to the body to block any compensatory shoulder movements. Passive and active rotation of the distal radius and ulna is then assessed and any associated crepitus noted. Supination is generally greater than pronation. Where pronation or supination is abnormal, the other joints of both upper limbs should be assessed. The functional significance of any reduction of range is dependent on the normality or otherwise of adjacent joints.

Angular deformity

The normal carrying angle varies with gender, averaging 10 degrees valgus for males and 13 degrees valgus for females. The angle can only be adequately assessed with the elbow in full extension. A flexion deformity may hide angulatory pathology, and hyperextension may give the impression of deformity.

Rotational deformity

Rotational deformity is often overlooked. If both shoulder joints are normal, asymmetrical ranges of rotation indicate humeral rotational deformity. This is assessed by standing behind the patient with the elbow at 90 degrees and the forearm behind their back. The patient bends forward with the shoulder held in full extension; each shoulder is maximally internally rotated. Increased internal rotation is measured as the angle between the forearm and the horizon of the back. There is frequently an increase in internal rotation associated with malunited supracondylar fractures.

Forearm length and radioulnar dissociation

Radial head pathology, including resection, subluxation and dislocation, may be associated with radioulnar dissociation. In the acute setting, with failure of the radial head, the line of injury may pass through the radiocapitellar joint, along the IOM to the distal radioulnar joint (DRUJ). As well as the obvious elbow injury (e.g. radial head fracture or dislocation), the DRUJ should be assessed.

If signs of DRUJ derangement occur in the presence of a radial head fracture or dislocation, acute longitudinal radioulnar dissociation (ALRUD) should be suspected. Mehloff has described a 'push–pull' manoeuvre, using X-rays to quantify the degree of longitudinal instability of the radius. Early diagnosis of this condition allows early treatment, and this improves the prognosis.

Secondary changes in the forearm bones occur if this problem arises prior to the cessation of skeletal growth. By placing the ulnar borders of both forearms together, the relative lengths of the foreams can be assessed.

Strength

There are four basic tests to assess strength about the elbow. This assessment is only a gross estimate and at present quantitative assessment is usually undertaken at a research level.

Flexion is tested with the elbow flexed to 90 degrees and the forearm in neutral rotation. Flexion is then resisted. At the same time, the biceps tendon should be observed for any loss of continuity. Extension is tested in a similar position, but in the reverse direction. If extension is very weak, then gravity should be excluded or the arm placed overhead and extension tested against gravity. Normally flexion is stronger than extension in the normal limb.

Testing forearm rotation is performed with the elbow flexed to 90 degrees and commencing in neutral rotation. Pronation and supination is resisted by fixing the forearm at the wrist. Normally, supination is slightly stronger than pronation.

Haemarthrosis and joint effusion

The position of maximal joint volume is 80 degrees of flexion. If a tense effusion or haemarthrosis is present, such as following an intra-articular fracture, the elbow will assume this position, to minimise discomfort. If the capsule has been breached, however, intra-articular pressure is released, haematoma and swelling are apparent and the range of comfortable movement is paradoxically increased. A small elbow joint effusion is identified by a loss of the sulcus of the infracondylar recess. The recess is sited distal to the lateral condyle, adjacent to the lateral aspect of the olecranon and the radial head.

Synovitis

Mild synovitis may be palpated in the infracondylar recess laterally. If the synovitis is extensive (e.g. inflammatory arthropathies), the proliferative synovium may track beneath the annular ligament and extend along the radial neck and interosseous membrane. It may occasionally produce a posterior interosseous nerve lesion and a soft tissue forearm mass. The same process can produce a large antecubital cyst or become intraosseous, resulting in loss of bone stock.

Erosive arthropathy frequently results in instability. It is usually due to loss of bony architecture and is thus associated with joint crepitus.

Bony impingement

To elicit impingement, the end point of elbow flexion or extension should be noted. A gentle push beyond that end point reproduces the symptoms.

Impingement of the olecranon process occurs in a variety of settings, including instability, osteoarthritis and following hyperextension injury (acute and chronic). In valgus instability, the impingement is generally posteromedial. Osteophytic encroachment of the olecranon fossa produces impingement wherever the osteophytes meet. Loose bodies may produce a similar result. To demonstrate posteromedial impingement a slight valgus load should be added to the extension force. Occasionally, loose bodies may be palpated, anteriorly or posteriorly.

Anterior impingement of the elbow occurs between an enlarged coronoid process and the obliterated coronoid fossa. Occasionally, the small radial fossa superior to the anterior aspect of the capitellum may fill with osteophytes, and impingement may occur with the radial head, in full flexion. The differentiation between anterior coronoid impingement and anterior radial head impingement is clinically very difficult and is best made radiologically.

Articular abnormalities involving the humeroulnar/radiocapitellar compartments

Diffuse anterior or posterior compartment osteophytosis as a result of osteoarthritis produces progressive loss of movement. Initially there is loss of full extension, due to both bony block, and also secondary capsular fibrosis. Pain in the mid-range of elbow movement is a late sign of osteoarthritis and is usually of an aching character. Multiple loose bodies suggest a diagnosis of synovial osteochondromatosis or, if the elbow is grossly deranged, a neuropathic joint.

Assessment of the articular surfaces is enhanced by considering the medial and lateral compartments separately. It is usually possible to clinically distinguish between radiocapitellar and humero-ulnar symptoms. When radiology shows diffuse pathology, it is important to determine which compartment, lateral or medial, is responsible for symptoms. If the symptoms are localised, significant benefit may be achieved by minor surgical intervention, which may avoid or postpone a major reconstruction; thus, the good relief of pain obtained with transhumeral ulna–humeral arthroplasty for elbow osteoarthritis.

Radiocapitellar joint

Valgus stress testing can provoke radiocapitellar symptoms. The site and extent of pathology can be assessed by the arc of crepitus on flexion extension. If the patient 'makes a fist', this increases the compressive force across the radiocapitellar joint. If this manoeuvre increases pain or crepitus, it indicates radiocapitellar symptoms. There may be tenderness along the joint line, and the anterior and posterior aspects of the capitellum may be palpated with the elbow extended and flexed, respectively; thus, some radiocapitellar lesions can be palpated.

Humeroulnar joint

Medial compartment (humeroulnar) articular lesions may be assessed by noting pain and crepitus throughout flexion and extension, particularly when performed against resistance in the plane of the arm/forearm. This may be achieved by asking the patient to hold a light weight in the hand while flexing and extending the elbow. The increased load increases the forces across the joint, compressing the surfaces. Gross loss of bony architecture can produce 'pseudo instability' in

the presence of intact collateral ligaments (e.g. rheumatoid disease).

Selective injection to differentiate diagnoses

Selective injections of local anaesthetic to specific sites about the elbow may be a useful diagnostic manoeuvre. Generally, the first step is to define the problem as either intra- or extra-articular. The elbow joint is most reliably aspirated and injected at the 'soft spot' (infracondylar recess), with the elbow flexed to 90 degrees. Small volumes (about 1–3 ml) of lignocaine (lidocaine) are necessary, to avoid diffusion and more distant anaesthetic effects. Accurate injection is essential.

The lateral aspect of the elbow has well-defined bony landmarks, and lends itself readily to these techniques. Accurate placement is more difficult anteriorly and anteromedially. To allow precision and to avoid the important vascular structures it is often helpful to use computed tomography (CT) or plain X-ray control (e.g. partial distal biceps rupture). The commonest use for this technique is in assessing lateral elbow pain.

Clinical settings in which injection techniques may be valuable are

1. Differentiating lateral elbow pain:
   - lateral epicondylitis
   - revision lateral release
   - posterior interosseous nerve entrapment
   - lateral cutaneous nerve of the forearm entrapment.
2. Other conditions:
   - radial tuberosity bursitis/partial biceps tendon tear
   - brachialis fasciitis
   - partial triceps avulsion
   - wound neuromas
   - differentiating extra- or intra-articular problems.

Functional assessment scores

American shoulder and elbow score is given in the Appendix 1 (p. 357).

Diagnostic imaging

The complex and highly constrained shape of the elbow makes plain X-ray assessment difficult. The importance of obtaining a true lateral cannot be emphasised enough. Anteroposterior (AP) views of the elbow with varus and valgus stress if demonstrating an increase of greater than 3 mm of joint space widening suggest instability. Oblique views of the radial head are helpful in assessing radial head pathology. The soft tissue planes are important in assessing the joint for an effusion/haemarthrosis or tendinous disruption. In the acute setting, if ALRUD is suspected, AP views of the whole forearm with axial traction and compression may be diagnostic.

Conventional tomography provides an easy form of assessment of joint congruity in the plane of motion, especially if there are metallic implants present. Arthrotomography (air ± contrast) is beneficial if the loose bodies are non-ossified.

CT scan is especially useful for small loose bodies and better definition of the internal architecture of the distal humerus, proximal radius and ulna. Occasionally three-dimensional reconstructions provide better assessment of complex periarticular deformities or fractures (e.g. preoperative assessment for traumatic proximal synostosis releases or complex osteotomies).

Ultrasound is useful for assessing the common flexor or extensor origins (e.g. epicondylitis or epicondyle avulsions) or epicondyle or condylar injuries in the growing skeleton. In addition, joint ganglions, effusions and synovitis are detectable. In the preoperative patient when planning a

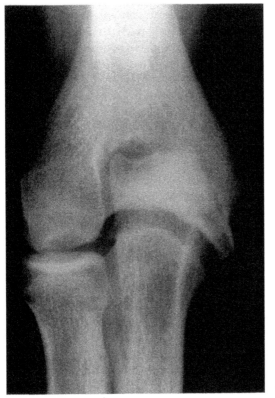

A

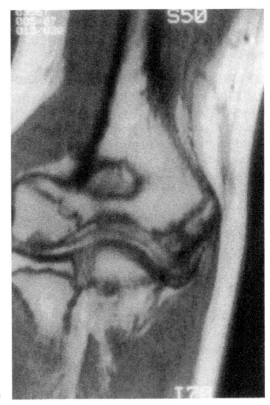

B

Figure 5.3 This 15-year-old boy sustained a supracondylar fracture of the distal humerus at age 6. He presented with activity related elbow pain and a flexion contracture. A: Plain X-ray demonstrates the 'fish-tail' deformity secondary to injury of the nutrient vessel to the trochlea. Note the associated osteochondritis dissecans (OCD) of the capitellum.
B: MRI demonstrates the abnormal architecture of the distal humeral epiphysis, the abnormal humeral articular surface, the OCD lesion of the capitellum and the sparing of the radius and ulna.

revision procedure (with the appropriate trans-ducers), the ulnar nerve can be mapped out for the surgeon to demonstrate its altered anatomical relationships or instability.

Magnetic resonance imaging (MRI) for the elbow is still being evaluated, but has a limited place. It is useful in the evaluation of ligament and tendon disruptions (especially partial lesions), osteochondral impaction injuries, avascular necrosis, partial and complete tendon disruptions and soft tissue lesions/masses (Fig. 5.3).[5]

Diagnostic elbow arthroscopy most frequently provides additional information for decision making, such as evaluating various chondral lesions, the synovium and subtle instabilities. It rarely provides a diagnosis in isolation of other findings.

REFERENCES

1. Morrey BF, Askew LJ, An KN, Chao EY: A biomechanical study of normal functional elbow motion.
2. Morrey BF, An KN: Articular and ligamentous contributions to the stability of the elbow joint. Am J Sports Med 11:315–19, 1983.
3. O'Driscoll SW, Morrey BF, Korinek S et al: Elbow subluxation and dislocation: a spectrum of instability. Clin Orth 280:17–28, 1992.
4. Hotchkiss RN, An KN, Sowa DT, Basta S, Weiland AJ: Pathomechanics of the proximal migration of the radius: an anatomic and biomechanical study. J Hand Surg 14:256–61, 1989.
5. Fritz RC, Steinbach LS: Magnetic resonance imaging of the muskuloskeletal system: part 3: the elbow. Clin Orthopaed Rel Res 324:321–39, 1996.

B. ELBOW TRAUMA

Jeff Hughes and Maureen Williams

ELBOW DISLOCATION AND INSTABILITY

A classification of elbow instability is given in Table 5.2.

Acute elbow dislocations usually result from a fall on to an outstretched hand. With simple dislocations the soft tissue lesion is extensive and usually involves disruption of the capsule, MCL, LCL, common flexor and extensor origins, brachialis and often a chondral injury to the trochlear, a 'shear' fracture (*not* avulsion as there are no soft tissue attachments to the tip of the coronoid) of a small flake of coronoid process and an impaction injury of the rim of the radial head and posterior capitellum.

The understanding of elbow instability is evolving. O'Driscoll and co-workers have presented a concept of elbow instability as a circle of soft tissue injury from lateral to medial, occurring in

Table 5.2 Classification of elbow instability

Acute
Simple (no associated fracture)
    Dislocation
    Subluxation ('perched dislocation')
Complex
    Fracture/dislocations (instability associated with fractures)

Chronic
Unreduced
Recurrent (dislocation/subluxation)
    Posterolateral rotatory
    Valgus
    Varus

three stages. This approach allows an appreciation of the different instabilities produced by various combinations of ligament injuries (Fig. 5.4).[1]

ASSESSMENT OF ELBOW INSTABILITY

Posterolateral rotatory instability (PLRI)

The lateral ulnar ligament (part of the LCL complex) is the primary posterolateral stabiliser.

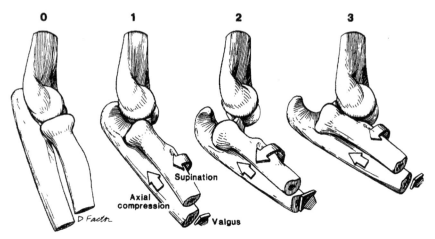

Figure 5.4 Elbow instability is a spectrum from subluxation to dislocation. The three stages illustrated correspond with the pathoanatomic stages of capsulo-ligamentous disruption. Forces and moments responsible for displacements are illustrated. 0, reduced; 1, posterolateral rotatory instability (PLRI); 2, perched; 3, dislocated. (Reproduced with permission from O'Driscoll et al.[1])

PLRI of the elbow is clinically demonstrated with the *lateral pivot shift test*.[2] The patient lies supine with the arm overhead. A combination of axial compression, as well as valgus and supination moments are applied to rotate and subluxate the humeroulnar joint. Maintain these forces from a fully extended position. When the elbow flexes past a certain point (usually 30–60 degrees), it reduces with a palpable clunk. Most people, however, demonstrate marked apprehension before allowing this degree of subluxation. This test is more dramatic and sensitive if performed as part of an examination under anaesthetic with fluoroscopic control.

A more subtle method of demonstrating PLRI is to position the patient as above, hold the elbow flexed at 90 degrees and fully supinate the forearm with no flex/extension of the elbow. A sulcus develops at the lateral joint line of the sigmoid fossa as the ulna rotates and lifts off the distal humerus, drawing the soft tissues into the opening joint space.

A plain X-ray may demonstrate an enlocated joint, but the presence of the 'telltale' shear fracture of the coronoid process in an 'elbow strain' suggests a 'perched dislocation' has occurred, which has then self-reduced.

Valgus instability

Valgus instability is due to anterior bundle MCL deficiency. The radial head is the main secondary valgus stabiliser of the elbow. Valgus stability is assessed with the trunk of the patient fixed and the shoulder maximally externally rotated. The elbow is flexed to 25 degrees to unlock the olecranon from the olecranon fossa and minimise the contribution of bony congruity to stability. As a valgus force is applied, the MCL is palpated and local tenderness and laxity noted.[3] This same manoeuvre is much more sensitive under X-ray control.

To distinguish between valgus instability and PRLI, the valgus stress test should be performed with the forearm pronated as this manoeuvre will obliterate any posterolateral instability, and allow the distinction to be made.

Varus instability

The RCL (part of the LCL complex) is the main varus stabiliser of the elbow. It is demonstrated by fully internally rotating the glenohumeral joint and flexing the elbow joint 30 degrees to unlock the olecranon. A varus stress is applied to the elbow, and any opening of the lateral joint space noted. The degree of laxity is best quantitated with X-ray control.

Management of acute simple dislocations

Posterior displaced elbow dislocations are best reduced with the muscles relaxed (under general anaesthetic). The elbow is held flexed at 30–40 degrees with the forearm supinated to allow the coronoid to pass forwards without injury to the trochlea chondral surface. With gentle longitudinal traction on the forearm, the olecranon is 'thumbed' distally and the elbow flexed up.

Ideally an assessment of the PLRI, valgus and varus instability under image intensifier is then undertaken. The stable range of passive flexion/extension with no valgus/varus stress is then identified and documented.

In most patients following reduction, there is a congruent stable arc of movement. In the initial rehabilitative phase there is mild instability of the joint, especially in full extension. If the patient is totally immobilised for 2–4 weeks, a post-traumatic stiff elbow can result.[4]

Early assisted/active mobilisation (without loading or stressing the joint) has reduced the incidence of stiffness and resulted in no increased instability.[5] This can be achieved by fitting an adjustable hinged splint and dialling in the 'safe' flexion/extension range at few days post-injury. Assisted active movements are commenced within a few days, along with elevation, ice and compression to reduce swelling. A full range of movement is allowed at 2–4 weeks. Protected motion is continued for 6 weeks. If at this stage there is a lack of full ROM, then a splinting programme, as per post-traumatic stiffness, is commenced (see below).

If the elbow is only stable with the forearm in full pronation (gross PLRI), then a cast brace with the forearm *fully* pronated is applied and full movements encouraged. This is applied for 3–6 weeks and then removed, and the extremes of flexion/extension obtained.

If the elbow is unstable, even with elbow flexed 60 degrees or in extremes of forearm rotation, this is an indication to undertake primary open surgical repair and/or apply a hinged elbow distraction device. Again, immediate mobilisation is commenced postoperatively. If a distractor is required, an axillary catheter for analgesia will be required to obtain early movement. The distractor is left *in situ* for 4–6 weeks.

COMPLEX FRACTURE/DISLOCATIONS

Dislocations with associated fractures often results in a poorer outcome. Commonly associated fractures include radial head, coronoid and olecranon fractures. The principle of management is immediate skeletal stabilisation and early joint mobilisation. The management of the individual fractures is outlined below.

COMMON ELBOW FRACTURES
Fractures for the distal humerus

Numerous patterns of elbow fractures have been described for the distal humerus. The AO classification has three main categories – A = non-articular, B = partial articular, C = articular – with 27 subtypes. Occasionally, immobilisation for undisplaced fractures is indicated, but is associated with a high incidence of flexion contracture. Displaced fractures, especially fractures involving the articular surface, are best treated with ORIF (Fig. 5.5); otherwise, post-traumatic osteoarthritis results in pain and stiffness. Frequently, tomography is required to define the extent of joint involvement. Anatomical reduction of the joint surface is mandatory.

The postoperative care is directed at preserving the reduction until union is established. Aggressive active mobilisation is avoided until 6–8 weeks. If early mobilisation risks the reduction, and if normal bony architecture has been achieved, then a staged soft tissue surgical release of contracture can reliably restore a functional range of movement.

Complications of these fractures include avascular necrosis (AVN) and non-union, heterotopic ossification, post-traumatic osteoarthritis and

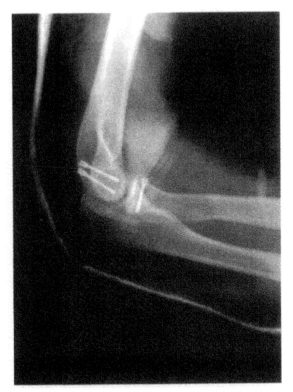

Figure 5.5 Intra-articular fractures usually require accurate ORIF to obtain good pain-free functional movement. This patient sustained a displaced fracture of the radial head and the capitellum, which were fixed with Herbert screws.

ulnar neuropathy. In the young patient, salvage options include distraction (±interposition) arthroplasty, elbow arthrodesis or revision osteotomy and bone graft. In the elderly patients, a semiconstrained arthroplasty restores good function in both the primary and salvage situation.

Coronoid fractures

Coronoid fractures have been classified into three types:[6]

- type I: shear fracture of the tip of the coronoid
- type II: less than 50% of the coronoid process involved
- type III: more than 50% of the coronoid process involved.

Type I fractures are treated as per a simple dislocation; however, occasionally delayed arthroscopic debridement of a prominent malunited coronoid fragment is required to prevent painful impingement in full flexion.

Occasionally, type II and usually type III result in gross elbow instability on the basis of loss of joint and ligament integrity and, if left unreduced, result in very poor outcomes. They are therefore managed by early ORIF or, if the soft tissues do not allow, application of a hinged elbow distractor. Again, early mobilisation is commenced postoperatively, as outlined previously.

These fractures have a high incidence of post-traumatic flexion contracture (even type I) and once stability is established a turnbuckle/extension splint regime may be required.

Radial head fractures

Radial head fractures can be classified into:

- type I: undisplaced fracture
- type II: fractures involving 30% radial head fractures with minimal displacement, angulation or depression
- type III: comminuted fractures of the head – (note: types I–III are not associated with elbow dislocation)
- type IV: dislocation of the elbow and MCL (±LCL) insufficiency in association with any of the above types.

Treatment of type I involves early mobilisation only (±aspiration of the haematoma for patient comfort); type II requires early ORIF and early mobilisation; and for type III early or delayed excision[7] has been advocated.

With type IV the fracture is treated on its merits as above; however, the MCL insufficiency is managed with a hinged splint to protect against valgus instability. Rarely, this fracture is associated with an IOM tear, which extends into the DRUJ (ALRUD). If this is suspected, all attempts to salvage the radial head are undertaken as no adequate salvage procedures exist for ALRUD following early or delayed radial head excision (Fig. 5.6). Reduction and temporary cross-pinning of the DRUJ in supination may be indicated for 3 weeks.[8]

Olecranon fractures

Early mobilisation is only possible if ORIF is performed. The commonest technique is tension

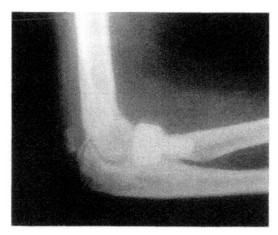

Figure 5.6 Radial head replacement. This patient sustained a grossly comminuted radial head fracture which was not able to be reconstructed. The distal radioulnar joint was noted to be unstable as well; thus, an occult ALRUD was suspected and a radial head replacement undertaken to prevent proximal migration of the radius.

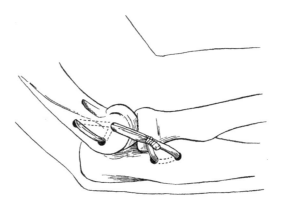

Figure 5.7 Lateral collateral ligament reconstruction using palmarus longus graft.

band wire fixation; however, more distal or complex fracture patterns may require a neutralisation plate. Once provisional wound healing has been achieved, early mobilisation out of a splint/sling is undertaken with no resisted triceps for at least 4–6 weeks.

CHRONIC INSTABILITY

Chronic unreduced dislocations

The clinical results of missed dislocations are variable. In some situations the elbow dislocation is accepted or if pain and loss of function are significant, then open reduction is indicated despite the potential for significant complications. The procedure frequently involves an anterior and posterior capsulectomy, MCL slide of the humerus, LCL repair and application of a hinged distractor device for approx 4–6 weeks. Immediate postoperative mobilisation as for a post-traumatic stiff elbow (see below) is the basis to restoring a 'functional ROM'.

Reconstruction for posterolateral rotatory instability (PLRI)[9]

PLRI instability should be considered if there has been a history of trauma (sprain or full dislocation), recurrent locking or clunking, generalised ligamentous laxity or if following a lateral elbow surgical procedure. It is not uncommon to have a post-traumatic stiff elbow in association with PLRI!

Reconstruction is indicated when there is symptomatic chronic instability. Most instability is intermittent in nature; however, a chronically subluxed joint has persistent pain. No strengthening or conservative therapy programme other than avoidance of precipitating activities or splinting (occasionally taping) the arm into full pronation is effective in reducing the instability symptoms. Reconstruction is contraindicated in the skeletally immature elbow.

The procedure involves insertion of a tendon graft (usually palmaris longus) (Fig. 5.7) through bone holes on the ulna (at the insertion of the annular ligament and on the supinator crest), to the isometric point on the lateral epicondyle, thus reconstructing the humeroulnar part of the LCL. At the same time, the lateral capsule is reefed and imbricated with a resorbable suture passed through the same drill holes to further splint the repair. Occasionally, primary repair only is indicated without the need for a tendon graft.

Postoperatively, the elbow is immobilised at 90 degrees and full pronation in a splint for 3 weeks; then a hinged splint with 30-degree extension block for 6–9 weeks or longer (depending on the degree of ligamentous laxity). A guide to the patient's tendency to develop contractures can be obtained from their response to immobilisation of the elbow on previous occasions. Light activities are allowed for further 3 months. As this is a static stabilising procedure, strengthening will not augment stability, but will only assist with restoration of function. Return to sports is allowed at 6 months.

Ongoing pain and flexion contracture is seen in some patients, especially those having had numerous procedures. A non-isometric reconstruction may be associated with restriction of elbow flexion.

Valgus instability reconstruction[10]

Many patients tolerate valgus instability to a significant degree; however, high-grade athletes undertaking throwing or raquet sports or valgus instability producing ulnar nerve symptoms may require reconstruction. Primary MCL repair is occasionally achievable in the acute presentation; however, most chronic instabilities require a tendon graft (palmarus longus). At the time of repair, all heterotopic calcification is excised; the tendon graft is sited to reproduce the anterior bundle of the MCL. The ulnar nerve is transposed if ulnar nerve symptoms are present.

Postoperatively, the elbow is immobilised at 90 degrees in neutral rotation in a locked hinged splint for 2 weeks; then full ROM as tolerated within a protective hinged splint for a further 6 weeks. At 3–4 months, gentle throwing is allowed, which is gradually upgraded, such that by 1 year full activities are allowed.

REFERENCES

1. O'Driscoll, Morrey BF, Korinek S et al: Elbow subluxation and dislocation: a spectrum of instability. Clin Orth 280:17–28, 1992.
2. O'Driscoll SW, Bell DF, Morrey BF: Posterolateral rotatory instability of the elbow. J Bone Joint Surg 73A:441, 1991.
3. Jobe FW, Start H, Lombardo SF: Reconstruction of the ulnar collateral ligament in athletes. J Bone Joint Surg 68A:1158, 1986.
4. Mehloff TL, Noble PC, Bennett JB, Tullos HS: Simple dislocation of the elbow in the adult. J Bone Joint Surg 70A:244, 1988.
5. Josefsson P, Gentz C, Johnell O et al: Surgical vs nonsurgical treatment of ligamentous injuries following dislocation of the elbow. J Bone Joint Surg 69A:605, 1987.
6. Regan W, Morrey B: Fractures of the coronoid process of the ulna. J Bone Joint Surg 71A:1348–54, 1989.
7. Broberg MA, Morrey BF: Results of delayed excision of the radial head after fracture. J Bone Joint Surg 68A:669–74, 1986.
8. Hotchkiss RN, Green DP: Fractures and dislocations of the elbow. In: Rockwood, Green (eds), Fractures in adults, 3rd edn, 1991.
9. O'Driscoll SW, Morrey B: Surgical reconstruction of the lateral collateral ligament. In: Morrey B (ed.), Master techniques in orthopaedic surgery – the elbow. New York: Raven Press, 1994.
10. Jobe FW, El Attrache NS: Treatment of ulnar collateral ligament injuries. In: Morrey B (ed.), Master techniques in orthopaedic surgery – the elbow. New York: Raven Press, 1994.

C. THE STIFF ELBOW

Jeff Hughes and Maureen Williams

PRINCIPLES OF PREVENTING POST-TRAUMATIC/POSTOPERATIVE ELBOW STIFFNESS

- Control of inflammation/oedema
- Adequate analgesia
- Restore functional range of movement (ROM)
- Restore strength and maintain ROM.

The elbow is frequently associated with the development of post-traumatic contracture due to multiple factors (propensity for the anterior and posterior capsule to become fibrosed and shorten, the collateral ligaments calcify and the formation of heterotopic ossification). The causes maybe classified into intra- and/or extra-articular. The classification given in Table 5.3 helps determine the approach to the restoration of elbow movement. Pain is usually not a prominent feature of post-traumatic stiff elbows. If present, then an intrinsic joint problem should be excluded.

Table 5.3 Classification of post-traumatic stiff elbow

Extra-articular:
    capsular fibrosis of anterior capsule and collateral
    ligaments
    heterotopic calcification
Intrinsic:
    intra-articular adhesions
    articular cartilage loss
    joint incongruity (gross joint trauma, malunion) (Morrey)[4]

Note: All intrinsic contractures are associated with some
form of extrinsic contracture.

PREVENTION

Not all post-traumatic contractures are prevent-
able; however, a number of simple measures are
associated with better outcomes following trauma.
Following an acute injury, the initial problem
is usually joint or bony instability; then, by 3–4
weeks it often becomes joint stiffness. Appropriate
splintage allows early *movement* and control of
swelling. This dramatically reduces the flexion
contractures associated with elbow immobilisation
after injury. If a contracture becomes established
and the joint is congruent, then a turnbuckle
programme (see below) can reduce the magni-
tude of the contracture.[1]

The minimal requirements for elbow function
are a *stable skeleton,* a *congruent articulation* and
joint stability (anterior bundle of MCL, LUCL
and annular ligament). If early movement may
compromise fracture fixation, then a period of
immobilisation to allow fracture union to occur,
followed by a staged surgical release, may be
preferable, as the results of surgical release in
patients where bony architecture has been accurately restored are good.

PREVENT HETEROTOPIC CALCIFICATION (Fig. 5.8)

The development of heterotopic ossification
(HO) is often associated with elbow stiffness.[2]
The incidence of heterotopic ossification following
elbow trauma has been reported to occur from
4.5% (Linscheid and Wheeler) to 20%. Other
factors that dramatically increase the incidence

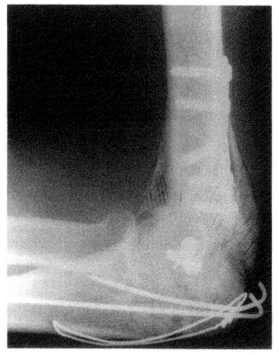

Figure 5.8 This patient sustained a closed head injury in
association with a fracture of the distal humerus, which
required ORIF. Postoperatively, the patient developed a
painless extra-articular bony ankylosis. A surgical removal
of the heterotopic ossification resulted in a full range of
movement.

include neural axis trauma, severe burns and
delayed operative treatment (from approx 3–12
weeks).

Nonsteroidal anti-inflammatory drugs (NSAIDs)
such as indomethacin have yet to be demonstrated to uniformly prevent HO in the elbow.
There is, however, enough anecdotal evidence to
recommend their use at the time of or immediately following injury in high-risk situations for
the prevention of HO. Instituting NSAIDs after
HO has occurred is ineffective.

*Early passive movement does not cause ectopic
bone!* However, if HO is occurring, it will be made
more symptomatic by passive mobilisation. An
appropriate routine is to commence the NSAID
immediately following surgery and continue
for approx 2 to 3 months. A standard dose of
indomethacin of 25 mg three times a day with
meals is used.

Conservative treatment

Recognition of the high-risk injury allows one to determine those patients who should be mobilised ± splinted or managed surgically. Those patients with major intra-articular pathology (e.g. large chondral defects, joint surface incongruity, impingement of surgical implants), severe or established contractures (greater than 6 months) and painful elbows are not candidates for non-operative measures. The principles of splinting and rehabilitation are the same as for the postoperative regimes given below.

Surgical treatment

The indications for surgical release depend upon the needs of the individual. Generally, a total ROM less than 80 degrees, a flexion contracture more than 40 degrees and/or a loss of flexion to only 115 degrees are the indications to consider a surgical release.

Operative treatment

Prior to surgical release an examination under anaesthetic (with image intensifier) is useful, as occasionally there is associated elbow instability present in a stiff elbow. Manipulation under anaesthetic of a post-traumatic stiff elbow is not to be recommended. It has a poor chance of providing increased movement and may result in significant complications (heterotopic bone, inflammation, neurological injury and periarticular fracture).

SURGICAL RELEASE OF THE STIFF ELBOW

Restoration of flexion/extension

The role of arthroscopic capsular release is still to be defined. It appears to be appropriate for moderate flexion contractures with pure anterior capsule pathology. It has been associated with major neurological complications.[3]

Combined loss of flexion and extension usually requires both open anterior and posterior capsulectomy (*not* capsulotomy, as this is associated with a significant recurrence of the contracture).[4] An anterior approach[5] can only address anterior pathology. A lateral approach allows anterior and posterior capsulectomy. A posterior incision with raised skin flaps allows a lateral approach to the anterior and posterior capsule and also allows access to MCL or ulnar nerve pathology. If patients have no intra-articular joint derangement, the prognosis for restoring a functional ROM is good.

The indications for use of an elbow joint distractor (distraction arthroplasty) include loss of greater than 50% of the articular surface of the humeroulnar joint, to maintain stability of a joint following an extensive release, following a significant osteo/chondroplasty of the humeroulnar joint and any interposition graft. The main advantage of a distractor is that it allows early mobilisation of the joint while the tissues heal. A distractor normally allows the elbow to be mobilised from 30 to 120 degrees without undue soft tissue impingement on the pins. An interposition arthroplasty (fascia lata) usually yields a functional elbow, but does not allow unrestricted loads compared to a normal elbow.[4]

Restoration of forearm rotation

The causes of loss of forearm rotation include annular ligament adhesions, malunions of the radial head and neck (camming), proximal radioulnar synostosis, radioulnar malunions, IOM contractures and disruptions of the DRUJ. Restoration of forearm rotation is a complex problem; patients often have multiple causes. Thus, surgery maybe required at a number of levels on the forearm.

With regard to excision of a post-traumatic synostosis, there is a significant recurrence rate, and full preservation of operative ROM is uncommon. Most retain approximately half of the ROM achieved at operation. Dynamic forearm rotation splints are especially good at maintaining this ROM as long as there is very little associated DRUJ pain. If patients have a combined forearm synostosis and restriction of flexion/extension, then the results of combined procedures are poorer.

POSTOPERATIVE CARE OF THE POST-SURGICAL ELBOW

Prevention of infection

Many patients have had multiple procedures and have an increased risk of sepsis. Perioperative infection, if it occurs, will dramatically limit the postoperative mobilisation, so all patients should have prophylactic antibiotics. This can be augmented by a regional venous infusion of cephalosporin when the tourniquet is applied. This results in high bone and soft tissue levels which are maintained for 24 hours.

Wound care/reduce swelling

Good haemostasis is mandatory. The tourniquet should be released at the end of the surgical release, and the surgical field compressed for 15 min to allow the tourniquet hyperaemia to settle. A careful haemostasis should then be performed. Transverse steristrips should be avoided as they produce shearing and blistering of the skin.

A compression dressing is applied, a protective splint fitted if ligament repair was required and the arm elevated. A cold compression cuff is also applied with the cold cycle being applied for 10–15 min every hour. Continuous cold therapy is suboptimal. Thereafter, the elbow is kept elevated at all times. A compression stocking is left on for a minimum of 2 weeks and only removed to perform flexion exercises or change dressings. The suture is removed at 2 weeks. A sequential limb compression pump (e.g., Masman pump) is used to further reduce swelling.

Good analgesia

Good pain relief is essential to achieving a good surgical result, as it allows early mobilisation of the elbow. The most effective pain relief is achieved with continuous axillary sheath infusion of local anaesthetic (bupivacaine). It usually provides a significant partial or complete anaesthesia and motor and sympathetic blockade of the arm distal to the axilla. It can be left *in situ* for 3–5 days. Pain management can be augmented with an intravenous PCA (narcotic) infusion. It allows early mobilisation of the elbow (day 1) for lengthy periods 20–24 hours a day. Following removal of the axillary catheter, regular paracetamol ± codeine is prescribed. An NSAID commenced at the time of surgery for HO prophylaxis also provides additional analgesia.

Early mobilisation/CPM (Fig. 5.9)

Early movement has been shown to reduce the incidence of post-traumatic flexion contracture. Early movement should not compromise any ligament or bone reconstruction; thus, the need to adequately splint the limb and modify the load to the elbow as tissues heal/unite. The range of motion (ROM) achieved at surgery is documented and used as a guide to the ROM to be achieved on the continuous passive movement (CPM) machine. Some situations will not allow the use of a CPM until there has been appropriate healing. Pain and swelling determine how quickly this ROM is achieved; however, maximum ROM is usually achieved within 1–2 days following a surgical release of a stiff elbow. There are a number of CPMs available (some being portable); however, the best movement appears to be achieved with those that take the elbow from full extension to full flexion. Some units combine supination and pronation.

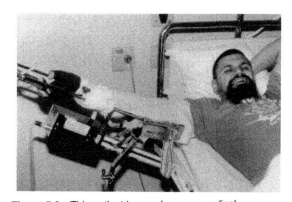

Figure 5.9 This patient has undergone a radical elbow release. An axillary catheter was inserted for postoperative analgesia and to allow early mobilisation on a CPM.

Restoration of function and exercise programme

Following removal of the axillary catheter (3–5 days) and prior to discharge, the patient is encouraged to use the arm with activities of daily living (ADL, e.g. meal times, washing and dressing). This begins the retraining of the whole limb (e.g. with a large flexion contracture the shoulder is often held protracted and this needs to be re-educated). After the application of ultrasound or heat, ROM exercises are taught:

1. Active assisted flexion, extension, supination and pronation. Flexion or extension ROM exercises are best performed at alternate sessions during the day. Pulley exercises are useful adjuncts.
2. Proprioceptive neuromuscular facilitation exercise, i.e. contract – relax (without maximal resistance) (Fig. 5.10). For example, to gain extension: isometric contraction of the biceps at the limit of the extension range is held for 3–5 seconds and subsequent relaxation is followed by stretch into extension for 5 seconds.
3. Static splinting into flexion or extension, as dictated by the arc of movement desired, is applied after exercises.

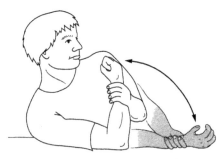

Figure 5.10 Contract and relax exercises. The patient applies heat to the elbow. They then position themselves with the armpit at bench height; the wrist is grasped and the elbow taken to just short of maximal extension. The patient then attempts to flex the elbow while resisting with the normal hand for a sustained period. The flexor muscles are then relaxed and a sustained passive stretch applied to the elbow into extension. This is repeated. The reverse is undertaken to progress with elbow flexion.

4. Cryotherapy is used following each session, and especially if haematoma or soreness persists.

Following discharge

5–14 days. Gentle active movements continued. The patient is instructed in a daily home programme, utilising the above techniques:

1. Reduce swelling: limb is maintained elevated as much as possible. Compression stocking at all times. If a sequential compression pump is available, it is applied 2–3 times a day for 30–40 min.
2. CPM is used three times a day for 2 hours at a time.
3. Exercises as above, in combination with NSAIDs and analgesics.

15 days. Sutures are removed and more aggressive static splinting is introduced if required:

- CPM 3 times a day for 1–2 hours, longer if possible, in the evening
- Exercises hourly for 5–10 min.

If pain increases with therapy, then upgrade NSAIDs and cold therapy, rest the joint and recommence when pain has settled. Increasing pain and warmth despite these measures suggests HO formation and a plain X-ray (soft tissue penetration) is indicated.

At 6 weeks, strength exercises are instituted (Fig. 5.11). Heavy loading of the elbow is then

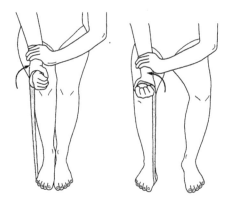

Figure 5.11 Strengthening exercises. Resisted arm rotation.

dictated by the ligament stability and the status of the articular surface documented at surgery. Table 5.4 gives a protocol following surgical release of the stiff elbow.

Table 5.4 Postoperative protocol following surgical release of the stiff elbow

Time	Treatment
Day of operation	Cryocuff Compression bandage Elevation in a sling above shoulder height Establish good analgesia (axillary catheter)
Days 1–5	CPM 20 hours/day Compression bandage/compression pump Assisted shoulder ROM exercises
Days 5–6	Removal of axillary catheter CPM 3 sessions/day Restoration of functional exercises Activities of daily living Shoulder and hand exercises Static splinting into extension is introduced
Day 7	Discharge with above regime and CPM
Days 14–21	Continue as above Reinforce the need to control swelling Continue use of heat and ice Static splinting into flexion with Velcro strap Alternate extension splinting Decrease reliance on CPM
Week 6	Commence light resisted strengthening
Week 8	Cease NSAIDs unless required for analgesia or turnbuckle regime

CPM = continuous passive movement, NSAIDs = non-steroidal anti-inflammatory drugs, ROM = range of motion.

Dynamic elbow distractor (Fig. 5.12)

This external fixation device of the elbow allows the elbow to hinge around its normal axis, while at the same time providing stability. Following application, a check AP/lateral X-ray is mandatory to confirm the elbow is reduced and the pins are in appropriate positions. The joint should be distracted approximately 5 mm. If there is any doubt about the reduction, lateral tomograms should be performed. The routine protocol for a surgical release is undertaken (axillary catheter, CPM). Pin-sites are inspected daily for skin tethering/sepsis and treated early. The device is left *in situ* for 4–6 weeks. Following removal of the distractor, a low-profile hinged elbow brace is worn for a further 6 weeks or longer if indicated.

Splints

Static splints (turnbuckle) (Fig. 5.13). These are used to regain and maintain the extremes of elbow flexion but especially extension. The splint is commenced at approximately 14 days. As these splints have highly efficient gear (e.g. JAS splint) or turnbuckle mechanisms they can apply large forces and therefore need to be supervised closely. If the patient finds that one arc of movement is being lost overnight, then the arm should be splinted in extension and flexion alternately at night.

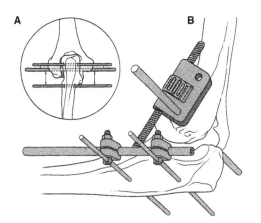
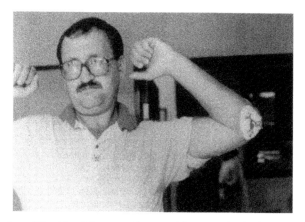

Figure 5.12 A dynamic elbow distractor stabilises an elbow (A), while at the same time providing a moderate degree of elbow flexion/extension and forearm rotation (B).

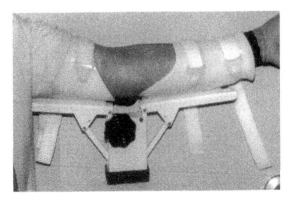

Figure 5.13 Adjustable 'turnbuckle' splints are used to produce elastic deformation of adhesions and capsular contractures. They usually require intermittent physiotherapy supervision to customise a stretching protocol. Additional measures such as analgesics, NSAIDs, heat and cold are usually instituted to allow progress to be maintained.

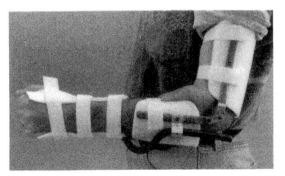

Figure 5.14 Dynamic forearm rotation braces are better tolerated if flexion/extension of the elbow is not sacrificed. Braces that splint the wrist seem to produce less pain at the DRUJ.

If the flexion splint causes the soft tissues to bunch and impede movement, then a simple adjustable Velcro strap around the wrist and upper arm will help regain flexion. Continued problems with joint swelling will tend to restrict the return of full ROM, especially flexion. The use of these splints invariably requires the use of hot and cold modalities, and often NSAIDs, to maximise and retain the gains. An overaggressive use of a splint may result in increased heat and pain in the joint, which can be settled by a short period of rest and cold therapy.

Dynamic forearm rotation splints. These require the elbow to be held flexed and an outrigger rotates the hand and distal forearm. The wrist is included to prevent rotation at the wrist, and the hand provides a more comfortable purchase to rotate the forearm (Fig. 5.14). The splinting

commences as soon as the soft tissues allow. The degree of tension is determined by the resistance to splinting and the discomfort felt at the DRUJ. The splint is alternated between pronation and supination intermittently through the day for 20–30 min a time. The most resistant movement may be splinted at night at a low tension.

Hinged splints. Postoperative splintage for 6 weeks is usually required in those patients undergoing a ligament repair or reconstruction. If there is ongoing instability, these may be a long-term solution.

If there is *valgus instability* and the *anterior bundle of the MCL ligament* requires protection, a hinged arm–forearm orthosis in neutral forearm rotation is used.

If there is *posterolateral rotatory instability* (*LUCL*), then forearm supination is avoided by placing the forearm in *pronation*. Combined MCL and LCL instability may require an elbow distractor/fixator device rather than an external splint.

REFERENCES

1. Green DP, McCoy H: Turnbuckle orthotic correction of the elbow flexion contractures after acute injuries. J Bone Joint Surg 61A:1092–5, 1979.
2. Classification and Heterotopic Ossification: Hand Clinics: Difficult Disorders of the Elbow and Forearm, Aug 1994.
3. Jones GS, Savoie FH III: Arthroscopic capsular release of flexion contractures (arthrofibrosis) of the elbow. Arthroscopy 9:277–83, 1993.
4. Morrey BF: Treatment of the post-traumatic contractures of the elbow: operative treatment, including distraction arthroplasty. J Bone Joint Surg 72A:601–18, 1990.
5. Urbaniak JR, Hansen PE, Beissinger SF et al: Correction of post-traumatic flexion contracture of the elbow by anterior capsulectomy. J Bone Joint Surg 67A:1160–4, 1985.

D. ELBOW RECONSTRUCTION AND ARTHROPLASTY

Jeff Hughes and Maureen Williams

OSTEOARTHRITIS OF THE ELBOW

Primary osteoarthritis is usually seen in middle-aged males, especially in heavy manual workers or amputees and paraplegics who 'use their arms as legs'. It frequently results in impingement of hypertrophic osteophytes and loose bodies in both the anterior and posterior compartments of the elbow. The patient complains of progressive restriction (initially extension then flexion) of movement, associated with painful end points. These symptoms can be addressed with a debridement of all loose bodies and osteophytes.[1,2]

The procedure does not address radiocapitellar disease or severe mid-range pain. The procedure is performed via a 5 cm posterior longitudinal triceps splitting approach. The posterior compartment is thoroughly debrided of degenerative osteophytes, then a foramenotomy is made to join the olecranon and coronoid fossae. The coronoid osteophytes are then removed via the foramin along with any loose bodies. Occasionally, if the flexion contracture is severe, the anterior capsule can be stripped from the humerus and folded down and excised (anterior capsulectomy), which allows better restoration of elbow extension, especially with postoperative turnbuckle splinting.

The postoperative protocol is as for a surgical release of the stiff elbow, although the axillary catheter is not always required and is usually left in for 2 days only. Resisted triceps exercises are avoided for 4 weeks. Improvement in extension and flexion is usually only moderate. NSAIDs are continued for both pain relief and control of inflammation, as osteoarthritic joints tend not to tolerate turnbuckle regimes without them.

Radial head excision

Complete radial head excision at the level of the annular ligament is preferable to partial excision. Indications include unsalvageable radial head fracture (Mason type III), inflammatory or osteoarthritis involving mainly the radiocapitellar articulation. Radial head excision is contraindicated with skeletal immaturity, acute or chronic longitudinal radioulnar dissociation (Esses–Lopresti lesion). Complications described following excision include wrist pain, weakness of grip and forearm rotation, proximal radioulnar impingement, valgus instability (due to unrecognised MCL deficiency), heterotopic calcification and late humeroulnar osteoarthritis.[3]

Passive assisted forearm rotation is commenced day 2 postoperatively. If a good ROM is not achieved by 2–3 weeks, a dynamic rotation splint should be considered.

TOTAL ELBOW ARTHROPLASTY (TEA)

Indications

The primary indication for TEA is pain. Secondary indications include restoration of movement and function. The commonest indication is rheumatoid arthritis and other inflammatory arthropathies. Other indications include salvage of post-traumatic elbow in the elderly patient, such as non-union/malunions of the supracondylar/intercondylar humerus and acute comminuted condylar fractures

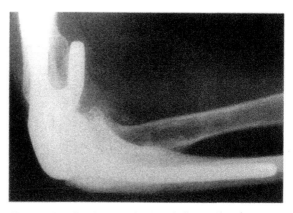

Figure 5.15 Semi-constrained total elbow arthroplasty. The Coonrad–Morrey III total elbow uses a 'floppy hinge' to minimise forces being applied to the implant and the cement bone interface. This reduces the incidence of aseptic loosening. Note the combination of biological (porous ingrowth) and cement fixation.

unable to be satisfactorily stabilised. Post-traumatic causes usually require a semi-constrained prosthesis to prevent instability.

Until the exact kinematics of elbow arthroplasties are established, they are best classified as:

linked (constrained, e.g. Stanmore, and semi-constrained, e.g. Coonrad–Morrey III[4] (Figs 5.15 and 5.16), GSB,[5] Pritchard–Walker) and *unlinked* (unconstrained or resurfacing arthroplasties), e.g. Souter–Strathclyde (cemented), capitocondylar (cemented), Questral (anatomical/uncemented) (Fig. 5.17) and Kudo III (uncemented).[6]

The surgical indications are more varied for semi-constrained arthroplasty, as the 'sloppy hinge' allows the use of TEA where the bone and soft tissue deficits would normally preclude an unconstrained arthroplasty (e.g. elbow ankylosis, post-traumatic).

The Coonrad–Morrey III prosthesis (Mayo clinic), although non-anatomical demonstrates well the evolution in TEA implant design in an attempt to reduce the common complications of TEA (such as implant loosening and instability). This is evidenced by:

1. a hinged articulation to prevent instability
2. a 'floppy hinge' to reduce load at the implant fixation interface
3. eccentric or condylar fixation (anterior flange with bone graft) and combined pore coat for 'biological fixation', rather than relying entirely on intramedullary fixation.

Custom implants may be required in tumour resection, revision arthroplasty, abnormal anatomy

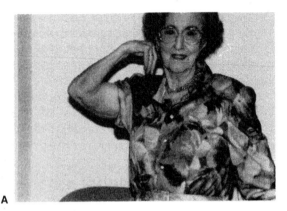
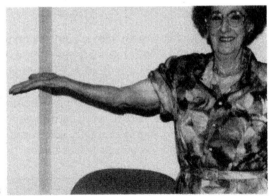
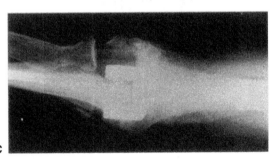

Figure 5.16 A–C: Although the commonest indication for TEA is the severely disabled patient with rheumatoid arthritis, salvage of the comminuted distal humeral fracture in the elderly patient is demonstrating good results. A semi-constrained total elbow prosthesis (Coonrad–Morrey) is usually required.

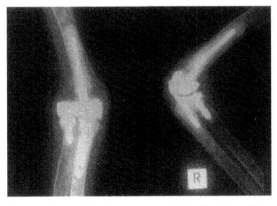

Figure 5.17 Unlinked or unconstrained arthroplasty. The Sorbie Questor total elbow reproduces the anatomical joint shape and axis of rotation of the normal elbow.

or if there has been compromise of the humeral shaft by a total shoulder prosthesis.

Contraindications

Sepsis, neurological deficit, absence of flexor and extensor muscle function, inadequate bone or soft tissue, inability of patient to comply with restrictions postoperatively.

POSTOPERATIVE CARE

Because of the quite superficial position of the arthroplasty and the sometimes poor wound healing over the olecranon, the priority immediately postoperative is to obtain good wound healing without sepsis. The arm is dressed in a compression dressing and a splint applied that allows the elbow to be nursed in a position of stability (if applicable) and without undue skin tension. The arm is elevated at all times and hand movements are commenced straight away. The drains are removed at 24–36 hours. At day 3 if the wound is healing well, assisted elbow flexion is begun.

If a large haematoma forms and threatens wound healing, then early evacuation in theatre with copious lavage, careful haemostasis, intravenous and regional antibiotics is recommended.

If a triceps approach has been utilised, then resisted extension movements are avoided for 6 weeks. Long term, if the olecranon is unduly prominent, the patient should be advised to wear a protective pad to prevent olecranon bursitis, which if it becomes infected can communicate directly with the arthroplasty.

Unlinked

The rehabilitation of unlinked prostheses is aimed at protecting the ligament repairs and preventing instability of the arthroplasty. The arm is splinted into 30–45 degrees of flexion. Initially, there is no need for intensive physiotherapy, other than the minimisation of swelling to promote wound healing.

Those patients with a severe preoperative flexion contracture (especially if post-traumatic) generally do not achieve full extension. If a stretching programme is going to be instituted postoperatively, the use of a semi-constrained prosthesis should be considered instead, as aggressive mobilisation into extension may produce irreversible posterior instability in unlinked arthroplasties.

Linked

Semi-constrained arthroplasties require minimal rehabilitation. Assisted active movements are commenced as soon as the wound is demonstrated to be healing (3–4 days). Flexion is obtained relatively easily with simple functional activities of daily living. Extension, if slow or resistant, can be improved with a splint. Strength exercises are avoided other than normal activities. A weight restriction of 3 kg is placed upon the arthroplasty.

REFERENCES

1. Morrey BF: Transhumeral elbow debridement or ulnohumeral arthroplasty. Primary arthritis of the elbow treated by ulnohumeral arthroplasty. J Bone Joint Surg 74B:409, 1992.
2. Kashwagi D (ed.): Outerbridge Kashiwagi arthroplasty for osteoarthritis of the elbow in the elbow joint. In: Proceedings of the International Congress, Kobe, Japan. Amsterdam: Excerpta Medica, 1986.
3. Karlson MK, Hasserius R, Besjakov J, Josefsson PO: Results of excision of the radial head after fracture. A 13–33 year follow-up. Twelfth Open Meeting American Shoulder and Elbow Surgeons, 1996.
4. Morrey BF, Adams RA: Semi-constrained arthroplasty for rheumatoid arthritis of the elbow. J Bone Joint Surg 74A:479, 1992.
5. Bell S, Gschwend N, Steiger U: Arthroplasty of the elbow: experience with the Mark III GSB prosthesis. Aust NZ Surg 56:823–7, 1986.
6. Kudo H, Iwano K, Watanabe S: Total elbow arthroplasty with a nonconstrained surface replacement prosthesis in patients who have rheumatoid arthritis. A long term follow-up study. J Bone Joint Surg 72A:355, 1990.

E. SOFT TISSUE INJURIES – EPICONDYLITIS AND BICEPS TENDON REPAIR

Mark Perko and Rosemary Prosser

EPICONDYLITIS

This common affliction is colloquially known as either tennis or golfer's elbow. It has been used loosely to describe pain about the epicondylar region of the elbow. It can be confused with a variety of conditions and should be clearly identified to avoid errors in diagnosis or treatment. It is a degenerative rather than an inflammatory condition of the tendinous extensor or flexor origin. The triceps insertion is rarely involved.[1,2]

Incidence

The peak incidence occurs in the third and fourth decades and is infrequently seen outside of this age group. That is not to state that medial or lateral elbow pain is not common in other decades of life but rather that other pathologies are more likely than epicondylitis. It is not confined to sport, as the name may suggest, but can occur with any activity or occupation requiring stressful or repetitive forearm use. In the vast majority of cases the condition is transient.

Differential diagnosis

Osteochondritis dissecans. This occurs in adolescents and is the most likely cause of lateral elbow pain in this age group. The pain is activity-related and may be associated with a loss of motion, particularly extension. It usually involves the capitellum but, rarely, the trochlea may be involved.

Articular injuries. There are a number of joint injuries which are related to sporting pursuits. They are associated with valgus or extension stresses such as in throwing and in racquet sports. This may result in osteochondral lesions and associated ligamentous avulsions or attenuations of the medial collateral ligament.

Primary degenerative arthritis. This is not necessarily an affliction of the elderly but often presents in the third and fourth decades more commonly in men.

Inflammatory arthropathy. Synovitis and an effusion are uncommon in isolation but can be seen in crystal arthropathies. They may also involve the adjacent bursae of the elbow.

Neural lesions. Entrapment neuropathies of the ulnar and radial nerves may cause pain about the elbow. Entrapment of the posterior interosseous nerve by the supinator arcade can cause similar symptoms. Ulnar nerve symptoms are more likely to be associated with joint lesions such as a medial ligament injury or medial joint osteophytes.

Constitutional factors. Some patients seem prone to various tendinopathies and stenosing tenosynovitis of the wrist and hand, which can present simultaneously.[3]

Referred pain. Cervical or shoulder pain will often radiate to the elbow and may mimic local pathology.

Pathology

The initiating event is not well understood, but tendon involvement is primarily a degenerative change and not an inflammatory one. The macroscopic appearance is that of greyish, oedematous and friable tissue similar to scar tissue and the microscopic appearance is that of invading fibroblasts with vascular granulation tissue usually termed angiofibroblastic hyperplasia. Inflammatory infiltrates are not an associated histological feature.

Clinical presentation and findings

The history of a single initiating event is uncommon and usually there is a gradual onset of symptoms. The pain can vary in intensity, is activity-related and can be severe enough to limit most activities. There is often a constant ache and the epicondyle can be very tender if knocked during daily activities. The clinical findings are those of specific local tenderness at the anterior aspect of the lateral epicondyle over the extensor origin or at the anterior aspect of the medial epicondyle.

The pain is precipitated by resisted finger or wrist extension, and resisted gripping in wrist extension with the elbow in extension in the case of lateral symptoms. Grip strength testing with the elbow in flexion and extension may provide useful objective data. Resisted forearm pronation or wrist flexion precipitates medial-sided symptoms. Loss of elbow motion is not usually a feature. Ulnar nerve symptoms can occur in association with medial epicondylitis.[4]

Treatment

The broad principles of treatment are rest or, more appropriately, avoidance of aggravating activities, use of physical modalities to promote healing and reduce swelling, and medical or surgical therapies and rehabilitation for return to activity.

Initial treatment

Resting the affected limb does not require immobilisation but should involve avoidance of aggravating activities. Technique correction for the sportsperson is important. Counter force splinting of the proximal forearm can also be of benefit in reducing pain.

Physical modalities may also facilitate reduction of swelling and promote healing. These may include cryotherapy, interferential therapy, laser therapy, electrical stimulation (high voltage galvanism[5]), pulsed electromagnetic field therapy and acupuncture.[6]

Medical therapies such as nonsteroidal anti-inflammatory agents (NSAIDs), either as a topical or oral medication, can often alleviate the pain associated with this condition.

An injectable corticosteroid preparation is often of great benefit if symptoms do not respond to physical modalities, topical or oral medication. The injection should be deep to the tendon and not subcutaneous, as this can lead to unsightly subdermal atrophy.

Rehabilitation programme

Splinting. Rehabilitation consists of a graduated programme of exercises, including stretching and strengthening, with a gradual resumption of activity. The use of counterforce splinting is recommended until satisfactory strength is regained. Counterforce splinting should perform effective constraint when the muscle is contracting and expanding in order to minimise compression of the neurovascular structures and allow dynamic muscle tendon function. The splint has been shown to lower extensor muscle force at the elbow in the serve and backhand of tennis players.[7]

Nirschl[8,9] cautions against the use of an immobilisation splint due to the disuse atrophy of the musculature caused by immobilisation. Short-term use of a wrist extension splint in severe cases has been reported in the literature.[5,10]

Exercise. Stretching techniques may be both passive and active, and may be augmented by cryotherapy. Resistive strengthening should not be commenced until there is appropriate pain-free musculotendinous length and pain-free active range of motion.

The aim of the strengthening programme is to improve endurance and tolerance to repetitive stress. Low resistance and a high repetition rate is recommended. Strengthening should be aimed at all aspects of muscle function. Eccentric, isometric and isotonic contraction with varied velocities should be utilised, particularly for the sportsperson.

The strengthening programme needs to be closely supervised and progressed. Epicondylitis is easily flared with overzealous exercise, particularly in the early stages of rehabilitation. Wrist exercises should be commenced with the elbow in flexion and progressed to elbow extension. Likewise, the forearm position can be progressed from supination to pronation. Total upper arm strength and mobility requires assessment and strengthening in deficit areas. Deficits in rotator cuff strength have been associated with epicondylitis. Nirschl[8] and Ellenbecker[5] recommend shoulder and scapular exercises in addition to elbow, forearm and wrist exercises.

Return to sport or work. On return to sport, technique correction and equipment review are important. A midsize racquet is recommended for tennis players.[11] Wide body frames and oversize racquets produce greater power and dampen vibration; however, they also produce greater shock up the arm with off-centre impact forces. A reduction in string tension is also recommended on return to sport.[6] A larger handle size is preferred, as it reduces the effort of grip and forearm extensor activity. Nirschl has recommended that the racquet handle size should be equal to the measurement from the top of the ring finger to the proximal palmar crease.

Increasing handle size on hand tools may also be beneficial for the manual worker. Alteration or modification of work activities or techniques may also be necessary; this needs to be done on an individual basis.

Associated joint and nerve irritation

Strong contraction of the forearm musculature transmits high compressive forces through the proximal radiohumeral joint. Radiohumeral joint stiffness and irritability may lead to degenerative joint changes. The treatment focus for patients with joint irritability may include joint mobilisation as well as massage and local physical modalities combined with reducing forces across the joint.

In long-standing epicondylitis, radial (posterior interosseus nerve) or ulnar nerve irritation may develop. This needs to be assessed and differentiated from entrapment neuropathy. Gentle neural mobilisation and transcutaneous electrical nerve stimulation (TENS) may become first-line treatment techniques in these patients.

Surgery

Surgery is indicated only for resistant cases where symptoms severely limit daily activities. The choice of surgical procedure remains controversial as most studies report good results with release of the tendon origin irrespective of whether a pathological lesion is sought. Ancillary procedures such as capsular release, posterior interosseous nerve or ulnar nerve release and denervation[12] are also reported. The necessity of these procedures, however, as a routine part of the surgical procedure, can be questioned unless dual pathology is thought to be present.

Postoperative therapy

The postoperative regime is similar to the conservative programme. Relative rest in a splint or bulky bandage for the first 3 weeks may be necessary. Gentle short arc exercises are commenced in the first week. Full active range is expected by the third week. The resting splint is replaced by a counterforce splint at this time. Gentle light resisted grip, e.g. foam ball squeezing, is also commenced. Light resisted activity may be started between weeks 5 and 6. Return to full sporting activity level takes an average of 4½ months.[11]

Specific tips

Patients with excessive inflammation or swelling will need to rest for a longer period and will only tolerate very slow progression. Close attention to progression of the strengthening programme is essential.

BICEPS TENDON INJURY
Incidence and presentation

Rupture of the distal biceps attachment is an uncommon occurrence and accounts for less than 10% of all biceps ruptures but, unlike rupture of the long head, the disability caused by distal rupture is much greater, especially for young active individuals. Repair is advisable in this age group. The injury has only been described in males. Partial rupture can also occur, but is rare, as is tendinitis of the biceps insertion. The mechanism of injury is usually an extension force applied to a flexed and supinated forearm. This can occur with a violent extension force such as in contact sports or, more commonly, in older patients the biceps gives way with a loud crack while carrying a heavy load. The patient will usually recall this snapping or tearing sensation in the forearm followed by pain. Extensive bruising in the forearm is common within a few days.

Clinical findings

On examination, bruising anterior to the elbow and in the forearm will be obvious and the muscle

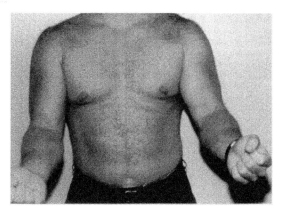

Figure 5.18 Patient with a recently ruptured left distal biceps, demonstrating retraction of the muscle into the arm.

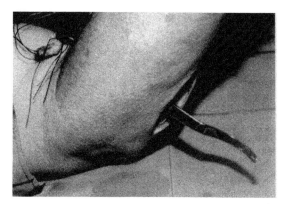

Figure 5.20 The biceps tendon is retrieved. The tendon is then passed down to the radial tuberosity and reattached with suture anchors or sutures through drill holes through the bone.

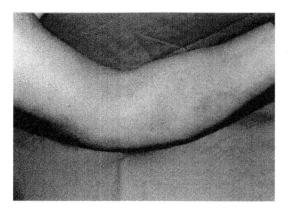

Figure 5.19 Bruising in the forearm is usually present.

belly is retracted into the upper arm (Figs 5.18 and 5.19). Bruising only above the elbow is more indicative of a rupture of the musculotendinous junction or muscle belly, which may not be amenable to surgical repair. The biceps tendon, which is normally easily palpable with resisted elbow flexion is absent, and the patient will have weakness of elbow flexion and forearm supination with resistance.

Treatment

The biceps accounts for 30–40% of elbow flexion and forearm supination strength.[13] There is also a 60–80% loss of elbow flexion and forearm supination endurance.[13] For individuals who are manual labourers or for those that require forearm strength, operative repair is preferable. The loss of strength is not compensated for by the remaining flexors or the supinator. Proximal retraction of the muscle produces an obvious cosmetic defect, and painful cramping may occur with any heavy exertion. Surgical repair should aim to reattach the biceps tendon to the radial tuberosity in order to restore both flexion and supination strength. This can be accomplished by a two-incision technique whereby the tendon is retrieved via a small incision in the arm and the tuberosity exposed by a muscle-splitting approach posteriorly (Fig. 5.20). The tendon is reattached with suture anchors or through drill holes in bone. Alternatively, an anterior exposure can be used; however, this procedure requires exposure of the anterior neurovascular structures and is more difficult. The cosmetic result also is inferior.[14–17]

Postoperative programme

Postoperatively, patients are managed in an elbow extension block splint at approximately 70–80 degrees from full extension (Fig. 5.21).

Early passive forearm rotation should be commenced within a few days of surgery.

Supination requires more attention than pronation. The patient is given a home exercise programme and supervised at regular intervals.

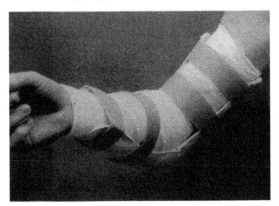

Figure 5.21 The elbow extension block splint worn for 5–6 weeks post-repair.

Oedema control and scar management are attended to using appropriate measures when necessary.

The timing of active motion will depend on the strength of tendon attachment. Attachment with suture anchors has greater strength than using sutures alone. At 3 weeks following suture anchor attachment, assisted active and active motion are introduced. These exercises include elbow flexion and extension and forearm rotation (Fig. 5.22). The extension block splint is maintained. The splint can be discarded after 5–6 weeks.

After removal of the extension blocking splint, a graduated strengthening programme is commenced. Further passive stretching and dynamic splinting may be used, if required, to obtain full extension and forearm rotation.

Specific tips

Full supination will be slow to achieve if full passive supination is not obtained in the first 3 weeks.

A graduated strengthening programme should include high- and low-velocity exercise,

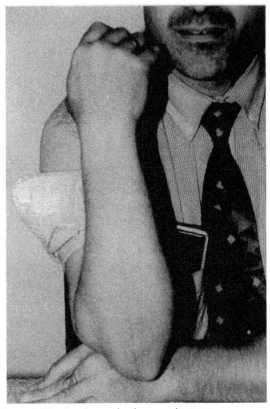

Figure 5.22 Passive supination exercises are commenced within the first week. This is progressed to assisted active supination at 3 weeks; passive supination is continued. This patient is 8 weeks following repair. He demonstrates full active supination; the forearm incision can also be seen.

particularly for athletes, as well as concentric and eccentric exercise.

Supination strengthening is best achieved with resistive exercise devices, e.g. weight well, Theraband, BTE (Baltimore Therapeutic Equipment) work simulator and work-hardening activities which include the use of screwdrivers and spanners.

REFERENCES

1. Goldie I: Epicondylitis lateralis humeri: a pathological study. Acta Chir Scand Suppl 339:7, 1964.
2. Nirschel RP, Petrone F: Tennis elbow. The surgical treatment of lateral epicondylitis. J Bone Joint Surg 61A:832–9, 1979.
3. Nirschel RP: Mesenchymal syndrome. Virginia Med M 96:659–62, 1969.
4. Gabel GT, Morrey BF: Operative treatment of medial epicondylitis: influence of concomitant ulnar neuropathy at the elbow. J Bone Joint Surg 77A:1065–9, 1995.

5. Ellenbecker TS: The elbow in sport: injury, treatment and rehabilitation. Champaign IL: Human Kinetics, 1997:89–119.
6. Patterson S: Surgical management of acute and chronic elbow injuries. In: Chan KM (ed.), Sports injuries of the hand and upper extremity. New York: Churchill Livingstone, 1995:181–4.
7. Groppel J, Nirschl R: A mechanical and electromyographical analysis of the effects of various counter force braces on the tennis player. Am J Sports Med 14(3):195–200, 1986.
8. Nirschl RP: Prevention and treatment of elbow and shoulder injuries in the tennis player. Clin Sports Med 7:289–308, 1988.
9. Nirschl R, Sobel J: Conservative treatment of tennis elbow. Phys Sports Med 9:43–54, 1981.
10. Coonard R, Hooper W: Tennis elbow: its course, natural history, conservative and surgical management. J Bone Joint Surg 55A:1177–82, 1973.
11. Nirschl RP: Muscle and tendon trauma. In: Morrey B (ed.), The elbow and its disorders. Philadelphia: WB Saunders, 537–52, 1993.
12. Wilhelm A: Tennis elbow: treatment of resistant cases by denervation. J Hand Surg 21B:523–33, 1996.
13. Morrey BF, Askew LJ, An KH, Dobyns JH: Rupture of the distal biceps tendon: biomechanical assessment of different treatment options. J Bone Joint Surg 76A:418–21, 1995.
14. Agins HJ, Chess JL, Hoekstra DV, Teitge RA: Rupture of the distal insertion of the biceps brachii tendon. Clin Orthop 234:34–8, 1988.
15. Baker BE, Bierwagen D: Rupture of the distal tendon of the biceps brachii. J Bone Joint Surg 67A:414, 1985.
16. Louis DS, Hankin FM, Eckenrode JF, Smith PA, Wojtys EM: Distal biceps brachii tendon avulsion: a simplified method of repair. Am J Sports Med 14:234–6, 1986.
17. Norman WH: Repair of avulsion of insertion of biceps brachii tendon. Clin Orthop 193:189–94, 1985.

6

The shoulder

A. FUNCTIONAL ANATOMY AND ASSESSMENT

Karen Ginn

FUNCTIONAL ANATOMY OF THE SHOULDER JOINT

Articular surfaces

The humeral head is spherical in shape, with a surface area approximately three times that of the glenoid fossa.

The small, pear-shaped glenoid fossa is very shallow, with an average concavity of 2.5 mm along its anteroposterior axis.

With only 25–30% of the humeral head in contact with the glenoid fossa in any joint position, the articular surfaces afford minimal bony constraint to shoulder joint movement.

The inherent bony instability of the shoulder joint is due to this lack of articular surface contact and not articular surface incongruity, since the humeral head and glenoid fossa have almost identical radii of curvature.

Glenoid labrum

The glenoid labrum is a wedge-shaped fibrous structure that forms a ring around the glenoid fossa, being firmly attached inferiorly but frequently loosely attached superiorly.

The shoulder joint capsule, the glenohumeral ligaments and the tendon of the long head of biceps brachii attach to it.

The presence of this labrum increases the depth of the glenoid cavity to 5 mm in the anteroposterior direction. By increasing the surface area of the glenoid cavity, the glenoid labrum makes a contribution to shoulder joint stability by increasing the contact area between the articular surfaces.

The flexible, fibrous structure of the labrum, its loose superior attachment and the common occurrence of degenerative labral lesions in those over 40 years of age need to be considered when assessing the relative significance of its role in shoulder joint function.

Joint capsule

The shoulder joint capsule attaches from the glenoid labrum to the anatomical neck and inferomedial shaft of the humerus.

It is very lax, allowing approximately 2 cm distraction between the articular surfaces. However, limited volume within the shoulder joint capsule, resulting in a relative vacuum within the joint, is believed to contribute to passive shoulder stability.

It is less than 1 mm in thickness, but is reinforced anterosuperiorly by the glenohumeral and coracohumeral ligaments and laterally by insertions from the four rotator cuff muscles.

Openings in the joint capsule connect the shoulder joint cavity to the subscapular bursa and to the synovial sheath surrounding the tendon of the long head of biceps brachii.

Ligaments

The relatively few ligaments at the shoulder joint provide stability at the extremes of shoulder range of motion.

The *coracohumeral ligament* is a thin, broad band that extends from the base of the coracoid process to the transverse humeral ligament between the tendons of supraspinatus and subscapularis, i.e. in the rotator interval. With the glenoid cavity correctly oriented slightly superiorly, the coracohumeral ligament is said to prevent inferior translation and limit external rotation of the humerus, between 0 and 60 degrees of abduction, although these roles remain controversial.

The superior, middle and inferior glenohumeral ligaments are anterosuperior thickening in the joint capsule. They all limit external rotation and offer some resistance to anterior dislocation of the humerus, the superior ligament being most effective in the adducted position with increasing contribution from the middle and inferior ligaments as abduction range of motion increases. The glenohumeral ligaments vary considerably in size and location and are sometimes absent leading to the speculation that they have limited functional significance.

The thick *coracoacromial ligament* passes between the coracoid and acromion processes of the scapula. It prevents superior dislocation of the humeral head but does not prevent superior translation. The large subacromial bursa functions to protect structures in the subacromial space, e.g. supraspinatus tendon, in the event of superior movement of the humeral head.

The *transverse humeral ligament* passes between the greater and lesser tubercles of the humerus and functions as a retinaculum for the long head of biceps brachii.

Rotator cuff muscles

The shoulder joint relies primarily on muscles to maintain functional joint stability. All of the muscles that move the shoulder joint play some role in compressing the humeral head into the glenoid cavity and thus contribute to increasing shoulder stability during movement.

The most important muscles performing this dynamic stabilising role are the four muscles of the musculotendinous rotator cuff: subscapularis, an internal rotator of the humerus; infraspinatus and teres minor, external rotators of the humerus; and supraspinatus, which has no definite action at the shoulder joint. The rotator cuff muscles take origin from the mobile scapula and their tendons splay out and interdigitate to form a common, continuous insertion into the lateral shoulder joint capsule and onto the tubercles of the humerus (Fig. 6.1).

The rotator cuff muscles combine to provide a balanced force to the humeral head to keep it accurately positioned in the glenoid cavity during all shoulder movements. For example, they must provide a coordinated, synchronised downward force to the humeral head during the initial phase of abduction in order to counteract the tendency for deltoid to translate it superiorly.

Contrary to popular belief, the supraspinatus muscle does not initiate abduction, but rather functions in this dynamic stabilising role throughout abduction range as part of the rotator cuff team.

By preventing unwanted humeral head translation, the rotator cuff muscles not only facilitate maximum available articular surface contact but also protect the glenoid labrum, shoulder capsule and ligaments from damage during movement.

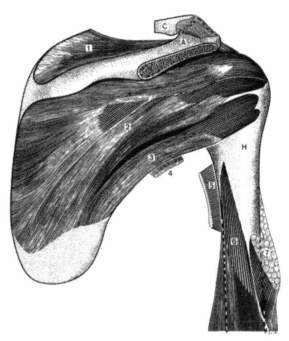

Figure 6.1 Posterior view of the right shoulder and the rotator cuff. (Reproduced with permission from Guyot J: *Atlas of human limb joints*. Berlin: Springer-Verlag, 1981.)

Scapulohumeral rhythm

Full-range shoulder movement requires not only movement at the shoulder joint but also upward rotation of the scapula. This rotation is necessary to position the glenoid cavity for optimal articulation with the humeral head and to maintain the mechanical advantage of many shoulder muscles.

Upward rotation of the scapula is produced mainly by the coordinated activity of the upper trapezius and serratus anterior muscles in early range, and upper and lower trapezius in later range, and is accompanied by movement of the clavicle at the sternoclavicular and acromioclavicular joints.

Scapulohumeral rhythm refers to the characteristic pattern of synchronised movement that occurs between the scapula and the shoulder and clavicular joints during shoulder movements. For example, during the initial 30 degrees of abduction, movement occurs predominantly at the shoulder joint with approximately 4 degrees

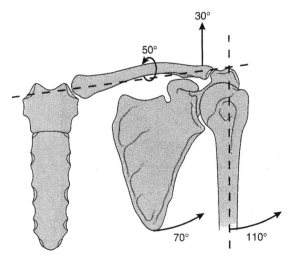

Figure 6.2 Movements of the scapula, clavicle and humerus that combine to produce normal scapulohumeral rhythm during abduction.

of humeral movement for every 1 degree of movement of the scapula. From 30 degrees to full abduction, the scapula rotates upwardly, and the shoulder joint and scapula contribute approximately 2 degrees for every 1 degree of scapula movement. Upward rotation of the scapula is accompanied at first by elevation of the lateral end of the clavicle produced by upper trapezius activity and then by posterior rotation of the clavicle produced as a result of tension in the coracoclavicular ligament (Fig. 6.2).

In order to achieve scapulohumeral rhythm all the relevant muscles moving the humerus and scapula must act synchronously to perform their mover and stabiliser roles. Muscle synchrony necessitates a high level of neuromuscular control, which entails the ability to recruit appropriate muscles at the correct time as well as the ability to suppress extraneous muscle activity.

ASSESSMENT OF THE SHOULDER

Interview

In addition to general and medical history information, the following questions are of relevance in determining the clinical diagnosis and management goals and strategies for shoulder dysfunction:

• **What symptoms are you having?** The most common symptoms of shoulder dysfunction are pain on movement and/or a feeling of instability, both of which indicate inadequate dynamic shoulder joint stability. Pain at rest and paraesthesia in the upper limb are uncommon symptoms of local mechanical shoulder dysfunction.

• **Where is your pain?** Shoulder pain is most commonly felt during movement over the antero-superior aspect of the shoulder joint line and/or on the lateral aspect of the arm.

• **Are you right or left handed?** Significant differences in strength have been demonstrated between dominant and non-dominant shoulders in some upper limb athletes. Knowledge of hand dominance may, therefore, be necessary to correctly interpret muscles tests in establishing a clinical diagnosis and treatment goals.

• **What activities/movements bring on your symptoms?** Aggravating movements identified by the patient will help to direct the physical examination. Information about the specific functional activities affected by the shoulder symptoms will aid in setting individually determined treatment goals as well as providing baseline functional data that can be used to evaluate the progress of treatment.

• **Can you lie on your affected shoulder?** Disturbance to sleep is a common complaint. Improvements in sleep patterns can provide a useful functional measure of treatment effectiveness.

• **When and how did your shoulder symptoms begin?** Knowledge of the mechanism of injury will aid a clinical diagnosis and efficiently guide the remainder of the examination, including the need for radiological assessment. There are two main diagnostic categories: symptoms resulting from a specific injury where a major aim of the examination is to identify the injured structures; symptoms resulting from repetitive stress to tissues characterised by insidious onset. In this second category the examination will be aimed at determining the physical characteristics that predispose to microtrauma injuries such as abnormal scapulohumeral rhythm, and external factors that may be aggravating the problem, such as poor sporting technique.

- **Have you had problems in either of your shoulders in the past?** Knowledge of the frequency and progress of previous episodes of shoulder problems, including the type and effectiveness of previous treatment, will aid diagnosis and help in setting long-term treatment goals and more immediate treatment strategies.

Physical examination

Because of the critical role played by muscles in shoulder mobility and stability, a major focus of the physical examination of the shoulder is the assessment of muscle function. Assessment of the shoulder muscles should include measurement of muscle length and strength, evaluation of the quality of the coordination between scapular and humeral movement and evaluation of the effectiveness of muscle groups as dynamic joint stabilisers.

Cervicothoracic screening

To eliminate the cervicothoracic vertebral column as a source of the shoulder problem, the following examination should be performed in an attempt to elicit shoulder symptoms:

- active full-range movements of the neck with overpressure if applicable
- passive accessory/physiological movements of the cervical and upper thoracic vertebral column joints
- neurological examination of the upper limb, including neural tensioning procedures.

Observation

Careful observation of shoulder symmetry and posture will help direct the physical examination and aid in the development of a clinical diagnosis:

- differences in muscle bulk may reflect muscle weakness or tightness
- increased scapular protraction is associated with decreased subacromial space height
- scapula 'winging' may indicate weakness of the serratus anterior or tightness of pectoralis minor.

Active movements

Active movements concurrently assess mobility, muscle length, strength and coordination and the patient's willingness to move. Many active movements are appropriate to assess shoulder function. The following selection would allow a thorough assessment of a majority of dysfunctional shoulders:

1. In standing:
   - abduction in the coronal plane
   - flexion in the sagittal plane
   - hand-behind-back
   - movement identified by the patient as particularly provoking symptoms.
2. In standing and/or supine:
   - internal and external rotation at 90 degrees abduction or flexion.

During active movements, the following information should be accurately recorded to aid in the establishment of a clinical diagnosis and to enable accurate evaluation of the effectiveness of the treatment implemented:

- The quality of the movement, i.e. are the various components of the shoulder complex moving in a smooth, coordinated manner and in the correct sequence. Following injury or as a result of pain, adaptive motor patterns often develop as the individual attempts to move his arm in the most effective way possible given the effects of the lesion. One of the most common adaptive motor patterns at the shoulder involves increased scapular range of movement or scapular movement earlier in range than normal (Fig. 6.3). Further examination will be necessary to determine the cause(s) of such abnormal coordination. Changes to optimal scapulohumeral rhythm, which can often be identified by careful observation of the expected biomechanical events, may have deleterious effects on shoulder joint mechanics, resulting in further symptoms.
- Reliable baseline measurements of the points in range where symptoms begin, where symptoms are eased and where the patient is not prepared to move further. The patient's perception of the reason for the limit to range of movement should be noted. As the limb is returned to the

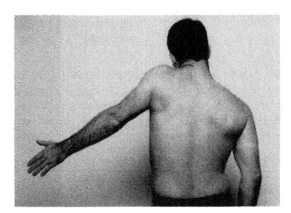

Figure 6.3 Abnormal scapulohumeral rhythm during abduction – early onset and excessive scapular elevation.

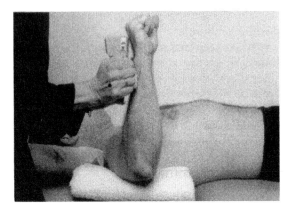

Figure 6.4 Assessment of external rotation isometric strength using a hand-held dynamometer.

starting position, the behaviour of the symptoms should again be recorded.

Palpation

Evaluation of tissue tension, structure size and joint tenderness by direct manual palpation will help to direct the rest of the physical examination and may serve as a tool to evaluate the effects of treatment. It is essential to compare the palpation findings at the affected shoulder to the uninvolved side as many structures/sites at the shoulder are normally tender, e.g. the bicipital groove and the coracoid process. Because similar palpation findings are common to many shoulder pathologies, the role of palpation in aiding a clinical diagnosis is limited.

Muscle length tests

To assess muscle length accurately, tests must be performed passively, with the patient well stabilised to isolate specific muscles or muscle groups and to eliminate the effects of muscle weakness and muscle incoordination on the range of motion. Information from the history will provide a guide as to the most relevant tests to be performed for each individual patient; however, the following muscles would commonly be tested as they are often tight in the dysfunctional shoulder:

1. In supine lying:
   - shoulder internal rotators – particularly subscapularis

   - shoulder external rotators, i.e. infraspinatus and teres minor
   - scapular elevators, i.e. upper trapezius and levator scapulae.
2. In side lying:
   - scapular protractors, i.e. serratus anterior and pectoralis minor.

Isometric muscle strength tests

Hand-held dynamometry has demonstrated acceptable reliability for measuring shoulder muscle strength.[26] As with the assessment of muscle length, information from the history will determine the most relevant muscle groups and the place in range to assess isometric strength. The following shoulder movements would commonly be assessed:

1. In sitting:
   - abduction in the scapular plane in full internal rotation – this position elicits maximal activity in supraspinatus.
2. In supine:
   - internal rotation
   - external rotation (Fig. 6.4)
   - abduction
   - protraction.
3. In prone:
   - retraction.

Interpretation of the results of isometric muscle tests, particularly in the presence of pain, needs some care. Because of the interdependence between scapular and humeral muscles during shoulder movements, maximal contraction of any muscle group will require contraction of other muscles to maintain adequate dynamic stability of both the scapula and the shoulder joint. Isolating specific muscle groups thus becomes difficult. In addition, pain produced during isometric strength testing may be the result of pathology in the muscle group supposedly being tested or may be due to trauma at the joint because other muscles cannot adequately perform their joint stabiliser function under the conditions produced by the testing procedure.

Special tests

Hawkins and Kennedy impingement test. This test is designed to assist in the diagnosis of impingement syndrome by approximating the greater tubercle and the acromion, thus compressing the subacromial structures. With the subject seated or standing, the shoulder is placed in 90 degree flexion and then fully internally rotated. The test is positive if the patient's pain is reproduced.

Jobe subluxation and relocation tests. These tests, which have been shown to be valid and reliable, are designed to assess the integrity of capsular and ligamentous structures and thus assist in the diagnosis of anterior shoulder instability. The patient lies supine with the affected arm over the edge of the plinth. The examiner positions the shoulder into 90 degree abduction and 90 degree external rotation and applies a posteroanterior glide to the humeral head – the subluxation test. The test is positive if the patient experiences apprehension and pain. The examiner then applies an anteroposterior glide to the humeral head – the relocation test. Reduction of apprehension and pain denotes a positive test.

FURTHER READING

Cook EE, Gray VL, Savinar-Nogue E, Medeiros J: Shoulder antagonistic strength ratios: a comparison between college-level baseball pitchers and non-pitchers. J Orthop Sports Phys Ther 8:451–61, 1987.
Inman VT, Saunders JB, Dec M, Abbott LC: Observations on the function of the shoulder joint. J Bone Joint Surg 26:1–31, 1944.

Matsen FA III, Fu F, Hawkins RJ (eds): The shoulder: a balance of mobility and stability. Illinois: American Academy of Orthopedic Surgeons, 1993.
Pagnani MJ, Warren RF: Joint stabilizers of the glenohumeral joint. J Shoulder Elbow Surg 3:173–90, 1994.
Schenkman M, De Cartata VR: Kinesiology of the shoulder complex. J Orthop Sports Phys Ther 8:438–50, 1987.

B. CONSERVATIVE MANAGEMENT OF ROTATOR CUFF, CAPSULITIS AND FROZEN SHOULDER

Craig Allingham and Jenny McConnell

The shoulder is especially prone to chronic overuse injuries because it sacrifices stability for mobility to allow us to freely manoeuvre our arms. As a result of the multifactorial nature of most shoulder problems, conservative treatment is usually the first option in management. Assessment plays a key role in identifying specific anatomical deficits (e.g. detached labrum) and any underlying causative factors which may be remote from the symptoms.

THORACIC SPINE AND SHOULDER MOVEMENT

- Full range of shoulder elevation is dependent on mobility of the thoracic spine.[1,2]
- Middle and lower trapezius reinforce the thoracic extensor muscles, and weakness in any of these will predispose to kyphosis and inefficient shoulder elevation.
- With age, thoracic kyphosis increases and thoracic mobility decreases by up to 35%.[3]

POSTURAL CONSIDERATIONS

- Forward or depressed shoulders disturb normal scapulohumeral rhythm (delaying upward rotation), predisposing to subacromial impingement and perhaps a decrease in total elevation.

- Downwardly rotated and protracted scapulae lengthen the lower trapezius resting length, reducing its efficiency and again predisposing to impingement.

ROTATOR CUFF CONDITIONS

Efforts have been made to identify specific entities of rotator cuff pathology: i.e. impingement syndromes, cuff tears and cuff laxity. More recently, inter-relationships between these conditions have been suggested[4] where one type of pathology may predispose to one or two of the others, resulting in a multiplicity of findings upon assessment with positive tests for ligament laxity, impingement and cuff lesions. Figure 6.5 represents this inter-relationship, showing the overlap between these pathologies, and the areas into which individual patients' presentations can be placed.

Once elements of the different pathologies are identified, the question of the need for surgery is addressed and the patient has made an informed decision to proceed conservatively, the clinician must try to attribute culpability as to which (if any) of the three rotator cuff problems is the primary cause of failure to heal. Despite this confession that shoulder pathology – especially the

overuse onset or degenerative types – is rarely discrete, each of the components will be discussed separately.

Impingement

Compression and abrading of soft tissues contained within the subacromial space occurs with repeated elevation or internal rotation of the humerus, especially under load or when fatigued.

Predisposing factors

- Anatomical – curved or hooked acromion, reducing the capacity of the subacromial space, or an expansive coracoid process, encroaching during movements in the sagittal plane.
- Postural.
- Tightness – flexibility imbalance in the rotator cuff/capsule complex, causing premature elevation of the humeral head during activity.
- Weakness – failure of the rotator cuff muscles to maintain centralisation of the humeral head under load.
- Trauma – impingement loading (e.g. fall onto elbow) with resultant subacromial tissue damage.

Structures damaged

Supraspinatus, infraspinatus, teres minor, biceps brachii (long head) and the subacromial bursa are all located in the impingement zone. Which structure sustains damage depends on the posture, activity and loading pattern demonstrated by the patient. More than one structure may be involved.

Signs and symptoms

- Painful arc during elevation or rotation.
- Pain lying on the shoulder overnight, easing when rolled off it.
- Aching at rest: eased with gentle, unloaded movement (easing inflammatory congestion).
- Sharp pain on unguarded movements.
- Tenderness below the acromion.

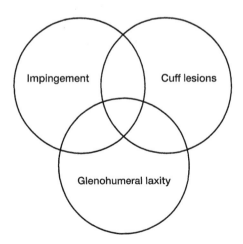

Figure 6.5 The inter-relationships between rotator cuff pathology. (Reproduced with permission from Allingham.[4])

- Positive impingement test(s) (preferred test is internal rotation in 90 degree flexion).
- Pain on strong isometric hold tests (failure to stabilise the humeral head under load during resisted supraspinatus, biceps or rotation tests).
- Positive findings of impingement (bunching of the tendons) observed during ultrasound investigation (should be compared with normal side as pain-free 'impingement' may be a normal finding).

Tendinitis

- Impingement represents compressive or shearing trauma to the tendons of the rotator cuff; however, tensile overloading can also damage the microstructure, with resultant inflammation and dysfunction.
- Shoulder tendinitis usually implicates the tendons of supraspinatus, infraspinatus/teres minor and biceps brachii. Pectoralis major and latissimus dorsi are occasionally involved.

Rotator cuff tears

The rotator cuff is subject to occasional high levels of one-off loading, usually in the younger patient, and to years of daily loading in activities of living, working and recreation in the older age group. The latter pattern predisposes to gradual weakening of the cuff, with resultant degenerative changes and loss of muscle strength due to age and changing lifestyle.

Structures damaged

- Tendons of supraspinatus, infraspinatus or biceps brachii (the last may be avulsed or it may pull the superior labrum from the glenoid rim, the SLAP lesion (superior labral anterior posterior lesion)).

Signs and symptoms

- Acute or acute-on-chronic traumatic episode often involving falling onto the arm, or

preventing a fall by taking body weight through the shoulder.
- Initial pain, which may ease with rest, but which becomes persistent upon returning to activity and with the irritation of the inflammatory process.
- Pain on heavy loading or overhead elevation.
- Aching pain even at rest, especially with the arm dependent.
- Inability to lift the arm overhead (not a reliable sign).
- Pain and weakness on resisted testing of the rotator cuff muscles.
- Tenderness at the site of the tear.
- Positive findings on ultrasound investigation, computer tomography (CT) arthrogram, magnetic resonance imaging (MRI) or arthroscopic procedure.

Conclusive diagnosis of a rotator cuff tear is notoriously difficult, as the tear may be in-substance (contained within the tendon margins), partial thickness or full thickness. Diagnostic testing is useful but not reliable, subsequent operative findings often being at odds with one's suspicions.

Rotator cuff and capsular laxity

Laxity of the rotator cuff can result from repetitive microtrauma (gradual lengthening of the anterior capsule in baseball throwers, for example), or from macrotrauma (post-subluxation), or may be due to a genetic collagen deficiency (e.g. Ehlers–Danlos syndrome). If the control imparted by the dynamic restraints of the shoulder joint cannot stabilise the humeral head, the laxity may present as an instability, with episodes of micromotion ('dead-arm') or macromotion (subluxation or dislocation). This is a capsular laxity where the dynamic ligament tensioning function of the cuff muscles may be less effective due to the capsular attenuation or damage.

Management consists of a progressive strengthening programme for the rotator cuff muscles, commencing in mid-range and moving toward the limits of range and speed of movement as control and strength improve. The Allingham protocol (see Table 6.1) can be adapted by adding resistance exercises for the shoulder rotators. This programme relies heavily on the compliance of the subject and any improvement in stability will only apply while the rotator cuff is active. Unanticipated trauma, even minor, may result in instability as the passive restraints remain lengthened.

CONSERVATIVE TREATMENT PRINCIPLES

- Effort must be made to identify causative factors (postural, biomechanical, anatomical) in shoulder pain.
- These are often remote (e.g. spinal pathology or poor core stability) and may involve inappropriate recruitment patterns and timing of particular muscles.
- Aims of treatment:

1. immediate decrease in symptoms
2. optimal loading of shoulder complex through range
3. balanced muscle activity and stabiliser synergy
4. adequate mobility of soft tissue and neuromeningeal structures.

Unloading – symptom reduction

Unloading refers to any strategy that establishes a 'recovery-friendly' environment by reducing stresses and barriers that presdispose glenohumeral conditions to chronicity. Without adequate unloading, treatment is severely handicapped.

Rest, postural correction, manual therapy (massage or grade two joint mobilisations), taping, mobilisation of thoracic spine and shoulder flexibility or strength exercises are all examples of unloading strategies which may reduce the tensile irritation on inflamed tissues.

Taping

The use of taping to unload brings benefits by:

1. repositioning the humeral head to centralise it in the fossa (see Fig. 6.6).
2. facilitating the deltoid and/or unloading connective tissue tension of the cervicobrachical fascia or neural structures (very useful for night pain).
3. inhibiting the upper trapezius (cross fibre taping), thereby facilitating the lower trapezius (Fig. 6.7).

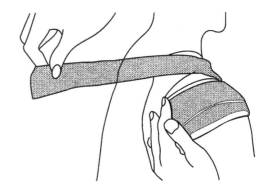

Figure 6.7 Application of the inhibitory tape across the fibres of upper trapezius. Firm tension is applied by pulling down on the tape.

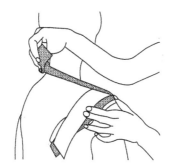 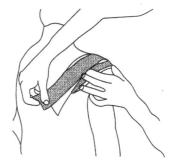

Figure 6.6 Repositioning tape for humeral head: first strip more lateral; second is over the acromion. Lift humeral head with thumb during application and continue tension with tape. Use hypoallergenic stretch tape (5 cm) on skin, and overtape with 38 mm rigid tape.

Normalise central posture and dysfunction

Mobilise stiff thoracic spine

- More effectively performed with the patient in sitting or side lying, thus avoiding the splinting effect of the ribcage on the plinth.
- Elements of shoulder elevation and fascial stretch or neural mobilising can be implemented during the spinal mobilisation procedure.
- Resisted external rotation of a stiff shoulder during mobilisation may help with capsular adhesions.
- Follow treatment with postural retraining and exercises to maintain any thoracic or shoulder mobility gains.

Mobilise stiff lumbar spine

- Shoulder mechanics can be affected by stiffness in the lumbar spine, especially if latissimus dorsi is tight.
- Mobilisation with the latissimus dorsi on stretch should precede home maintenance exercises.

Restore force couple synergy

Scapulothoracic junction

- Asymmetry on movement of the *scapulothoracic junction* (scapulohumeral rhythm) often indicates inappropriate compensatory muscle activity whereby the scapular elevators are initiated excessively or early in range, thereby placing the lower scapular muscles (lower trapezius and serratus anterior) at a recruitment disadvantage and reducing their ability to effectively control the scapula.
- The fibres of lower and middle trapezius must be activated to rotate the glenoid cavity upwards. This delays impingement and reduces the rotator cuff demand to control the head of humerus (in later range).
- Training focuses on patient awareness of posture and scapular position. 'Lift your sternum up' is a useful cue.

- A biofeedback machine is a useful learning tool in the early stage, with dual channels monitoring upper and lower trapezius simultaneously.
- Tactile feedback, visual feedback (via mirrors or direct video loop) can also help with the trapezius retraining. Stretching of shortened scapular elevators, mobilising of a tight scapulothoracic junction and taping to inhibit the elevators are useful adjuncts to treatment.

Glenohumeral cuff synergy

- Rotator cuff activity serves to centralise the humeral head in the glenoid fossa, preventing unwanted micromotion which may predispose to impingement (upward motion) or instability (anterior motion).
- An adduction-based programme, progressing from isometric near neutral to isotonic through range, appears effective in developing this control;[5] see Table 6.1.
- In addition to the neuromuscular training, subacromial congestion can be eased by the rhythmic pressure changes during the exercise/rest cycle of isometric exercise.
- This exercise is best combined with active scapular depression and sternal elevation to optimise the thoracic posture and inhibit recruitment of the already overactive scapular elevators.
- An optimal starting position is vital, so posture must be corrected and positional taping may help in the early stages (see Fig. 6.6)
- The exercise must be performed pain-free.

Functional retraining

- When the clinician is satisfied from the patient's reports and observations of movement in the clinic that the posture and mechanics of the upper quadrant are more 'normal', or at least less disturbed, a programme of progressive strengthening, flexibility and control exercises is incorporated into the programme.

Table 6.1 Shoulder rehabilitation – the Allingham Programme

Criteria for inclusion:
- must be able to execute resisted adduction without pain or tricking
- must have respected healing time post-trauma or surgery.

Stage	Activity
1. Posture	• Great attention to posture of thoracic spine, cervical spine, scapulothoracic and glenohumeral joints must be paid before commencing this programme • Optimal biomechanics of the glenohumeral joint cannot be achieved otherwise
2. Isometric adduction – neutral	• Adduction in the coronal or scapular plane using a pillow or bolster between the arm and ribcage (Fig. 6.8) • Maximal effort provided there is no pain • Ensure scapula is not elevated during execution by insisting on active depression if necessary • Ten repetitions for 8–10 seconds each
3. Isometric adduction – through range	• Isometric adduction at increasing points through range of elevation (various planes) up to 90 degrees • Again, avoid scapular elevation. Dosage as above
4. Isotonic adduction	• Adduction through range using pulleys or elastic resistance (Fig. 6.9) • Arm is concentrically adducted from outer range, and then eccentrically abducted from the adducted position • Must be done with no pain • Increased resistance will often reduce pain, by placing increased demands on glenohumeral adductor/downward glide force vectors • Range used and resistance offered depends on competent scapular control at each level of progression • Dosage is to fatigue of scapular control, pain or 15–20 repetitions, whichever comes first • Increase resistance if not fatiguing under 20 repetitions
5. Adduction plus external rotation	• Starting in the neutral (adducted) position with pillow or bolster as above • Maximal adduction is performed then combined with isometric (first) and then isotonic external rotation of the glenohumeral joint (Fig. 6.10) • Isotonic external rotation is done using pulleys or elastic resistance • Again, no pain during the exercise and attention to posture is required • Progression from isometric to isotonic, and the amount of isotonic resistance is dependent on competent scapular control • Progress to resisted rotations in outer ranges of abduction up to 100 degrees; more for swimmers and throwers
6. Brachiating	• Pull-up/step-up exercises introduced, whereby the arm is used to reach up in front and pull up body weight as the subject steps upwards at the same time (Fig. 6.11) • This exercise utilises the adductor/extensor group in its climbing action, for which it has evolved but may be underutilised in daily activity • Progress the lift provided by upper body by lessening the push from the legs • Remember scapular control
7. Core stability	• As needed, include exercises for core stability to improve control of lumbopelvic area in both open and closed-chain activities. Target transversus abdominus, gluteals and multifidus • This control is necessary to optimise the scapular and glenohumeral control
8. Shoulder hardening	• Progressive resistance exercise programme for all shoulder muscles (Fig. 6.12) • Gym-based and medium term at least (3–6 months)
9. Functional retraining	• Specific sport/occupational retraining, integrating the gains made throughout the programme into the specific movements and resistances of the subject's activities
10. Stretch shortening cycle	• Retraining of this eccentric/concentric action common to many throwing and racquet sports (Fig. 6.13) • Must have achieved 80% strength of uninjured side • Must be able to control scapula (quality of movement) during execution and complete pain-free • High-speed, low-dose exercises starting with bilateral work, progressing to unilateral • Quality of movement is vital and any fatigue or pain will undermine the end result

- These exercises begin with general trunk and pelvic stabilisers (lunges, abdominal curls, butt squats, trunk rotations), and upper back exercises (weighted rowing, prone flies, pull downs), progressing to light then heavy resistance exercises for the shoulder and arm using free weights, exercise tubing or hydrotherapy.
- At all times correct posture, core stability and normal scapular mechanics must be maintained.
- Eccentric exercises for tensile tendinitis has been advocated as providing optimal training stimulus for fibroblastic collagen repair,[6] and should be included in later rehabilitation. These are progressed by speed and/or external resistance.
- Later in rehabilitation the retraining becomes more activity-specific as determined by the intentions of the patient. Loading,

speed of movement, repetitions, rest periods and complexity are manipulated to simulate occupational, recreational or sporting activities for which the patient is being retrained.

The Allingham programme is shown in Table 6.1.

Principles of management – rotator cuff tears

Conservative management of a confirmed rotator cuff tear is dependent on the age, activity level, history and aspirations of the patient. For the younger subject with an acute tear, surgical repair is most likely to return them to near their previous level of function. For the degenerative tears in mid-to-later life, conservative management is the usual course of treatment until proven inadequate.

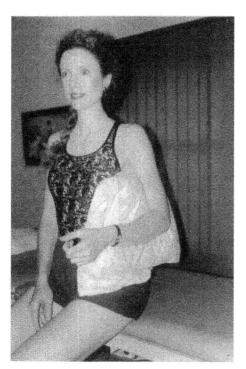

Figure 6.8 Isometric adduction: combined adduction of shoulder with depression of scapula in neutral. Must have cushion or bolster between arm and trunk (stage 2).

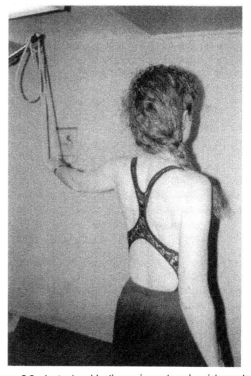

Figure 6.9 Isotonic adduction: using external resistance to train the adductors and/or extensors of the shoulder (stage 4).

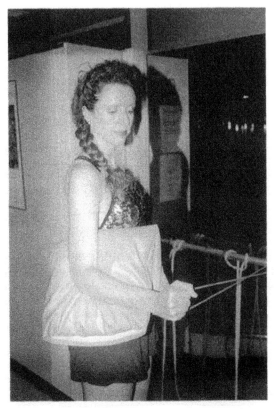

Figure 6.10 Isometric adduction with external rotation: introducing control of the humerus during isotonic rotation to strengthen posterior cuff (stage 5).

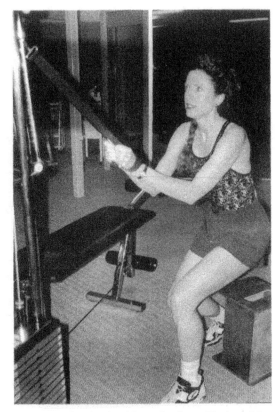

Figure 6.11 Brachiating: bilateral pull-up of body weight from sitting (stage 6).

Conservative management for rotator cuff tears comprises:

1. Unloading for pain modulation – taping, massage, postural advice, rest, medication, etc.
2. General strengthening of the upper body:
   - a progressive exercise programme to increase strength and control around the scapula and shoulder (see Table 6.1)
   - avoid any painful ranges or extremes of movement
   - where indicated, start with bilateral activities, gradually moving to unilateral work and incorporating movements utilising the injured cuff tendon(s) through their normal range as available.

The emphasis is on slow progressions because the quality of a degenerative cuff is quite poor; thus, a prolonged period of protection may be indicated.

CAPSULITIS/FROZEN SHOULDER

- The literature fails to describe capsulitis as a discrete entity, and it may exist as a prodromal first stage of adhesive capsulitis or frozen shoulder.
- The spontaneous onset of shoulder and upper arm pain is characterised by extreme limitation of range, initially by pain, and later by stiffness.
- Night pain is common and may disturb sleep.
- The aetiology of the condition is unknown, but it is common in postmenopausal females and post-thoracic surgery patients;

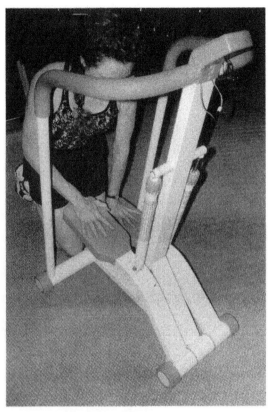

Figure 6.12   Shoulder strength and endurance work: building an aerobic base. Non-weight bearing reciprocal press exercise on stepper (stage 8).

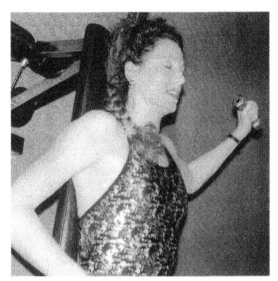

Figure 6.13   Stretch-shortening work: drop back plyometrics to train at the cocking/acceleration transition for throwing (stage 10).

emotional stress may also be a predisposing factor.
- Histopathological changes have been noted – fibrosis of the capsular structures, loss of intracapsular volume, fibroblastic proliferation and histochemical changes in the connective tissues.[7]
- Typically, a self-limiting condition which may take up to 2 years to resolve.

Diagnosis

Diagnosis of capsulitis often tends to be one of exclusion and natural history. Differential diagnosis should include:

- trauma (macro or micro) with a demonstrable mechanical or structural lesion

- cervical spine lesions
- thoracic spine lesions
- cardiac or visceral referral
- neurovascular
- neuromeningeal
- Pancoast's tumour.

Commonly, the time taken to complete the investigations allows opportunity for the condition to progress to the fibrotic stage when the 'diagnosis' of frozen shoulder is obvious, having developed from the capsulitis.

Frozen shoulder: management

Stage one – pain but still mobile

- Pain relief in initial stages; sometimes taping helps perhaps by decreasing neural tissue reactivity.
- Nonsteroidal and/or analgesic medication, or physical pain relief using TENS.
- Intra-articular steroid injections.
- Thoracic spine mobilisation and postural correction.
- Active exercise and gentle isometric strength work within pain limits.

Stage two – stiffness more than pain

- Thoracic spine, scapular and glenohumeral joint mobilisation and exercises to at least maintain ranges, and perhaps improve them.
- Massage, myofascial releases and stretches can reduce secondary connective tissue dysfunction.
- Aggressive mobilisation may prove counterproductive in terms of patient compliance.
- Hydrodilatation, particularly for patients with more than 100 degrees of abduction (L Watson, pers. comm.), and manipulation under anaesthetic,[8] usually combined with steroid infiltration of joint space – both followed by immediate joint mobilisation routines – have been shown to be of benefit.
- Any therapy if pursued for long enough will appear to be responsible for recovery when it spontaneously occurs.

CONCLUSION

Effective management of shoulder problems hinges on analysing the problem and understanding the environment in which the joint is acting. Therapy should be aimed at precipitating the changes that will optimise that environment. Once accomplished, the reconditioning phase of training continues to ensure all the stabilising muscles are fatigue-resistant and able to cope with the demands of work, sport and leisure.

CASE STUDY.

A case study illustrating the principles of management is now given:

A 58-year-old male fell onto his right shoulder and subsequently had difficulty lifting the arm. On examination, flexion was limited to 110 degrees, abduction to 50 degrees and external rotation to 25% of the uninjured side. External rotation was markedly weak (grade 3-). An ultrasound study revealed a tear in the supraspinatus tendon. Treatment involved taping the humeral head into a centred position and mobilising the thoracic spine. Range of motion improved to 170 degrees flexion and 130 degrees abduction. External rotation strength improved to grade 4. After 4 months, full pain-free range was achieved and planned surgery was cancelled. Review at 6 months showed complete functional return (even skiing).

REFERENCES

1. Kapandji I: The physiology of the joints, Vol 1, Upper limb, 2nd edn. Edinburgh: Churchill Livingstone, 1970.
2. Ayoub E: Posture and the upper quarter. In: Donatelli R (ed.), Physical therapy of the shoulder. New York: Churchill Livingstone, 1987.
3. Crawford H, Jull G: The influence of thoracic form and movement on ranges of shoulder flexion. Proceedings MPAA 7th Biennial Conference, 1991.
4. Allingham CM: Regional considerations: the shoulder. In: Zuluaga M et al. (eds), sports physiotherapy: applied science and practice. Melbourne: Churchill-Livingstone, 1995.
5. Allingham CM: The sporting shoulder: course notes, Redsok Seminars, Maroochydore, 1996.
6. Curwin S, Stanish D: Tendinitis: its etiology and treatment. Toronto: Collamore Press, 1984.
7. Owens-Burkhart H: Management of frozen shoulder. In: Donatelli R (ed.), Physical therapy of the shoulder. New York: Churchill Livingstone, 1987.
8. Kelley M, Clark W (eds): Orthopedic therapy of the shoulder. Philadelphia: JB Lippincott, 1995.

FURTHER READING

Falkel J, Murphy T: Shoulder injuries. In: Malone T (ed.), Sports injury management. Baltimore: Williams & Wilkins, 1988.

C. FRACTURES

David Sonnabend and Jill Allen

Fractures about the shoulder girdle include injuries to the clavicle and scapula but the commonest site of bony disruption is the proximal humerus (Fig. 6.14).

FRACTURES IN CHILDHOOD

Before skeletal maturity, the humeral head may separate through the physeal plate, often taking a piece of metaphysis with it in a 'Salter–Harris type 11' pattern. These fractures can frequently be reduced by *manipulation*. Sometimes a flap of periosteum between the fragments, a displaced biceps tendon or the buttonholing of bone through the overlying deltoid muscle may prevent closed reduction. In these cases, *open surgical reduction* is generally easily stabilised by simple internal fixation, such as the use of Kirschner wires. While anatomical reduction is attractive, it is far from essential.

The proximal humerus in the paediatric patient has an extraordinary potential for remodelling. Because of the enormous range of movement in the human shoulder, *residual bony deformity even after skeletal maturity is compatible with normal shoulder function.*

FRACTURES IN EARLY ADULTHOOD

In early adulthood, proximal humeral fractures usually result from relatively high-energy injury (Fig. 6.15), and may present in a polytrauma setting. With the attainment of middle age, the abductor mechanism (rotator cuff tendons and their greater tuberosity insertions) may fail either

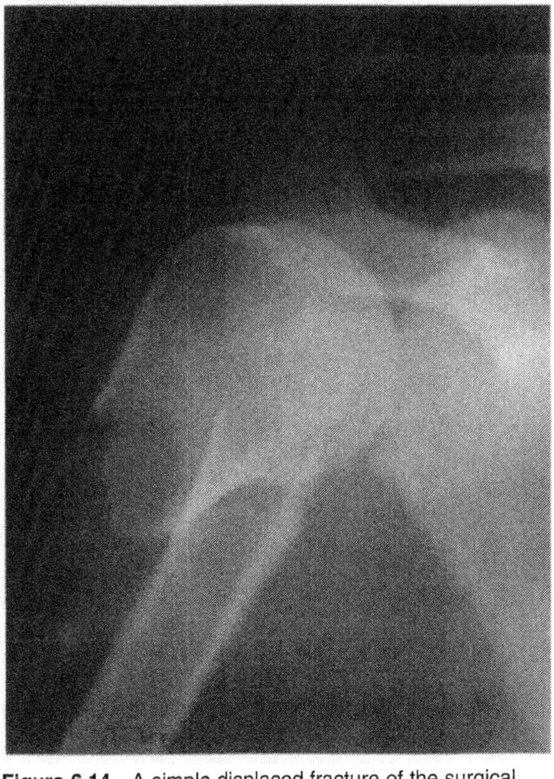

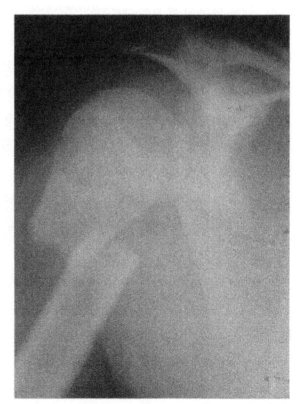

Figure 6.14 A simple displaced fracture of the surgical neck of the humerus – suitable for internal fixation if closed reduction unsuccessful.

Figure 6.15 Proximal humeral fracture. The associated scapular fracture implies a 'high-energy injury'.

through the tendon, with resultant rotator cuff disruption, or by avulsion of the greater tuberosity.

FRACTURES IN OLDER AGE

With further ageing, the by now osteoporotic bone of the greater tuberosity becomes the weak link in the chain, and *greater tuberosity avulsion* is not uncommon. In the elderly, *fractures of the surgical neck of the humerus* are almost as common as fractured hips, and like them, often result from minor trauma to an osteoporotic skeleton. Not surprisingly, they are more common in women. They are frequently impacted, and in the absence of concurrent dislocation or tuberosity fracture, *generally do not require surgical intervention*.

ANATOMICAL CLASSIFICATION AND SIGNIFICANCE

The blood supply of the proximal humerus is somewhat precarious, and may be jeopardised in certain fracture patterns. Proximal humeral fractures have been classified according to how many 'fragments' are present.

To be classed as a separate fragment, a fracture line must result in at least 45 degrees of angulation or 1 cm of fracture separation.[1] Although possibly a little simplistic, the classification of proximal humeral fractures into two-, three- and four-part patterns is very useful in deciding treatment.

TREATMENT

Operative

The blood supply to the humeral head enters through the neck of the humerus and both tuberosities. If both tuberosities and the humeral neck are fractured, as in the 'four-part pattern' (Fig. 6.16), then the blood supply to the head is very much at risk. *Avascular necrosis* of the humeral head is an unhappy problem. In this setting, many surgeons choose primary humeral head hemiarthroplasty for four-part fractures (Fig. 6.17). One possible exception is the impacted valgus fracture of the humeral neck, which even

if technically 'four-part', rarely produces avascular necrosis. The role of humeral head hemiarthroplasty in three-part fractures is not as well established. In the elderly osteoporotic patient, or in the grossly displaced three-part fracture, many clinicians opt for *hemiarthroplasty*. Gentle osteosynthesis with careful attention to preserving the remaining humeral head blood supply is the alternative. *The emphasis is on stability and preservation of vasculature rather than on restoration of anatomical normality.*

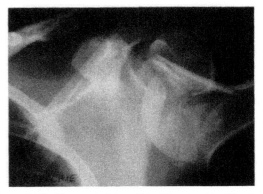

Figure 6.16 Four-part dislocation of the shoulder. Greater and lesser tuberosities are both widely displaced, as is the humeral head. Hemiarthroplasty is indicated, as humeral head is avascular.

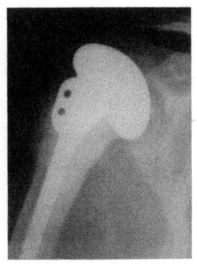

Figure 6.17 Humeral head hemiarthroplasty for four-part fracture. Greater and lesser tuberosities are both 'back in place', and rotator cuff should function well.

Non-operative

Important considerations in the treatment of shoulder fractures include the use of *slings* or other forms of immobilisation, and the *timing* of passive and active mobilisation.

While a collar and cuff may be easier to apply, it is frequently inappropriate for proximal humeral fractures, many of which become impacted at the time of injury. While this bone-to-bone apposition is maintained, fracture healing occurs. If the fracture becomes disimpacted, not only is inherent stability lost and reduction altered, but a gap may occur, a prelude to non-union. *With a collar and cuff, the weight of the arm acts to distract the fracture.* A triangular sling has the opposite effect, with the elbow resting on a surface which prevents its downward displacement, maintaining impaction and helping stability and bone union. Different considerations apply in the treatment of humeral shaft fractures, where the weight of the hanging arm may be used to straighten an angulated fracture.

Mobilisation – when and how

Prolonged shoulder immobilisation following trauma, be it unintentional or surgical, often leads to severe *stiffness. It is easier to retain movement than to regain it.* Following trauma, shoulder mobilisation could be commenced as early as is possible without jeopardising fracture stability and healing. Non-union of humeral neck fractures is not uncommon, and its treatment is difficult and often unsatisfactory. Striking a balance between early mobilisation to avoid stiffness and careful immobilisation to minimise risk of non-union is not easy.

Some authorities[2] advocate *gentle mobilisation*, initially by pendular exercises, as early as is tolerated. It is claimed that this does not increase the non-union rate, but this has not always been the authors' experience. Certainly, where a two-part humeral neck fracture is impacted and relatively stable, early mobilisation is optimal. In non-impacted comminuted three-part fractures of grossly osteoporotic bone, it is inappropriate. Several manoeuvres may help *determine when mobilisation can safely begin.* It is often possible to feel the humeral head through the deltoid, especially in a thin patient. Palpation then allows the examiner to detect any movement at the fracture site when the arm is abducted or rotated. If no movement occurs, and X-rays show a suitable fracture pattern, early mobilisation is appropriate. Alternatively, examination of the shoulder under image intensifier (fluoroscopy) control helps determine when a humeral neck fracture is sticky enough to be mobilised.

NON-OPERATIVE TREATMENT – SPECIAL CONSIDERATIONS

Greater tuberosity fractures

The rotator cuff tendons attach to the greater tuberosity. Contraction of the cuff musculature (supraspinatus, infraspinatus and teres minor) pulls on the tuberosity. If that tuberosity is broken from the humeral head, contraction of the cuff muscles can further displace the tuberosity. Thus, fracture patterns which include a displaced greater tuberosity fracture (Figs 6.18 and 6.19) can be made worse by active shoulder mobilisation

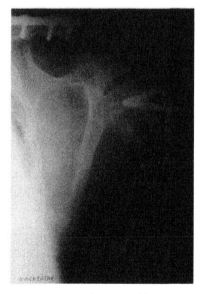

Figure 6.18 High-energy fractures of humerus and clavicle. The greater tuberosity fragment is displaced from the head, which in turn is displaced from the shaft – a 'three-part fracture'.

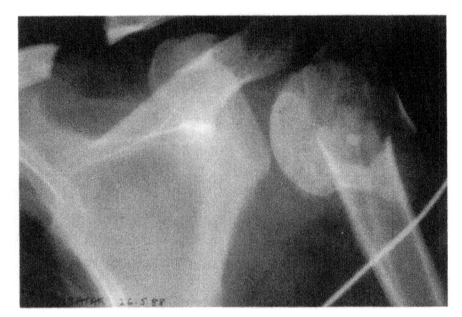

Figure 6.19 Internal fixation of the fracture shown in Fig. 6.17. A blade plate holds the humeral fractures firmly and allows early mobilisation.

before the fracture is 'sticky'. Gentle passive mobilisation however, particularly in the lines of pull of the cuff muscles, should not worsen any displacement. Consequently, greater tuberosity fracture is not a contraindication to passive mobilisation, other than into internal rotation.

Lesser tuberosity fractures

Lesser tuberosity fractures are rare 'in isolation' but not uncommon as components of three- or four-part fractures. With the subscapularis tendon attached to the lesser tuberosity, active internal rotation and passive external rotation are likely to displace the tuberosity. When considering whether or how to mobilise a fracture involving the tuberosities involving the humeral head, these factors should be considered.

Secondary impingement

The main problem associated with displaced fractures of the greater tuberosity is secondary impingement. The tuberosity is displaced upwards and backwards, and in its 'new position' may catch on the undersurface of the mid and posterior acromion. Simple anterior acromiplasty does not correct the problem. To decide whether open reduction is warranted, examination under fluoroscopy may help. An approximate rule of thumb is that *displacement of 1 cm or more on an anteroposterior radiograph requires re-reduction.*

OPERATIVE TREATMENT – SPECIAL CONSIDERATIONS

Where a fracture has been treated operatively, the surgeon should have a good idea of the fracture stability. *Liaison between therapist and surgeon and discussion with the patient are essential.*

In the majority of humeral head and neck fractures, treatment is non-operative. The factors outlined above must be considered, and each case must be treated on an individual basis. Blanket rules are inappropriate and dangerous. Many impacted fractures can be mobilised passively as soon as pain subsides. *Most humeral neck fractures can be mobilised passively by at least the 3-week mark.*

Progression to active-assisted and then active exercises needs to be individualised. In all cases, the aim is to mobilise as early as possible, progressing from passive to active-assisted and then active as quickly as possible without jeopardising fracture stability or bone union. As outlined in Chapter 2H, most of the mobilisation is performed by the patient, initially with help from family or friend, and ideally under the direction of a caring and attentive therapist.

If progress is inadequate (e.g. apparent non-union or failure to mobilise), the treating clinician should be reintroduced into the equation as soon as a problem is recognised. In this setting, ongoing inappropriate physical therapy further prejudices the end result and may turn an easily treated delayed union into an almost unsalvageable non-union.

SPECIFIC TIPS

- Liaison between physiotherapist and surgeon is vital.
- Careful passive movement, e.g. pendular movements, can be started before complete union to prevent stiffness.
- After union, an individual home treatment programme, monitored by the therapist, assists full recovery.

REFERENCES

1. Neer CS: Displaced proximal humeral fractures (Parts I & II). J Bone Joint Surg 52A:1077–103, 1970.

2. Resch H, Beck E, Bayley I: Reconstruction of the valgus-impacted humeral head fracture. J Shoulder Elbow Surg 4(2):73–80, 1995.

D. ROTATOR CUFF PATHOLOGY

David Sonnabend and Jill Allen

ANATOMY

The tendons of supraspinatus, infraspinatus and teres minor blend together near their insertion to the greater tuberosity to form a single tendinous 'cuff'. This cuff sits over the top and back of the humeral head, with its deep surface blending with the underlying capsule of the shoulder joint. This 'blending' is so complete that in adults the capsule and cuff form a single layer. Anteriorly, the tendon of subscapularis blends similarly with the capsule of the shoulder joint, as it extends laterally to attach to the lesser tuberosity, and is sometimes also included in the 'definition' of the rotator cuff. Inferiorly, no tendon blends with the shoulder capsule.

FUNCTIONAL CONSIDERATIONS

The prime function of the rotator cuff is to hold the humeral head down, and in apposition to the glenoid surface. This enables the deltoid and other shoulder girdle muscles to move the humeral head around a centre of rotation. Without the rotator cuff, deltoid contraction pulls the humeral head upwards instead of rotating the arm, and this causes the humeral head to abut on the undersurface of the acromion, and lose its articulation with the glenoid. The normal cuff runs under the coracoacromial arch, a 'half tunnel' produced by the undersurfaces of the coracoacromial ligament and the acromion. If the humeral head rises or the supraspinatus outlet (the half tunnel) is encroached on by acromial spur formation, the cuff can rub on the undersurface of that coracoacromial arch, producing the so-called *impingement syndrome.*

CUFF PATHOLOGY

- Impingement.
- Interstitial cuff disease.
- Partial-thickness cuff tear (articular or bursal side).
- Cuff lamination.
- Full-thickness tear.

Most rotator cuff disease is probably multifactorial. Interstitial cuff degeneration, possibly due to local ischaemia, can result in cuff damage and failure. A weak rotator cuff may allow proximal migration of the humeral head, with resultant secondary subacromial impingement. Similarly, primary impingement from above by an acromial spur may damage the cuff. The tendon may be injured by overuse, either chronic or on a 'one time' basis. Other specific diseases may also involve the rotator cuff, including *calcific tendonitis* (acute or chronic) with associated inflammation. Acute calcific tendonitis may be extraordinarily disabling. Any condition which affects synovium can involve the subacromial (subdeltoid) bursa, with secondary effects on the underlying rotator cuff. Ongoing cuff disease and impingement may result in partial or full-thickness cuff tear.

SYMPTOMS OF CUFF DISEASE

Pain from the rotator cuff is typically *severe at night*, and inability to sleep is often the patient's main complaint. The pain is exacerbated by forward reaching and overhead activity, which involves contraction of the spinati in particular.

CLINICAL PRESENTATION

The pain of subacromial impingement typically occurs in the *mid-arc of forward flexion*, and interferes with various activities of daily living and overhead sport. Patients may be able to push a full wheelbarrow with their arms by their side, but lifting a tea cup to a shelf may be agonising. Carrying the shopping may be easy, but serving a tennis ball impossible. Driving a car may be painful, whereas playing golf may not pain the dominant arm.

CUFF TEARS

Rotator cuff tears may be partial or full thickness. They may commence on the bursal (dorsal) or articular (deep) surface of the cuff, or may begin as interstitial disease which extends through the cuff. Arthroscopic and MRI studies suggest that the commonest sequence of events might be a deep surface rim rent of the anterior portion of the supraspinatus insertion, extending to become a full-thickness disruption. *Most lesions appear to start anteriorly*, just behind the biceps tendon.

The exact *incidence* of cuff tear in the community is not known. The incidence of cuff tears rises with age. Cadaver studies suggest that as many as 50% of people above the age of 70 might have full-thickness cuff tears. Many are probably asymptomatic.

Cuff tears may produce pain, weakness or both. When the tear involves mainly supraspinatus, a strong anterior deltoid can to some extent compensate, allowing some overhead activity. As the tear extends into infraspinatus, weakness of external rotation also arises. Tears may extend posteriorly, to effectively detach all of supraspinatus. If the tear continues even further, infraspinatus is also defunctioned. Prolonged 'defunctioning' of a muscle results in wasting, and large long-standing tears of supraspinatus are accompanied by palpable and often visible *wasting* of that muscle belly. If infraspinatus is also wasted, this implies a very large and long-standing tear, and does not auger well for repair or rehabilitation. Some rotator cuff tears are also accompanied by subscapularis disruption.

The ability of people to use the shoulders in the presence of full-thickness cuff tears varies enormously. People who work overhead, such as painters, plasterers and electricians, find cuff pathology severely disabling. Strenuous housework also places considerable demands on the rotator cuff. Repetitive forward-reaching at a keyboard may even make desk work difficult for people with significant cuff pathology.

CLINICAL ASSESSMENT OF CUFF DISEASE

- History – assess mode of onset and duration of symptoms. Long-standing cuff tears may retract, making repair difficult.
- Assess specific difficulties, especially occupational and sporting.
- Ask the patients what bothers them most. Minor disability and 'nuisance value'

symptoms may not warrant the prolonged inconvenience of formal rotator cuff repair.

PHYSICAL EXAMINATION

- Check for visible or palpable wasting of the spinati.
- 'Impingement testing': In the impingement test, the humeral head is pushed upwards beneath the acromion. If the rotator cuff is inflamed, catching beneath the humeral head and the acromion produces pain as the arm is forward flexed through the midarc. The pain may be exacerbated by internal rotation of the shoulder.
- Check for pain on active cuff contraction against resistance. This suggests interstitial cuff damage. Weakness of external rotation suggests infraspinatus involvement, implying a large tear.
- Is the long head of the biceps torn? The biceps tendon is often involved in the impingement process beneath the coracoacromial arch, and disruption of the long head of biceps is not uncommon in this setting.

Subscapularis should be assessed by Gerber's lift-off test.[1] If this is not possible, then in a thin patient, the strength of internal rotation in adduction may be tested by resisted pressing of the hand onto the anterior abdomen.

TREATMENT OF ROTATOR CUFF DISEASE

Impingement and tendinopathy

The diagnosis of impingement is essentially a clinical one, suggested by nocturnal shoulder pain, pain in the mid and upper range of forward flexion and abduction, and difficulty with overhead activities. The impingement sign, described above, is positive, and an injection of local anaesthetic into the subacromial bursa, the impingement test, temporarily relieves pain. X-rays may show a type-3 (hooked) acromion, or a spur on the undersurface of the anterior acromion, encroaching on the subacromial space. This is best seen on the outlet view. MRI and ultrasound may support the diagnosis, but are not infallible. Ultrasound, in particular, is very observer-dependent.

Treatment of subacromial impingement

Initial treatment of impingement includes alteration or restriction of particularly painful activities (e.g. overhead shots at tennis). One or two injections of steroid to the subacromial space may reduce inflammation and associated swelling, breaking the cycle of impingement and swelling.

Exercises? what and why:

- The mainstay of non-operative treatment is exercise. Posterior capsule stretching, inner range internal and external rotator strengthening and scapular stabilising exercises are important.
- A tight posterior capsule holds the humeral head higher than normal, and posterior capsule stretching reverses this, increasing the subacromial space.
- The shoulder rotators, especially subscapularis and infraspinatus, have a downward component to their vector, and increased tone in those muscles also lowers the humeral head. Subscapularis is most active in the inner range of internal rotation.
- Strong scapular stabilisers enable more of the forward flexion and abduction arcs to be performed by scapulothoracic movement. This reduces the required range of glenohumeral movement in those directions, thus reducing 'exposure' to impingement.

Tendinopathy

Impingement involves movement of the cuff beneath the arch. If static cuff contraction against resistance is painful, this suggests 'intrinsic' cuff pathology. This diagnosis may be supported by changes on ultrasound, or especially by MRI scan. If intrinsic cuff pathology (tendinopathy) is suspected, the exercise regime should also include supraspinatus stretches.

The specific exercises are described below. When commencing patients on exercises for cuff disease, it is important to tell them that the first week or two of exercises may increase their discomfort. If possible, they should persist with their programme for 8–10 weeks before assessing its efficacy.

Cuff tears may be repaired by tendon-to-tendon suture or by repair to bone. If these techniques do not suffice, tendon transfers are occasionally used. Subscapularis may be advanced superiorly to close a cuff defect. Rarely, latissimus dorsi may be transferred to help depress the humeral head and allow some external rotation or abduction. In these cases, special rehabilitation considerations apply.

Non-operative treatment of rotator cuff tears

The pain comes from the damaged tendon tissue itself, (intrinsic) and from impingement of the deranged tendon beneath the coracoacromial arch. The latter can in part be relieved by the same measures which are used for subacromial impingement of the intact cuff. This regime of capsule *stretching*, *rotator strengthening* and *scapular stabilising* exercises, and *occasional subacromial steroids*, may suffice. Certainly many people have asymptomatic full-thickness rotator cuff tears that do not require surgery. These non-operative measures may, however, hide a deteriorating situation, or delay operative intervention, while a large cuff tear retracts and becomes irreparable. Judgement is required in deciding between operative and non-operative regimes.

How long to persist with non-operative treatment

There is no urgency about surgery in the absence of full-thickness cuff tears. At least *3 months* of conservative measures should be trialled before any consideration is given to intervention. In the presence of a significant full-thickness tear, conservative management should be persisted with if results are clearly forthcoming, or if the patient is not a suitable candidate for surgery.

Surgical treatment of cuff disease

Decompression

Enlargement of the subacromial space is the key to correcting impingement. Resection of the coracoacromial ligament and removal of the undersurface of the anterior third of the acromion, together with the associated acromial spur, is referred to as 'acromioplasty'. It is a reliable and effective procedure, which can be performed either by open surgery or arthroscopically. The former is somewhat more precise, but involves detachment and reattachment of part of the anterior deltoid, which needs to heal postoperatively before active rehabilitation exercises can be undertaken.

This usually means a 2- or 3-week period of passive exercises only. Arthroscopic decompression does not involve deltoid detachment, and allows immediate active postoperative mobilisation.

Cuff repair

When a cuff tear is repaired, early tendon healing takes at least 6 weeks and, during that period, passive mobilisation is recommended. As cuff healing progresses, patients advance to *active assisted*, *active* and finally *active resisted* programmes, outlined below. Some cuff tears are repaired under tension, and require postoperative splinting in abduction to allow initial healing. In this setting, help may be required in lowering the arm to the side gradually, possibly in stages, before active mobilisation commences (see Postoperative therapy section).

The biceps and subscapularis tendons are occasionally involved in subacromial impingement and cuff tear. If the biceps tendon is significantly deranged, tenodesis in the bicipital groove allows more distal biceps function (elbow supination and flexion) to continue. If a *biceps tenodesis* has been performed however, it is effectively another form of tendon reattachment to bone. Six weeks of protection are then required before the elbow can be straightened (actively or passively) or active flexion and supination undertaken. Whereas most patients undergoing shoulder surgery are encouraged to keep their elbow, hand and wrist mobile, patients undergoing *biceps* tenodesis need to be protected for the first 6 weeks.

If subscapularis is repaired, either 'in isolation' or as part of a large cuff repair, active internal and passive external rotation need to be avoided for the first 3 weeks postoperatively, and then introduced gradually: this minimises strain on the repair.

CONSERVATIVE THERAPY FOR ROTATOR CUFF TEARS

- Not all patients are candidates for cuff repairs; neither do all tears require surgery.
- Relief from pain can often be achieved by easing the associated cuff impingement between the humeral head and the coracoacromial arch.
- A programme of *capsular stretching* and *rotator strengthening exercises* (spinati and subscapularis) can widen the 'gap' through which the tendon passes, relieving impingement on the tendon.
- *Scapular stabilising* exercises may reduce the need for glenohumeral movement by reducing scapulothoracic function.
- A regime of exercises for the patient to follow for a few minutes 5 times a day. While initially the symptoms may be exacerbated, continuing the programme for 6 to 8 weeks and avoiding overarm activity can result in a more comfortable lifestyle.

POSTOPERATIVE THERAPY FOLLOWING ROTATOR CUFF REPAIR

Before commencing therapy, discuss the operative procedure with the surgeon. Relevant factors such as the size of the tear and the condition and tension on the cuff will modify rehabilitation.

Splintage

- A sling, often with a body strap.
- As above, with the inclusion of a small abduction pad.
- Abduction frame or cushion.

The arm is immobilized for 6 weeks in one of the above devices. The abduction support may be removed at 2–4 weeks, if the patient can bring the arm down to the side without a pulling sensation. This should be done slowly and carefully so the repair is not put at risk.

During this period, passive movement only is permitted in the form of forward flexion, demonstrated by the physiotherapist to a family member or friend. The elbow is also flexed and extended and the patient encouraged to do hand exercises. This is made more comfortable for the patient if the shoulder is warmed first, either by a hot water bottle or warm shower, two or three times a day. In the absence of family the patient is instructed in pendulum exercise.

From 6–12 weeks. The sling is discarded and pulley exercises commenced. An explanation of a pulley system is given to the family prior to this time so that one can be erected at home. Initially, all the work is controlled by the opposite limb, with the operated arm moving as a passenger.

Sometimes a sling can replace the handle of the pulley until the arm is comfortable in the outstretched position. The pulley should be used 3 or 4 times a day. The foot can 'drive' the pulley if the opposite arm is non-functional.

During this time the patient starts active assisted movements with the arm being lifted by the opposite limb. Active movement from the elbow allows for activity at table or bench height, as long as the elbow is kept tucked in at the waist.

The patient may begin to use the arm actively, only and without resistance. Stretching exercises and the use of the pulley are continued alone at home. Driving is resumed gradually, depending on the size of the tear. Therapy visits during this time are only continued if the shoulder is unacceptably stiff.

From 12–20 weeks. The patient returns to therapy to begin a progressive strengthening programme that includes the use of resistant elastic tubing and light weights for the spinati and deltoid muscles. Scapulothoracic exercises are also commenced. These exercises are continued for the next few months until the tendon repair has reached full strength.

This regime is conservative, as resisted exercises are not introduced until significant tendon healing has occurred. Maximal realignment of the collagen fibres may take 9 months. Many practices are more aggressive in their return to strengthening exercises, but we prefer caution until time has elapsed for realignment of collagen fibres following tendon healing.

Specific tips

- It is important that the patient understands, before surgery, that the lengthy rehabilitation period may take up to 6 months.
- An oversized shirt or blouse will be needed to fit over the immobiliser.
- A protocol sheet outlining the postoperative therapy helps the patient prepare for the various stages.

THERAPY FOR ARTHROSCOPIC ACROMIOPLASTY (WITHOUT CUFF REPAIR)

A sling is worn for comfort for first few days, with gentle active assisted and pendulum exercises begun on day 1.

Active movements in all directions, except abduction, are carried out for the *first 6 weeks*. If the patient shows signs of stiffness, a pulley should be used at home. Monitoring of range by the therapist during this period may help.

At 6 weeks, progressive strengthening exercises with the use of elastic tubing and light weights are started. These may be started earlier if tolerated.

Pain at the anterior acromial-deltoid margin is sometimes experienced for a while. This is because some of the deltoid fibres are cut during surgery.

REFERENCE

1. Gerber C, Krushell RJ: Isolated ruptures of the tendon of the subscapularis muscle. Orthop Trans 14:261, 1990.

E.   ARTHROPLASTY

David Sonnabend and Jill Allen

Shoulder replacement was a relatively uncommon procedure until the 1970s. The work of Charles Neer established both *total shoulder replacement* and *humeral head hemiarthroplasty* (Fig. 6.20) as reliable and important procedures. The commonest indication for total shoulder replacement is glenohumeral arthritis, including rheumatoid and osteoarthritis. Humeral head hemiarthroplasty is used in various situations: shoulder reconstruction following four- and sometimes three-part fractures; in cases of avascular necrosis; and for a variety of salvage situations, including malunion and non-union of proximal humeral fractures.

Early dissatisfaction with arthroplasty related to frequent unsatisfactory results, with stiffness and poor function. More recently, the importance of soft tissue handling intraoperatively, careful muscle

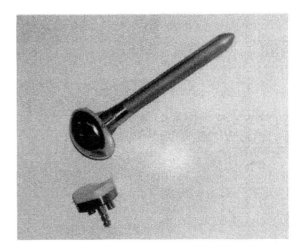

Figure 6.20   The metal joint.

balancing and fastidious attention to rehabilitation have resulted in dramatically improved results. More than with any other joint, *individualised and careful postoperative rehabilitation* is essential if the results of arthroplasty are to be optimised.

Early carefully supervised aggressive mobilisation is critical. Unlike hips and knees, where early postoperative stiffness can be overcome by long-term exercise, early stiffness following shoulder arthroplasty can be largely irreversible. Patient, surgeon and therapist must all appreciate the importance of the early postoperative weeks, and work together towards a common goal. Each patient's rehabilitation needs to be individualised, and details of findings at operation, including tissue strength and prosthetic stability, all contribute to the rehabilitation plan. In this regard, detailed communication between surgeon and therapist is critical.

THERAPY FOR TOTAL SHOULDER REPLACEMENT INCLUDING HEMIARTHROPLASTY

Sling. A sling is worn for 1 week. It is retained and worn for comfort. During this period, the patient may remove the sling while lying in bed or sitting in a chair.

Day 2. Passive forward flexion and external rotation are commenced, together with the use of a pulley. Safe range of external rotation is discussed with the surgeon first. Hand and elbow movements are demonstrated and continued throughout.

Day 7 or earlier. On removal of the sling, active exercises are commenced. Pulley work continues and some gentle isometrics help to strengthen the muscles. It may be safe to start active work earlier, if it is comfortable.

The active exercises introduced are climbing up a wall, using the rings on wall bars and some 'hanging' to increase the forward flexion range. The range often does not quite return to full, but at least 130 degrees of forward flexion and 30 degrees of external rotation (pain-free) can generally be expected, enabling most patients to carry out normal daily functional activities.

Day 28. Gradual progression to strengthening exercises for all muscles while maintaining stretching exercises. Care should be taken with those patients with rheumatoid arthritis or tenuous rotator cuffs. The use of a wall-mounted wheel encourages circumduction, with the height and tension being gradually increased.

Week 8. The first 8 weeks are paramount for the future of the new shoulder, but with continuing exercising, range and strength improve for months postoperatively.

Specific tips

- A wall-mounted wheel helps to regain shoulder circumduction.
- As with any joint replacement, antibiotics should be commenced immediately in the event of any infection such as a tooth abscess.
- Important to know if the rotator cuff is intact when gauging the range and strength of movement.

F. ARTHRODESIS

David Sonnabend and Jill Allen

Shoulder arthrodesis is a relatively uncommon procedure. It involves fusion of the humeral head to the glenoid socket, eliminating glenohumeral movement. Although two-thirds of normal 'shoulder movement' occurs at the glenohumeral joint, approximately one-third occurs at the scapulothoracic articulation. If a patient has good scapular motors, he can obtain useful shoulder movement in the presence of a glenohumeral fusion.

FUSION POSITION

Just where scapular movement can position the upper arm in space depends on the 'position of fusion'. In general, surgeons aim for a position of approximately 20 degrees of abduction, 30 degrees of forward flexion and 40 degrees of internal rotation relative to the trunk. The usual aim is to position the arm so that the *hand can, with elbow flexion, be brought to the mouth.* However, varying patient shapes and requirements determine the 'optimal position' for any one case.

When the arm is resting by the patient's side, fusion with greater abduction than 20 degrees allows more movement of the shoulder. However, when the arm is resting by the patient's side, it forces the scapula more medially than is comfortable, increasing parascapular discomfort.

INDICATIONS FOR ARTHRODESIS

Bone and joint infection, particularly tuberculosis, was once the commonest indication for shoulder arthrodesis. With improved antimicrobial therapy and effective shoulder replacement techniques, arthrodesis is now generally reserved for patients with paralytic problems. These include proximal brachial plexus palsies, where elbow and hand function is often normal. In patients with more extensive plexus palsies, arthrodesis may be performed primarily for comfort, or to augment the value of partial distal function, following tendon transfer, or reinnervation of a paralysed biceps, to restore elbow flexion. The ability to 'position the arm in space', even if it is only to be used as an 'assist arm', is often important. Where a paralysed flail shoulder hangs in inferior dislocation, the associated pain is often relieved by arthrodesis of the joint in a reduced position.

SCAPULAR CONTROL AND PHYSICAL THERAPY

To use a shoulder arthrodesis to best advantage, a patient *needs good scapular control*. Reasonable,

scapular control is a prerequisite for shoulder arthrodesis. As the surgical procedure is generally followed by several months of prolonged splint immobilisation, previously strong scapular motors may waste during the convalescent period. Once bony union has been achieved, usually by 10 weeks postoperatively, instruction and practice in using scapular motors to position the arm and hand in space are invaluable.

Splintage

The shoulder is immobilised for 8–10 weeks postoperatively, subject to clinical and radiological progress.

Therapy

While the shoulder is splinted, begin gentle active elbow, wrist and finger movements. Following splint removal, and subject to X-ray review, scapulothoracic exercises are commenced (see Chapter 6H).

Specific tip

Two-thirds of shoulder movement is glenohumeral and one-third is scapulothoracic. The patient will have a much reduced range of movement after the glenohumeral joint is fused. Therapy goals should be focused on obtaining the maximum range of scapulothoracic movement.

G.   INSTABILITY

David Sonnabend and Jill Allen

CLASSIFICATION

Classification of shoulder instability (Table 6.2) is according to direction, aetiology and voluntary or involuntary nature.

Frequency and ease of recurrence, together with degree of reduction, should be noted. Any concurrent axillary nerve palsy should be recorded.

Table 6.2 Classification of shoulder instability

Direction	Aetiology	Mechanism
Anterior	Non-traumatic	Voluntary
Posterior	Traumatic	Involuntary
Inferior	Trauma: major or repetitive	Habitual
Multidirectional		

Predisposing factors such as ligamentous laxity, abnormal humeral neck version or shoulder hypoplasia may coexist.

The commonest form of instability is *post-traumatic anterior instability*. Here, the humeral head is displaced anteriorly and inferiorly by combined abduction and external rotation of the shoulder. The initial episode is often the result of considerable violence, such as in the sporting arena. Subsequent dislocations may occur with increasing ease. The main static stabiliser is the inferior glenohumeral ligament. This is a condensation of the anterior portion of the shoulder capsule, between the neck of the humerus laterally and the anteroinferior labrum and adjacent glenoid neck medially.

PATHOLOGY OF ANTERIOR INSTABILITY

With the arm forced into abduction external rotation, the humeral head moves downwards and forwards. The inferior glenohumeral ligament may become stretched or be torn from its insertion. The *Bankart lesion* is a *capsulolabral disruption* at the medial end of the inferior glenohumeral ligament. As recurrences occur, *the ligament and adjacent capsule become increasingly stretched.* Sometimes the effect of a dislocation is purely that of capsular stretch. On rare occasions, the capsule may be avulsed laterally from the humeral neck rather than medially.

ANATOMICAL CONSIDERATIONS

The glenohumeral ligaments are condensations or thickenings of the capsule rather than *discrete bands.* Another important concept is that of the rotator interval. This is the gap between the superior glenohumeral ligament and the capsule underlying the anterior margin of supraspinatus. The biceps tendon runs beneath that interval, which is in effect an anatomical discontinuity of the anterosuperior capsule. The concept of a pathologically widened rotator interval is important in understanding multidirectional instability (see below).

When the humeral head, displaced beneath and in front of the anteroinferior glenoid, is pressed back on that glenoid by muscle contraction, a dent is sometimes produced in the posterosuperior portion of the humeral head, the *Hill–Sachs lesion.*

NERVE PALSY

The axillary nerve courses downwards and laterally across the subscapularis muscle belly, to wind beneath the glenoid neck on its way to the quadrilateral space posteriorly. The course of the nerve is somewhat variable. As the humeral head dislocates, the nerve may be severely stretched. It is not uncommon to find partial or complete *axillary nerve palsy* following anterior shoulder dislocation. The nerve should be examined prior to any closed reduction for both medical and medicolegal reasons. Most axillary nerve palsies associated with shoulder dislocation are caused by reversible neuropraxia and are transient. If there is no clinical evidence of nerve recovery 3 weeks after dislocation, nerve conduction studies are warranted. A torn axillary nerve can be treated by cable grafting, and should not be neglected.

CUFF TEARS WITH DISLOCATION

Most dislocations occur in young athletic patients, and are associated with capsular stretch, capsulolabral (Bankart) lesions or both. Primary dislocations in older patients are often associated with rotator cuff tears rather than capsulolabral or capsular injury: in this age group, the cuff is 'the weakest link in the chain'. When patients over age 40 are unable to actively abduct their arm after a traumatic dislocation, a major rotator cuff tear is more likely than an axillary nerve palsy.

MULTIDIRECTIONAL INSTABILITY

Some patients with systemic ligamentous laxity suffer from multidirectional shoulder instability (MDI). Their humeral head may be abnormally displaced anteriorly, posteriorly or inferiorly, depending on the forces applied. Sometimes, physical examination may suggest MDI, but symptomatic instability may be unidirectional only.

POSTERIOR INSTABILITY

Posterior dislocation is uncommon. It typically occurs when the shoulder is flexed, adducted and internally rotated, and a direct posterior force is applied along the line of the humerus. Locked posterior dislocation, requiring reduction under general anaesthesia and often by open surgery, may follow major trauma. The force involved in epileptic seizure or electrocution is an important cause. *Posterior subluxation*, however, is frequently more subtle in its presentation, sometimes resulting from repetitive minor trauma such as a much loved golf swing.

VOLUNTARY DISLOCATION

The one group of shoulder instabilities which needs to be carefully separated from the rest is that of voluntary instability. The patient develops a 'party trick'. By selectively contracting certain muscles while relaxing others, the shoulder is dislocated in an obvious and easily reproduced manner. These dislocations tend to occur in 'atypical positions', often with the arm by the side. The importance of picking these cases lies in recognising that they are not suitable candidates for surgical stabilisation. Whether wilful or not, these patients need to first overcome their psychological need to dislocate, often with professional help. The condition may be seen in adolescent girls, who may 'outgrow their problem' as they mature.

Sometimes an instability which begins as a voluntary problem in adolescence persists as an involuntary phenomenon. Treatment is then as for any other recurrent involuntary instability.

TREATMENT – ANTERIOR INSTABILITY

Matsen has proposed the acronyms *tubs* and *ambri* (Table 6.3) to summarise the nature and treatment of various anterior shoulder instabilities. In traumatic anterior dislocation, the instability is generally unidirectional, often associated with a Bankart lesion, and best treated surgically. Atraumatic dislocations are often associated with some element of multidirectional instability, which is frequently bilateral, and rehabilitation is usually appropriate. When surgery is required,

Table 6.3 Anterior shoulder instabilities

Tubs	Ambri
Traumatic	Atraumatic
Unilateral	Multidirectional
Bankart	Bilateral
Surgery	Rehabilitation
	Inferior capsular shift

inferior capsular shift is generally the procedure of choice.[1]

Surgery for instability

Surgery for anterior shoulder instability aims to restore anatomical normality where possible. Bankart avulsions should be repaired and, where only one or two dislocations have occurred, this is frequently sufficient. Multiple recurrences often result in additional capsular stretch, and in these cases, that too should be corrected, by one of the various capsular tightening procedures, such as *Neer's capsular shift*.[2] The inferior capsular pouch is eliminated by shifting the lateral insertion of the anterior and inferior capsule proximally. Concurrent closure of the rotator interval is an important part of this procedure.

Various suture anchors have been designed to help capsulolabral repair. *Arthroscopic repair* is technically difficult but certainly possible. To date, the reported results of arthroscopic repair have varied enormously. This may be because concurrent capsular tightening is not as easily performed arthroscopically. Many surgeons recommend arthroscopic repair of Bankart lesions for the first-time dislocator, but open repairs, with concurrent capsular tightening, in cases of recurrent dislocation.

Selection for surgery

Selection for surgery may be difficult. Traumatic anterior dislocation in young sporting patients (less than 25 years) almost always proceeds to recurrent instability. The prognosis for older, less-sporting first-time dislocators is better and, in these patients, initial non-operative treatment is appropriate.

TREATMENT – POSTERIOR INSTABILITY

Open surgical repair of anterior instability is generally successful in more than 95% of cases. Surgery for posterior instability has a higher failure rate, reaching over 50% in some series. The procedures used are similar to those for the anterior scenario. They include capsulolabral repair where appropriate, capsular tightening procedures, and various bone block and osteotomy procedures.

CONSERVATIVE THERAPY FOR SHOULDER INSTABILITY

Following reduction of shoulder dislocation, or in the case of joint laxity, the patient follows a programme of progressive *exercises for a period of 6–8 weeks*:

- *A sling* is worn for 2 weeks following dislocation. During this time, gentle *pendulum exercises and isometrics* are carried out to prevent stiffness and muscle wasting. Forward flexion is then encouraged together with closed external rotation (the elbow tucked in) to 20 degrees.
- *At 2 weeks*, inner range strengthening is commenced and in the case of anterior instability the posterior capsule is stretched.
- *At 4 weeks*, outer range strengthening is carefully introduced.

Throughout rehabilitation, importance is placed on the *scapulothoracic muscles*, beginning with shoulder bracing and progressing to chin-ups and floor push-ups.

THERAPY FOLLOWING SHOULDER STABILISATION

Anterior stabilisation

Splint. Patient wears a sling with a body binder for 3 weeks. The body strap is removed twice a day to allow pendular movements with the elbows flexed and supported. Occasionally, an abduction splint instead of a binder is used by throwing athletes, to minimise capsular

contracture, or by patients with simultaneous cuff repairs to reduce strain on the repair.

3 weeks. The body strap is removed and the patient continues pendular movements with the arms outstretched. Closed external rotation to neutral position or just beyond is encouraged. If the patient is over 25 years of age or demonstrates excessive stiffness, this should start at 2 weeks. Between 3 and 5 weeks, the sling can be removed in the home and while the patient is sitting.

5 weeks. The sling is discarded and active forward flexion in supine is commenced after warming the shoulder. Characteristically, the patient is extremely apprehensive for fear of the shoulder 'coming out'. A slow introduction, with frequent breaks for warming and relaxation, is important in regaining the patient's confidence that the shoulder is now stable.

External rotation to 25 degrees is encouraged. It often takes a few weeks to regain reasonable forward flexion.

8 weeks. Resisted exercises with elastic tubing for infraspinatus are commenced together with gentle scapulothoracic exercises.

10 weeks. Resisted exercises for subscapularis, supraspinatus and deltoid muscles are included together with upgrading scapulothoracic work, including sitting push-ups and rowing. Stretching is continued in patients showing untoward stiffness in forward flexion or external rotation.

16 weeks. Strengthening exercises are further upgraded, with the use of light weights in all directions. The patient now attempts full abduction with open external rotation.

Next few months. This period is devoted to strongly building up all the shoulder and scapulothoracic muscles, including floor push-ups and chinning the bar. Proprioceptive exercises (Chapter 6H) are particularly important, as these nerves may be damaged during the phase of recurrent dislocation or at surgery. Ball throwing and catching and floor push-ups on a rubber beach ball improve the sense of shoulder awareness, and are strongly emphasised, particularly for throwing athletes.

Up to 6 months postoperatively. Swimming breast stroke before overarm is advised while gradual inclusion of outer-range exercises are introduced. Contact sports and activities such as skiing, horse riding and rock climbing should not be resumed until at least 6 months postoperatively.

Specific tip

Patients are usually young. Following surgery, they are often very apprehensive on removal of the sling, remembering previous dislocations, so it is important to verbally reassure the patient before treating that the shoulder is now stabilised and that the exercises, carried out correctly, will *not* lead to dislocation.

Posterior stabilisation

Splintage. The shoulder is immobilised in 20 degrees of closed external rotation, ideally with the elbow just behind the coronal plane. The splint is prepared prior to surgery, and is worn for 6 weeks.

At 6 weeks. The splint is removed to allow for gradual internal rotation.

Procedure. The procedure follows that of anterior stabilisation, except that the internal rotator muscles are strengthened before the external rotators.

Multidirectional stabilisation

Rehabilitation moves more slowly than for unidirectional instability. Stretching exercises are limited, whereas strengthening exercises are as previously mentioned.

Specific tip

If the shoulder is unstable, or recently stabilised, surfing has three rules:

* do not surf alone
* do not surf in big seas
* do not surf in the last hour before dark.

If the shoulder dislocates, there is only one arm with which to paddle and keep afloat and no way of signalling distress.

REFERENCES

1. Matsen FA: In: Rockwood CA (ed.), The shoulder, Vol. 1. Philadelphia: WB Saunders, 1990:541.
2. Neer CS, Foster CR: Inferior capsular shift for involuntary inferior and multidirectional instability of the shoulder. J Bone Joint Surg 62A:897–907, 1980.

H. SHOULDER EXERCISES

Jill Allen

GLENOHUMERAL EXERCISES
Passive range of movement

Forward flexion

* Using a pulley system, draw the impaired arm upwards by pulling downwards with the opposite arm (Fig. 6.21).
* With the patient lying in supine, the physiotherapist, family or friend raises the arm (Fig. 6.22).

* The patient grasps the top of the door with both hands and gently sags at the knees (Fig. 6.23).

External rotation

* With the patient lying in supine, a strap holding the upper arm to the chest wall to keep the elbow in and with both elbows at right angles, a stick between the hands is used to push the forearm outwards (Fig. 6.24).
* Holding the door jamb with the elbow tucked in, pivot body outwards (Fig. 6.25).

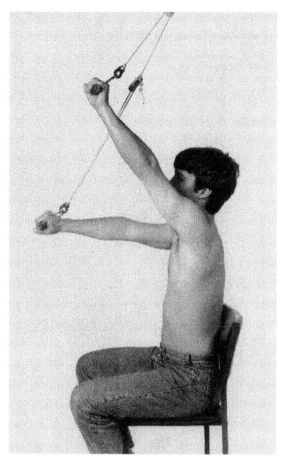

Figure 6.21 Use of a pulley to gain passive forward flexion.

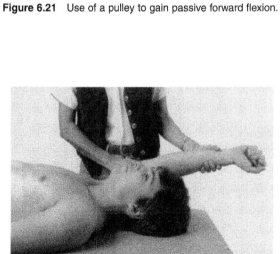

Figure 6.22 Increasing forward flexion with patient in supine.

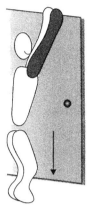

Figure 6.23 With both hands, hang from the top of the door and sag at the knees to increase elevation.

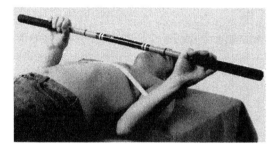

Figure 6.24 With upper arm belted to chest wall, externally rotate shoulder using baton.

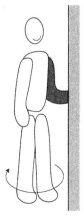

Figure 6.25 To externally rotate, hold door jamb, keep elbow tucked in, pivot on feet to turn body away.

Internal rotation

Pull arm up behind back using a towel or stick grasped in the opposite hand.

Extension

Holding stick between hands, push affected arm backwards.

Abduction

Abduction is often not advisable, because of the risk of subacromial impingement.

Capsule stretching

Anterior capsule. With arms raised against open doorway (or corner of room), step backwards and lean forwards.

Posterior capsule. Grasp elbow of impaired arm with opposite hand and pull upper arm across chest under the chin.

Inferior capsule. Grasp elbow of affected arm with opposite hand and draw it behind the head.

Superior capsule. In sitting position, grasp the seat of the chair with the hand of the affected arm and lean over to the opposite side. The stretch can be increased by tucking a pad up under the arm.

Pendulum

- Lean forwards, supporting elbows with hands, and rock arms back and forward.
- Lean forwards, letting the arm hang down, and make circles with the palm facing forwards and backwards.

Active assisted range of movement

Forward flexion

- Use the pulley, as in passive mode, but gradually introduce a more active role for the affected arm.
- Stand with stick between the hands and lift it upwards.
- Interlock fingers of hands and stretch arms towards the ceiling.

- Climb up the wall or slide the soapy hand up the tiled wall of the shower.

Other movements

Other movements can be achieved by gradually taking over a more active role with the stick exercises (Figs 6.26–6.28).

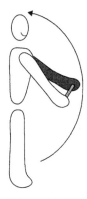

Figure 6.26 Lift an 18-inch stick over your head.

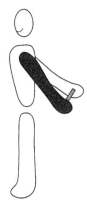

Figure 6.27 Hold an 18-inch stick behind your back and lift it as high as you can.

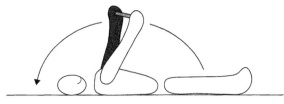

Figure 6.28 Hold an 18-inch stick between your hands and carry it over your head.

Transition from active assisted to active exercises

This transition can generally be made by allowing the patient use of the arm but with the elbow tucked into the side. A useful hint, readily understood, is to pretend there is a £50 note tucked into the axilla.

Active range of movement

All movements are carried out actively without the aid of a stick or the opposite limb, but without resistance, force or repetitive action.

Resisted range of movement

Using tubing

There are many types of resistant tubing. The cheapest and most convenient is the inner tube from a bicycle wheel. This can be cut into various strips to allow for progression in strength. It may be attached to a bar, a door handle or by feeding it through an open door and then closing the door. The latter has the added advantage of placement at various heights to allow for inner- and outer-range exercises.

Abduction. With the tube fixed at waist height and standing side on, grasp the tube and pull outwards, taking care not to go above shoulder height.

Adduction. As above, but facing in the opposite direction.

External rotation. Again, standing sideways but with the elbow tucked in, pull the tubing out from the waist.

Internal rotation. As above, but facing in the opposite direction, pull the tubing across to the opposite waist.

Deltoid

- Anterior: with the elbow bent and back to the door, push tubing forward.
- Middle: with the elbow bent, stand sideways and abduct arm.
- Posterior: with the elbow bent and facing the door, pull tubing backwards.

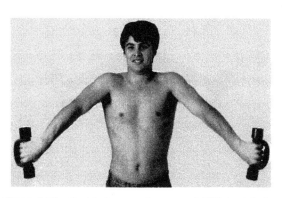

Figure 6.29 Resisted range of movement. With back to the door, holding light weights, pronate the arm up to shoulder height, 30 degrees forward at the body plane to strengthen supraspinatus.

Supraspinatus. With back to the door, holding light weights, pronate the arm so the thumb points downwards and lift the arm up to shoulder height, 30 degrees forward at the body plane (Fig. 6.29).

Later stage of rehabilitation

Use the tube in free form outer-range movements, making use of diagonal planes and increase the resistance.

Using light weights (0.5–2.0 kg)

External rotation. Lie on side with the affected arm uppermost and elbow tucked in; lift the weight up to waist height.

Internal rotation. As above, but with the affected arm underneath; lift the weight up to the opposite waist.

Biceps. Do bicep 'curls' but with the arm in external rotation to allow the long head of biceps to stabilise the anterior humeral head.

Later stage of rehabilitaton. Use the weights in free form movements, making use of diagonal planes and increase the loading (Figs 6.30 and 6.31).

Isometrics. Simply done by pushing either the fist, palm, back of hand or elbow against a solid object.

Circumduction

In the final stage of rehabilitation for most shoulder procedures, excluding arthrodesis and

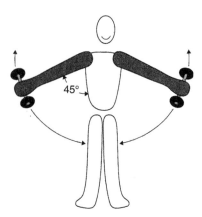

Figure 6.30 Resisted range of movement. With arms pronated, hold a 3 lb (1.35 kg) weight in each hand, lift to shoulder height 45 degrees forward of your body and down again to strengthen supraspinatus.

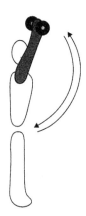

Figure 6.31 Resisted range of movement. Lift a 3 lb (1.35 kg) weight up above your head.

anterior and posterior instability, a fixed wall wheel with adjustable height and tension can help to regain final strength and mobility.

SCAPULOTHORACIC EXERCISES

As one-third of shoulder movement is controlled by the scapulothoracic muscles, these exercises should be included in the rehabilitation of all shoulder procedures. They are particularly important in the retraining of normal shoulder function, as invariably patients hitch their shoulders while striving for increased mobility.

- *Brace* shoulders.
- *Shrug* shoulders – with or without resistance.
- *Prone lie* on bench and 'hoist' weights with elbows bent.
- *Rowing*: using a machine or simulated by pulling backwards on two fixed lengths of tubing.
- *Push-ups*:
    standing
    sitting
    modified on hands and knees
    military style on hands and feet.
- *Chin-ups*: on a strong bar.

PROPRIOCEPTIVE EXERCISES

Following surgery, proprioceptive sense is often lost. The patient needs to relearn the position of the shoulder in space.

Ball throwing and catching. Start slowly, using a large soft ball and progress to fast catching and throwing of a small ball such as a squash ball. Later, introduce simultaneous running and catching.

Push-ups. Floor push-ups with the hands supported on a large rubber ball. For athletes, progress to a one arm push-up.

Bat and ball exercises. Patient plays on a court or hits up against a brick wall. Table tennis is an excellent sport.

'Tripod and challenge'. The patient is supported in an 'all threes' position, the good arm being held behind the back and the therapist exerts quick random pressure in all directions (Fig. 6.32). Progress to standing on one foot, bend over and place opposite hand on the floor. This can be made more difficult by placing a wobble board under the hand.

APPLICATION OF THERAPY

1. Moist heat applied to the shoulder preceding exercises: either hydrocollator pad or a hot shower.
2. Exercise sessions should be short and frequent. e.g. 2 hourly and length as tolerated.

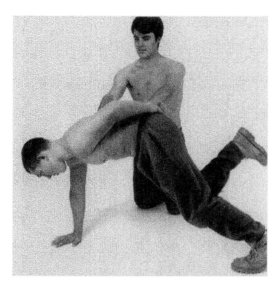

Figure 6.32 Patient resisting pressure to proprioception.

3. Do not push through pain. However, the exercises may cause a mild but short-lasting discomfort.
4. Patient should obtain the basic needs: e.g. pulley, stick, belt, ball, tubing, weights and soft ball for hand exercises.
5. The physical and mental ability of each patient to cope with surgery and therapy should be assessed and the treatment should be individualised. Family support is also important.
6. With an uneventful procedure and rehabilitation period, frequent visits to the physiotherapist are unwarranted (and expensive!). Far better if the patient is motivated to undertake his own recovery. This can be achieved by:

   • careful explanation pre- and postoperatively
   • time taken to listen to the patient's questions
   • the handing out of well-prepared sheets of diagrams and instructions
   • regularly scheduled appointments to review and progress treatment
   • availability of the therapist to take phone calls of concern between visits
   • assurance that the surgeon and therapist will liaise, preferably with the patient, if a problem occurs.

7. The physiotherapist should liaise with the surgeon as each procedure varies and, while there is an ordered regime, there are often precautions that should be heeded. There is no set recipe for rehabilitation.

HYGIENE AND CLOTHING

• Axillary discomfort and odour while wearing a sling or support can be alleviated by a family member applying warm water and absorbent powder while passive movement is being carried out. Using a hairdryer helps.
• An alternative sling can be used under the shower once the wound has healed.
• Clothing should be oversized for dressing ease. Front opening with Velcro fastening replacing buttons helps independence. Velcro can also replace shoulder seams.
• Using a cross-over bra or taping the straps behind can relieve pressure on the scar in female patients.

7

Upper limb nerve injuries and conditions

A. PERIPHERAL NERVE INJURIES

Doug Wheen

PATHOLOGY

Peripheral nerves are composed of extremely elongated nerve cells whose nuclei lie centrally in the spinal cord for motor nerves and in the dorsal root ganglion for sensory nerves. The peripheral nerves themselves are composed of sensory, motor and sympathetic axons and their support structures including basal lamina, Schwann cells, fibroblasts and a rich vascular network. Axons are generally grouped together into bundles or fascicles, each being surrounded by vascular connective tissue (endoneurium). Several fascicles may be grouped and surrounded by perineurium; these groups are then enclosed by epineurium, resulting in a complete peripheral nerve (Fig. 7.1).

Peripheral nerves may be injured by many factors, including pressure, burns, traction, direct laceration and other mechanical forces. Seddon[1] classified such injuries on a functional basis and, subsequently, Sunderland[2] has further classified these injuries on a structural level (Table 7.1). Ischaemia, metabolic disturbance and various drugs may also block peripheral nerve function.

Following axonal severance, significant changes occur in the cell in preparation for repair. At the site of injury, axons degenerate up to several nodes of Ranvier proximal to the lesion. Axonal sprouting then occurs, varying with the type and severity of the lesion. Under the influence of various biochemical mediators,[3–11] there is some attempt at targeted axonal guidance towards the distal nerve end. In the distal stump, wallerian degeneration takes place, including disintegration of the axon and phagocytosis of the myelin. Schwann cells multiply and endoneural collagen production increases, causing shrinkage of the distal tubules with time. As axonal sprouting bridges the zone of injury, some sprouts may connect with distal Schwann cell tubes and eventually connect to target (sensory or motor) organs. These successful axons then enlarge and mature and, dependent upon the original structure, may remyelinate. Many of the excess axon sprouts are deleted.

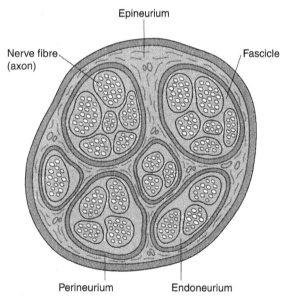

Figure 7.1 Structure of the normal peripheral nerve.

Table 7.1 Injury classification

Seddon	Sunderland	Features
Neurapraxia	Type I	Demyelination with fascicles intact. Examples: Saturday night palsy, tourniquet palsy. Spontaneous remyelination generally results in recovery over weeks to months
Axonotmesis	Type II	Loss of axonal continuity with preservation of endoneural tubes. Example: traction injury. Wallerian degeneration of axons occurs and recovery requires axonal regeneration and peripheral reinnervation. Axons should reinnervate correct targets. Muscle atrophy likely
Neurotmesis	Type III Type IV Type V	Perineurium intact with fibrosis++ Perineurium disrupted, epineurium intact Complete division of nerve and its structures. Example: laceration. Operative repair needed.

Axon growth rates in adults may average 1–2 mm per day but are dependent upon many factors.[12,13] This is a very complex and metabolically demanding process.

Successful regrowth depends upon many factors such as survival of the cell body, suitable local wound conditions, absence of infection, correct axonal alignment, time from injury to repair as well as biochemical mediators. These latter include neurotrophic factors such as nerve growth factors (NGFs) from the target organs and local tissues, neurite promoting factors such as laminin, and chemotactic (neurotropic) factors. Correct axonal alignment may provide contact guidance for the axon. The only factors currently able to be influenced by the surgeon are optimisation of local wound conditions, minimisation of nerve gapping and crude axonal alignment. Experimental studies into the manipulation of NGFs and neurotropic factors at the repair site may allow improved axonal regeneration in the future. These factors may be particularly useful in association with synthetic nerve conduits (see below). However, the current results of nerve repair are dependent primarily on the time from injury to repair and accuracy of axonal orientation.

Following nerve injury, and until mature nerve regeneration occurs, the distal part will suffer loss of its motor, sensory and sympathetic supply in the distribution of the injured nerve or nerves. Absence of motor supply results in distal weakness, muscle wasting and long-term irreversible damage to neuromuscular junctions. Abnormal postures and movement may result in skin, muscle, ligament and joint fibrosis and contracture. Loss of sensory and sympathetic supply causes loss of sweating, skin atrophy and loss of the all-important protective pain sensation. Repetitive or unrecognised trauma of an anaesthetic part, particularly in the presence of contractures, may cause infections, ulcers and Charcot joints.

NON-OPERATIVE TREATMENTS – PERIPHERAL NERVE INJURIES

Not all nerve injuries require operative repair. Neurapraxia and axonotmesis may be expected to recover spontaneously with time. However, all injuries should be assessed and intervention considered with the following aims:

1. To prevent problems during the period of reinnervation. Education, orthoses for limb and digit protection and splintage to prevent skin, muscle and joint contractures may be required. Strict care must be taken in the application of supportive or corrective splints in anaesthetic parts.
2. To monitor nerve recovery. Progress is evaluated by routine clinical tests such as an advancing Tinel sign, muscle testing and sensory mapping.
3. To assist recovery of all functions. Therapy may involve muscle strengthening exercises, desensitisation of hypersensitive areas, sensory re-education in cases of incomplete or incorrect sensory recovery and measures to relieve cold intolerance.
4. To assess functional difficulties. Advice should be given regarding appropriate functional orthoses or tool assistance. Functional and activities of daily living (ADL) assessment is particularly relevant at the time of any planned reconstructive procedures.

OPERATIVE TECHNIQUES IN NERVE INJURIES
Nerve exploration and neurolysis

Open wounds with clinical signs of nerve injury should be explored. The wound is debrided and extended as necessary to allow full visualisation. If the nerve is macroscopically intact, then the wound is treated appropriately and expectant treatments as outlined above should be instituted. Measures for scar minimisation may be needed. If a nerve is explored late following failure of recovery of either a closed nerve injury or open neurapraxia, external neurolysis to remove scar or any extrinsic compression from the nerve may be needed. Internal or intrafascicular neurolysis[14] is more rarely done as recurrent and more severe fibrosis may result in a poor outcome.

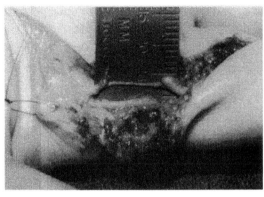 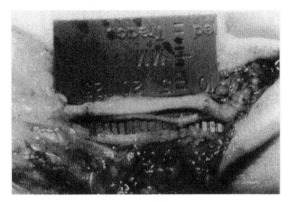

Figure 7.2 A, B: Traumatic 1-cm nerve gap within a digital nerve repaired using a sural nerve graft.

Nerve repair[15-19]

The essence of primary nerve repair is to optimise the factors for nerve recovery that are within the surgeon's influence. The wound should be adequately debrided. All surrounding tissues should be healthy following resection of damaged tissues. Flap coverage of the wound may be needed. The nerve exploration and repair must be done with magnification and microsurgical techniques. The nerve ends are geographically oriented and repaired with minimum tension.[20,21] An epineural repair aligns the intraneural fascicles by external sutures and minimises the amount of intraneural scarring and foreign body suture. Grouped fascicular repair may align axon bundles more accurately at the price of greater intraneural dissection and suture material. Neither method has been shown to give a superior outcome. Neither type of repair is suitable for all injuries. A combination of epineural and fascicular repair may be used if appropriate. Suture material may be minimised by the use of tissue glues.[22] Most primary nerve repairs are splinted for 2–3 weeks postoperatively to prevent nerve repair disruption.

Nerve grafting[23-26]

A nerve gap may arise in injuries where there is primary nerve loss or in cases of delayed nerve repair where the nerve ends have retracted. These gaps may be bridged using nerve grafts

harvested from other body regions (autografts). Grafts allow tension-free repairs, may reduce the need for postoperative splintage and allow early mobilisation of adjacent joints. A nerve graft brings Schwann cells, neural basal lamina and possibly a blood supply to the defect. However, there is loss of fascicular orientation across the nerve graft segment and the addition of an extra anastamosis compared to primary nerve repair (Fig. 7.2). There may be donor site morbidity such as scarring, sensory loss or neuroma formation. Popular donor sites are the sural nerve for nerve trunk defects and the medial cutaneous, lateral cutaneous or posterior interosseous nerves of the forearm for digital nerves. However, the latter donor often has a very small diameter and little fascicular material.

The radial sensory nerve is also a donor option, particularly in cases of multiple nerve injuries where it may also have been injured. Both the radial nerve and sural nerve may be taken as vascularised nerve grafts[27-33] if the recipient bed is poorly vascular. With forethought, some free flaps such as the lateral arm flap may also be harvested to contain nerve that may be used to bridge a defect.

Nerve conduits (Fig. 7.3A)

To avoid the donor site morbidity associated with nerve grafts, several biological and synthetic conduits have been devised to aid regeneration across nerve gaps. These include silicone tubes,

Nerve conduit

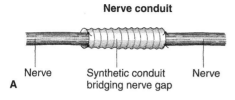

Nerve   Synthetic conduit   Nerve
A   bridging nerve gap

End-to-side neurorraphy

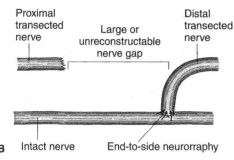

Proximal   Distal
transected   Large or   transected
nerve   unreconstructable   nerve
         nerve gap

B   Intact nerve   End-to-side neurorraphy

Figure 7.3 A: An absorbable polyglycolic acid tubular nerve conduit. B: The technique of end-to-side neurotisation.

absorbable polyglycolic acid tubes and freeze–thaw muscle basal lamina grafts.[34–57] All techniques are in early evaluation but suffer from a lack of Schwann cells in the conduit matrix. They are not suitable for large defects.[58–60] Exciting future developments may be conduits that provide a suitable scaffold as well as the necessary biological mediators and Schwann cells.

Nerve allografts[61–72]

Nerve allografts have rare application in general nerve surgery at the present time, although they have been used in occasional cases.[73–76] Potentially they may suffer from ongoing fibrosis associated with chronic rejection. It will be fascinating to assess the long-term sensory and motor nerve recovery in the nerve allografts that are part of the recently performed hand transplantation procedures.[77–80]

End-to-side neurotisation
(Fig. 7.3B)[81–89]

Recent work has suggested that the problem of large or non-reconstructable nerve gaps may be sometimes overcome by end-to-side anastamosis of the distal nerve stump to an adjacent intact nerve. Some very encouraging early results are reported, although this procedure seemingly contradicts many established dogmas of nerve injury, recovery and repair. The procedure is simple, avoids the morbidity of donor autograft harvest and may become a standard procedure in future years.

Nerve transfer and innervated flaps[90,91]

For example, in cases of long-term anaesthesia following median nerve injury, innervated fingertip pulp may be transferred from the ulnar nerve territory to the thumb. Although this type of operation has fallen into some disfavour due to the difficulty of adequately spatially re-educating the cerebral cortex, it may be appropriate in some cases.

Neuroma surgery

Symptomatic neuroma formation remains a problem in many patients following injury or repair. Neuromas may cause substantial patient disability, with pain, hypersensitivity, dystrophy and disuse. Neuromas of the digital nerves and of the terminal branches of both the radial nerve and the dorsal branch of the ulnar nerve enjoy a particularly bad reputation.[92] Treatment is often difficult. An excellent recent review of the pathology and treatments of transection neuromas is provided by Herndon.[93] The major problems remain the inability to prevent axonal sprouting following nerve injury,[2] the lack of deep tissue in the hand in which to bury neuromas (Fig. 7.4) and the functional mobility of hand structures. Surgery may be indicated. Many procedures have been advocated and fall into the following categories:

1. Simple transfer of the neuroma to a non-contact area or deep tissue.
2. Simple excision of the neuroma. The results of this treatment have never been surpassed in a large series.[94]

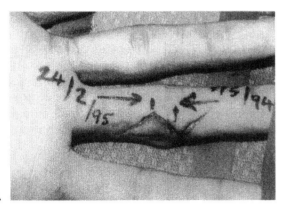
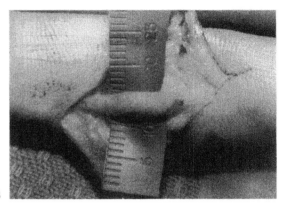

A

B

Figure 7.4 A, B: Case of a superficial symptomatic digital nerve neuroma in-continuity. This patient suffered lacerations of the nerve in 1994 and 1995. There is no deep tissue in which to bury such a neuroma within the digit. Surgical options include resection and restorative grafting or resection and deep proximal burial. A satisfactory outcome may still not be achieved.

3. Excision and restorative nerve grafting.
4. Excision and attempts to prevent axon sprouting by physical or chemical means: this is singularly unrewarding.
5. Excision and transfer to remote or deep tissue such as muscle or bone. Tethering and traction on the neuroma is probably the reason for some poor results following bone implantation[95] and interosseous muscle implantation[96,97] of neuromas in the hand.
6. Excision and capping of the nerve by either vein or silastic caps is not currently favoured.
7. Excision and vein implantation was popular in our unit.[98] However, with wider usage, several cases have required reoperation, and the overall results have not been convincingly superior to simple excision and burial.

Following any neuroma surgery, desensitisation techniques should be trialled (below) and general measures as outlined in Chapter 7E.

Other procedures in nerve reconstruction following injury

In cases of inadequate muscle recovery or following the development of joint contractures, tendon transfers, contracture release and flap repairs may be necessary. These procedures are covered in Chapters 7D and 2J.

POST-INJURY AND POSTOPERATIVE MANAGEMENT

Therapy principles

A denervated part will suffer loss of sensation, loss of autonomic control and sweating and loss of normal muscle excursion, balance and power. Trophic changes occur. Tissue is likely to suffer injury from minor trauma or pressure. Skin, muscle, ligament and joint contractures may occur due to adoption of abnormal postures.

Further to standard assessment, it is important to:

- assess and prevent potential problems associated with denervation, such as ulceration or contracture
- maintain appropriate postoperative positions to minimise the tension on any nerve repair
- replace or enhance any deficient motor function and assist assessment for any necessary tendon transfer
- treat any established problems such as contracture.

General therapy measures[99–104]

Sensory assessment and charting

Accurate assessment using static or moving two-point discrimination and Semmes–Weinstein

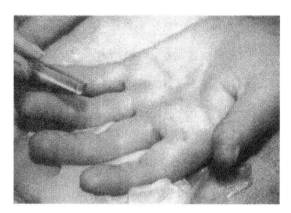

Figure 7.5 Monofilament sensory evaluation.

monofilament testing is necessary and may be done serially to assess progress (Fig. 7.5). Results should be charted diagrammatically. Commercial computer software is available to generate simple maps and assist with record keeping and archiving. A standard grading system such as the MRC system should be used.

Muscle testing and charting

All denervated muscles are assessed according to the MRC or similar system. Progress serial charting is done by a single therapist where possible. Before recovery, all joints are kept supple by appropriate passive range of movement (ROM). As muscles recover, specific exercise and strengthening programmes are tailored. Prior to tendon transfers the strength and excursion of potential donor muscles is assessed and appropriate strengthening programmes undertaken (see Chapter 7D).

Functional and ADL assessment

Splints may be devised to enhance or replace lost functions during the period of denervation. It is vital that all splints are comfortable and that the patient is trained to assess any potential for friction, blistering or ulceration in splints employed on anaesthetic parts. Many patients will not use splints outside of the office or therapy room unless they are functionally relevant.

Postoperative scar management and treatments

These measures are employed for surgical wounds (see Chapter 1B).

Treatment of joint contractures

These treatments are best prevented by appropriate early or postoperative splintage and movement. Patients must do a home exercise routine to maintain joint passive ROM. Established contractures are treated by conventional means (Chapter 2J). The amount of force applied to anaesthetic limbs must be carefully monitored to prevent skin breakdown due to splintage. Patients are instructed to regularly check anaesthetic areas for any redness or early signs of skin breakdown.

Desensitisation

Desensitisation is particularly applicable to digital nerve and fingertip injuries. The response to desensitisation treatments is very individual and treatment may be successful in only up to 50% of patients. In some patients treatment may worsen sensitivity and pain. It should then be ceased. Ideally, desensitisation therapy should be undertaken by the patient in at least 6-min episodes more than 6 times per day. It is most useful to brush the hyperaesthetic part against materials of different textures. Compliance is improved if the textured items are readily available. We have found that commercially available textured rods were often forgotten by patients. Textured clothing, the patient's hair or facial whiskers are useful and available materials. In very hypersensitive fingertip injuries, occlusive dressings that allow movement and use are often useful (e.g. OpSite or Coban).

Sensory re-education[105]

These techniques aim to restore central sensory perception to normal levels. Re-education may only commence if the patient has at least diminished protective sensation present. There also needs to be central cerebral coordination. Therefore, responsiveness and adaption may reduce with age. We have found the regular manipulation of various readily available textures and small objects to be the most useful technique, as has also been suggested by MacKinnon and Dellon.[105] This should be done for short periods (5–6 min) frequently (6×) during each day.

Specific therapy interventions

Median nerve injuries

There is sensory loss to the thumb and radial digits of the hand. In a low lesion (distal forearm, wrist or palm), there is loss of thumb abduction and opposition, resulting in poor pinch grip and longer-term adduction contracture of the thumb metacarpal (Fig. 7.6A). In higher injuries, there is also weakness of forearm pronation and wrist, finger and thumb flexion (pronator teres and quadratus, flexor digitorum superficialis (FDS), ½ flexor digitorum profundus (FDP), and flexor pollicis longus (FPL)).

Traction on a repair should be minimised postoperatively by splinting of the elbow in flexion and the wrist in the neutral position. It is inadvisable to splint the wrist in flexion, particularly in zone 4 and zone 5 combined flexor tendon and median nerve injuries. These injuries always result in significant postoperative scarring and tethering. Wrist flexion splintage may result in a difficult to correct wrist flexion contracture. This is a poor functional position and also increases pressure on the median nerve in the carpal tunnel. It also promotes palmar subluxation of the median nerve and flexor tendons if the carpal tunnel has been released. If needed, the digits are splinted in the position of safe immobilisation (POSI) position. It is important to maintain thumb abduction. After 3 weeks, splints are worn intermittently or at night only. Subsequently, passive ROM of all joints is maintained, while nerve recovery is awaited.

Hand function is greatly enhanced by an opposition strap or hand-based thermoplastic splint to position the thumb in abduction and opposition. (Fig. 7.6B,C).

Specific tip. It is sometimes difficult to maintain adequate thumb metacarpal position with a strap only. In that case, a thermoplastic reinforcement (Fig. 7.6D) or a thermoplastic splint moulded circumferentially around the palm may be better. Many patients do not need (and will not wear) such a splint if they can achieve functional opposition by trick movements or if there is adequate ulnar nerve innervation of flexor palmaris brevis (FPB).

A first web space C-splint should be worn at night to prevent adduction contracture. In the presence of established contracture, a dynamic splint may be required. This should provide abduction and pronation torque to the carpometacarpal (CMC) joint, taking care to avoid stretching the ulnar collateral ligament of the metacarpophalangeal (MP) joint of the thumb.

If functional opposition can be achieved, the patient should use the hand, but must be vigilant to avoid trauma to the anaesthetic digits. This could develop into chronic ulceration (see Fig. 7.6A). Patients must not smoke cigarettes using anaesthetic digits.

Radial nerve injuries

The most common injuries are below the triceps innervation. There is loss of wrist, finger and thumb extension. Loss of wrist extension results in marked hand weakness and difficulty achieving a functional grip (Fig. 7.7A) despite the presence of normally innervated flexor muscles.

Following primary operative repair, tension is usually minimised by elbow flexion and wrist and finger extension in the early phase. Subsequently, a wrist extension splint may be all that is required to achieve excellent functional use despite the loss of extrinsic finger (MP joint) extensors. The provision of static wrist extension by splintage coupled with active intrinsic extension of the interphalangeal joints will generally allow excellent functional use of the hand.

Specific tip. Simple extension splints are often well tolerated with excellent patient compliance. It is better to apply the splint dorsally rather than volarly (Fig. 7.7B–D) as it is difficult to avoid loss of wrist extension or 'pull-out' with a volar splint. If pull-out continues to be a problem, a circumferential splint is a further option.

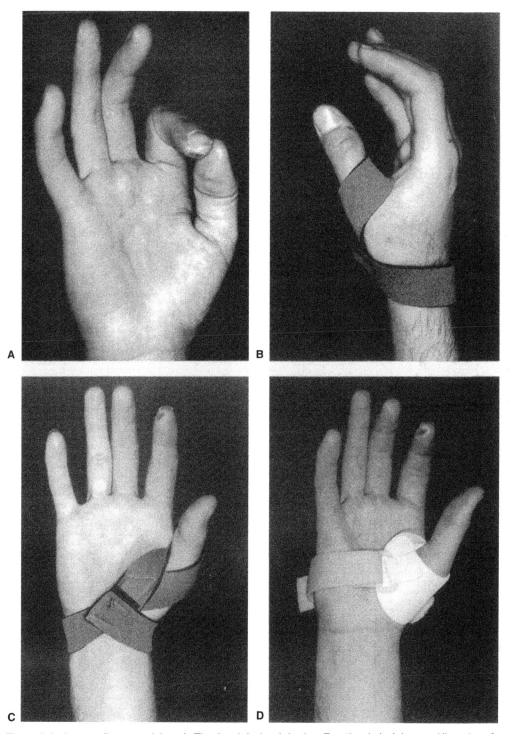

Figure 7.6   Low median nerve injury. A: The thumb lacks abduction. Functional pinch is poor. Ulceration of the index tip is due to anaesthesia and must be avoided. B, C: This opposition strap provides excellent functional abduction. D: An alternative thermoplastic bolster to provide thumb opposition.

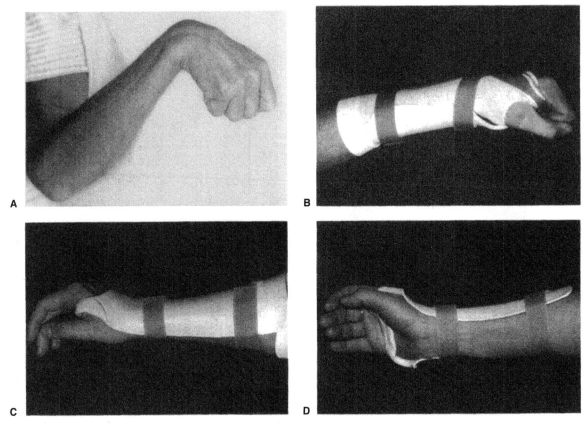

Figure 7.7 Radial nerve injuries. A: Without wrist extensor power, the wrist collapses into flexion with grip. The power of digital flexion is severely impeded in this position. B: A volar wrist extension splint tends to lose correction due to 'pull-out', as seen by the gapping between the palm and the splint with grip. C, D: Application of a simple dorsal wrist cock-up splint restores good function with less problem due to pull-out.

It is possible to allow wrist movement by harnessing the tenodesis effect (Figs 7.8 and 7.9). This also avoids the problem of over-strengthening the flexors.[106] Figure 7.8 demonstrates an outrigger tenodesis splint utilising static orthotic string. This is the easiest to construct as the tension of each digit can be individually adjusted. Figure 7.9 shows a lower-profile and seemingly simpler similar tenodesis splint. The digital loops are moderately difficult to balance correctly but it does provide a very satisfying end result. We rarely use dynamic extension outrigger splints in the treatment of radial nerve palsies. They are more bulky, more difficult to construct, require more ongoing maintenance and are not as well tolerated by patients as the above simpler splints. In a dynamic extension outrigger splint, the wrist needs to be held in 30 degrees of extension. There is a danger of development of extension contracture of the MP joints if the patient does not flex these joints adequately and regularly.

In low radial nerve injuries, the only deficit is loss of sensation over the dorsum of the first web space. More problematic is the common occurrence of painful neuromas at the site of injury, which can be quite refractory to all treatments. The problems are reduced, but not eliminated, by primary nerve repair where possible.

Ulnar nerve injuries

There is sensory loss to the ring and little fingers. In a low lesion (distal forearm, wrist or hand), there is loss of intrinsic muscle power. The long

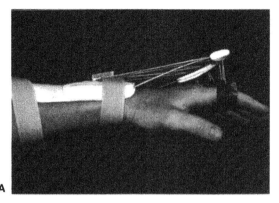
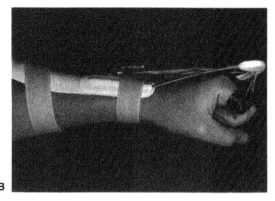

A   **B**

Figure 7.8   Tenodesis splintage in radial nerve palsy. A, B: This splint is well tolerated and provides excellent function.

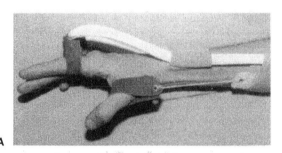

A

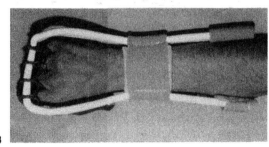

B

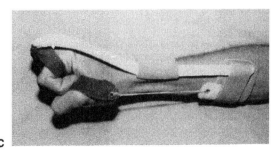

C

Figure 7.9   A–C: This comfortable and low-profile splint can be surprisingly difficult to construct, particularly to achieve correct balance of the digital loops. However, if successfully achieved, the functional result and patient compliance are excellent.

flexor tendons are intact and marked clawing of the ring and little fingers will result. Functionally, there is a combination of poor cylindrical grip and lack of power pinch, as well as the sensory deficit.

In higher lesions (arm, elbow or proximal forearm), the ulnar side of FDP tendons will also be denervated. Paradoxically, despite the larger number of muscles denervated, the clinical deformity and degree or clawing is usually less severe.

Postoperative minimisation of traction on an ulnar nerve repair should be discussed with the operative surgeon, as the required joint position will depend on the level of injury and if any transposition has been undertaken at the elbow. Distally, a neutral wrist position with MP joint flexion and interphalangeal (IP) joint extension (POSI) is usual.

Subsequently, hand function is enhanced and the development of proximal interphalangeal (PIP) joint contracture minimised by use of a simple figure of eight MP extension block anticlaw splint manufactured from flat strips of thermoplastic (Fig. 7.10).

Specific tip. The splint should be made with maximum MP joint flexion or it will not maintain sufficient MP correction to enable PIP extension, as the thin material is somewhat springy. The splint edges need to be bevelled proximally and distally to avoid pressure points and friction with digital extension. As shown, the splint can be extended around the thumb metacarpal to maintain adequate thumb web abduction in cases of combined

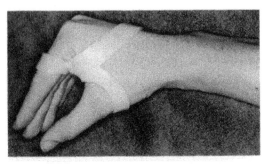

Figure 7.10 Lateral view of a low-profile anticlaw digital splint combined with thumb opposition support for a case of combined median and ulnar nerve palsy. These low-profile splints are very well tolerated. The only problem may be fatigue breakage due to constant use by the patient.

median and ulnar nerve palsy. The proximal dorsal part of the splint may need to be cut and fastened with an adjustable Velcro strap if there is a significant amount of intrinsic wasting. This allows the splint to be eased over the more prominent MP joints and then snugged around the metacarpals. These splints are low profile and provide good functional improvement. Patient compliance is usually excellent, the main problem being splint breakage due to overuse fatigue. We recommend against the use of a metacarpophalangeal joint flexion spring splint. It results in active strengthening of the extensor digitorum communis (EDC) instead of just allowing EDC redistribution of the extensor force to the PIP joints.

REFERENCES

1. Seddon H: Three types of nerve injury. Brain 66:237–88, 1943.
2. Sunderland S: Nerves and nerve injuries, 2nd edn. New York: Churchill Livingstone, 1978.
3. Bartlett PMM: Nerve growth factors. Todays Life Science March:12–21, 1991.
4. Bennett TM, Dowsing BJ, Austin L, Messina A, Nicola NA, Morrison WA: Anterograde transport of leukemia inhibitory factor within transected sciatic nerves. Muscle & Nerve 22(1):78–87, 1999.
5. Dowsing BJ, Morrison WA, Nicola NA, Starkey GP, Bucci T, Kilpatrick TJ: Leukemia inhibitory factor is an autocrine survival factor for Schwann cells. J Neurochem 73(1):96–104, 1999.
6. Lundborg G: A 25-year perspective of peripheral nerve surgery: evolving neuroscientific concepts and clinical significance. J Hand Surg (Am) 25(3):391–414, 2000.
7. Lundborg G, Dahlin L, Danielsen N, Zhao Q: Trophism, tropism, and specificity in nerve regeneration. J Reconstr Microsurg 10(5):345–54, 1994.
8. Seckel BR: Enhancement of peripheral nerve regeneration. Muscle & Nerve 13(9):785–800, 1990.
9. Seniuk NA: Neurotrophic factors: role in peripheral neuron survival and axonal repair. J Reconstr Microsurg 8(5):399–404, 1992.
10. Sondell M, Lundborg G, Kanje M: Vascular endothelial growth factor has neurotrophic activity and stimulates axonal outgrowth, enhancing cell survival and Schwann cell proliferation in the peripheral nervous system. J Neurosci 19(14):5731–40, 1999.
11. Terris DJ, Cheng ET, Utley DS, Tarn DM, Ho PR, Verity AN: Functional recovery following nerve injury and repair by silicon tubulization: comparison of laminin-fibronectin, dialyzed plasma, collagen gel, and phosphate buffered solution. Auris, Nasus, Larynx 26(2):117–22, 1999.
12. Buchthal F, Kuhl V: Nerve conduction, tactile sensibility, and the electromyogram after suture or compression of peripheral nerve: a longitudinal study in man. J Neurol Neurosurg Psychiatry 42(5):436–51, 1979.
13. Seddon H: Surgical disorders of the peripheral nerves. Baltimore: Williams & Wilkins, 1972.
14. Rhoades CE, Mowery CA, Gelberman RH: Results of internal neurolysis of the median nerve for severe carpal-tunnel syndrome. J Bone Joint Surg (Am) 67(2):253–6, 1985.
15. Sunderland S: The anatomic foundation of peripheral nerve repair techniques. Orthoped Clin N Am 12(2):245–66, 1981.
16. Terzis JK: Clinical microsurgery of the peripheral nerve: the state of the art. Clin Plast Surg 6(2):247–67, 1979.
17. Terzis JK, Sun DD, Thanos PK: Historical and basic science review: past, present, and future of nerve repair. J Reconstr Microsurg 13(3):215–25, 1997.
18. Watchmaker GP, Mackinnon SE: Advances in peripheral nerve repair. Clin Plast Surg 24(1):63–73, 1997.
19. Gelberman RH: Operative nerve repair and reconstruction. Philadelphia: JB Lippincott, 1991.
20. Millesi H: Peripheral nerve surgery today: turning point or continuous development? J Hand Surg (Br) 15(3):281–7, 1990.
21. Millesi H: Forty-two years of peripheral nerve surgery. Microsurgery 14(4):228–33, 1993.
22. Maragh H, Meyer BS, Davenport D, Gould JD, Terzis JK: Morphofunctional evaluation of fibrin glue versus microsuture nerve repairs. J Reconstr Microsurg 6(4):331–7, 1990.
23. Millesi H, Meissl G, Berger A: The interfascicular nerve-grafting of the median and ulnar nerves. J Bone Joint Surg (Am) 54(4):727–50, 1972.
24. Millesi H. Nerve grafting. Clin Plast Surg 11(1):105–13, 1984.
25. Millesi H: Progress in peripheral nerve reconstruction. World J Surg 14(6):733–47, 1990.
26. Millesi H: Techniques for nerve grafting. Hand Clin 16(1):73–91, viii, 2000.

27. Breidenbach W, Terzis JK: The anatomy of free vascularized nerve grafts. Clin Plast Surg 11(1):65–71, 1984.

28. Breidenbach WC, Terzis JK: The blood supply of vascularized nerve grafts. J Reconstr Microsurg 3(1):43–58, 1986.

29. Breidenbach WC, Terzis JK: Vascularized nerve grafts: an experimental and clinical review. Ann Plast Surg 18(2):137–46, 1987.

30. Breidenbach WC: Vascularized nerve grafts. A practical approach. Orthoped Clin N Am 19(1):81–9, 1988.

31. Doi K, Tamaru K, Sakai K, Kuwata N, Kurafuji Y, Kawai S: A comparison of vascularized and conventional sural nerve grafts. J Hand Surg (Am) 17(4):670–6, 1992.

32. Taylor GI: Nerve grafting with simultaneous microvascular reconstruction. Clin Orthopaed Rel Res 133:56–70, 1978.

33. Terzis JK, Skoulis TG, Soucacos PN: Vascularized nerve grafts. A review. Int Angiol 14(3):264–77, 1995.

34. Benito-Ruiz J, Navarro-Monzonis A, Piqueras A, Baena-Montilla P: Invaginated vein graft as nerve conduit: an experimental study. Microsurgery 15(2):105–15, 1994.

35. Bora FW Jr, Bednar JM, Osterman AL, Brown MJ, Sumner AJ: Prosthetic nerve grafts: a resorbable tube as an alternative to autogenous nerve grafting. J Hand Surg (Am) 12(5 Pt 1):685–92, 1987.

36. Chiu DT, Janecka I, Krizek TJ, Wolff M, Lovelace RE: Autogenous vein graft as a conduit for nerve regeneration. Surgery 91(2):226–33, 1982.

37. Doolabh VB, Hertl MC, Mackinnon SE: The role of conduits in nerve repair: a review. Rev Neurosci 7(1):47–84, 1996.

38. Francel PC, Francel TJ, Mackinnon SE, Hertl C: Enhancing nerve regeneration across a silicone tube conduit by using interposed short-segment nerve grafts. J Neurosurg 87(6):887–92, 1997.

39. Fullarton AC, Glasby MA, Lawson GM: Immediate and delayed nerve repair using freeze-thawed muscle allografts. Associated long-bone fracture. J Hand Surg (Br) 23(3):360–4, 1998.

40. Gattuso JM, Glasby MA, Gschmeissner SE, Norris RW: A comparison of immediate and delayed repair of peripheral nerves using freeze-thawed autologous skeletal muscle grafts – in the rat. Br J Plast Surg 42(3):306–13, 1989.

41. Gilchrist T, Glasby MA, Healy DM et al: In vitro nerve repair – in vivo. The reconstruction of peripheral nerves by entubulation with biodegradeable glass tubes – a preliminary report. Br J Plast Surg 51(3):231–7, 1998.

42. Glasby MA: Nerve growth in matrices of oriented basement membrane: developing a new method of nerve repair. Clin Anat 3:161–82, 1990.

43. Glasby MA: Interposed muscle grafts in nerve repair in the hand: an experimental basis for future clinical use. World J Surg 15(4):501–10, 1991.

44. Glasby MA, Carrick MJ, Hems TE: Freeze-thawed skeletal muscle autografts used for brachial plexus repair in the non-human primate [see comments]. J Hand Surg (Br) 17(5):526–35, 1992.

45. Hall SM, Enver K: Axonal regeneration through heat pretreated muscle autografts. An immunohistochemical and electron microscopic study. J Hand Surg (Br) 19(4):444–51, 1994.

46. Lawson GM, Glasby MA: A comparison of immediate and delayed nerve repair using autologous freeze-thawed muscle grafts in a large animal model. The simple injury. J Hand Surg (Br) 20(5):663–700, 1995.

47. Lenihan DV, Carter AJ, Glasby MA: An electrophysiological and morphological comparison of the microwave muscle graft and the freeze-thawed muscle graft. Br J Plast Surg 51(4):300–6, 1998.

48. Lundborg G, Rosen B, Abrahamson SO, Dahlin L, Danielsen N: Tubular repair of the median nerve in the human forearm. Preliminary findings [see comments]. J Hand Surg (Br) 19(3):273–6, 1994.

49. Lundborg G: Neurotropism, frozen muscle grafts and other conduits. J Hand Surg (Br) 16(5):473–6, 1991.

50. Lundborg G, Rosen B, Dahlin L, Danielsen N, Holmberg J: Tubular versus conventional repair of median and ulnar nerves in the human forearm: early results from a prospective, randomized, clinical study. J Hand Surg (Am) 22(1):99–106, 1997.

51. Mackinnon SE, Dellon AL: Clinical nerve reconstruction with a bioabsorbable polyglycolic acid tube. Plast Reconstr Surg 85(3):419–24, 1990.

52. Molander H, Engkvist O, Hagglund J, Olsson Y, Torebjork E: Nerve repair using a polyglactin tube and nerve graft: an experimental study in the rabbit. Biomaterials 4(4):276–80, 1983.

53. Mountain RE, Glasby MA, Sharp JF, Murray JA: A morphological comparison of interposed freeze-thawed skeletal muscle autografts and interposed nerve autografts in the repair of the rat facial nerve. Clin Otolaryngol Allied Sci 18(3):171–7, 1993.

54. Norris RW, Glasby MA, Gattuso JM, Bowden RE: Peripheral nerve repair in humans using muscle autografts. A new technique. J Bone Joint Surg (Br) 70(4):530–3, 1988.

55. Terada N, Bjursten LM, Dohi D, Lundborg G: Bioartificial nerve grafts based on absorbable guiding filament structures – early observations. Scand J Plast Reconstr Surg Hand Surg 31(1):1–6, 1997.

56. Walton RL, Brown RE, Matory WE Jr, Borah GL, Dolph JL: Autogenous vein graft repair of digital nerve defects in the finger: a retrospective clinical study. Plast Reconstr Surg 84(6):944–9; discussion 950–2, 1989.

57. Zhao Q, Lundborg G, Danielsen N, Bjursten LM, Dahlin LB: Nerve regeneration in a 'pseudo-nerve' graft created in a silicone tube. Brain Res 769(1):125–34, 1997.

58. Glasby MA, Gilmour JA, Gschmeissner SE, Hems TE, Myles LM: The repair of large peripheral nerves using skeletal muscle autografts: a comparison with cable grafts in the sheep femoral nerve. Br J Plast Surg 43(2):169–78, 1990.

59. Hems TE, Glasby MA: The limit of graft length in the experimental use of muscle grafts for nerve repair [see comments]. J Hand Surg (Br) 18(2):165–70, 1993.

60. Lawson GM, Glasby MA: Peripheral nerve reconstruction using freeze-thawed muscle

grafts: a comparison with group fascicular nerve grafts in a large animal model. J Roy Coll Surg Edinb 43(5):295–302, 1998.

61. Berger A, Lassner F: Peripheral nerve allografts: survey of present state in an experimental model of the rat. Microsurgery 15(11):773–7, 1994.

62. Best TJ, Mackinnon SE, Midha R, Hunter DA, Evans PJ: Revascularization of peripheral nerve autografts and allografts. Plast Reconstr Surg 104(1):152–60, 1999.

63. Comtet JJ, Revillard JP: Peripheral nerve allografts. I. Distinctive histological features of nerve degeneration and immunological rejection. Transplantation 28(2):103–6, 1979.

64. Evans PJ, Mackinnon SE, Best TJ et al: Regeneration across preserved peripheral nerve grafts. Muscle & Nerve 18(10):1128–38, 1995.

65. Evans PJ, MacKinnon SE, Midha R et al: Regeneration across cold preserved peripheral nerve allografts. Microsurgery 19(3):115–27, 1999.

66. Frazier J, Yu L, Rhee E, Shaw L, LaRossa D, Rostami A: Extended survival and function of peripheral nerve allografts after cessation of long-term cyclosporin administration in rats. J Hand Surg (Am) 18(1):100–6, 1993.

67. Jensen JN, Mackinnon SE: Composite tissue allotransplantation: a comprehensive review of the literature – part III. J Reconstr Microsurg 16(3):235–51, 2000.

68. Jensen JN, Mackinnon SE: Composite tissue allotransplantation: a comprehensive review of the literature – part II. J Reconstr Microsurg 16(2):141–57, 2000.

69. Jensen JN, Mackinnon SE: Composite tissue allotransplantation: a comprehensive review of the literature – part 1. J Reconstr Microsurg 16(1):57–68, 2000.

70. Katsube K, Doi K, Fukumoto T, Fujikura Y, Shigetomi M, Kawai S: Nerve regeneration and origin of Schwann cells in peripheral nerve allografts in immunologically pretreated rats. Transplantation 62(11):1643–9, 1996.

71. Midha R, Evans PJ, Mackinnon SE, Wade JA: Temporary immunosuppression for peripheral nerve allografts. Transplantation Proc 25(1 Pt 1):532–6, 1993.

72. Pollard JD, Fitzpatrick L: An ultrastructural comparison of peripheral nerve allografts and autografts. Acta Neuropathologica 23(2):152–65, 1973.

73. Mackinnon SE, Hudson AR: Clinical application of peripheral nerve transplantation. Plast Reconstr Surg 90(4):695–9, 1992.

74. Marmor L: The repair of peripheral nerves by irradiated homografts. Clin Orthopaed Rel Res 34:161–9, 1964.

75. McLeod JG, Hargrave JC, Gye RS et al: Nerve grafting in leprosy. Brain 98(2):203–12, 1975.

76. McLeod JG, Hargrave JC, Gye RS et al: Letter: Nerve grafting in leprosy. Lancet 1(7950):95–6, 1976.

77. Dubernard JM, Owen E, Herzberg G et al: Human hand allograft: report on first 6 months [see comments]. Lancet 353(9161):1315–20, 1999.

78. Jones JW, Gruber SA, Barker JH, Breidenbach WC: Successful hand transplantation. One-year follow-up. Louisville Hand Transplant Team [see comments]. N Engl J Med 343(7):468–73, 2000.

79. Lee WP, Mathes DW: Hand transplantation: pertinent data and future outlook. J Hand Surg (Am) 24(5):906–13, 1999.

80. Lundborg G: Hand transplantation [editorial]. Scand J Plast Reconstr Surg Hand Surg 33(4):369–71, 1999.

81. al-Qattan MM, al-Thunyan A: Variables affecting axonal regeneration following end-to-side neurorrhaphy. Br J Plast Surg 51(3):238–42, 1998.

82. Fortes WM, Noah EM, Liuzzi FJ, Terzis JK: End-to-side neurorrhaphy: evaluation of axonal response and upregulation of IGF-I and IGF-II in a non-injury model. J Reconstr Microsurg 15(6):449–57, 1999.

83. Liu K, Chen LE, Seaber AV, Goldner RV, Urbaniak JR: Motor functional and morphological findings following end-to-side neurorrhaphy in the rat model. J Orthopaed Res 17(2):293–300, 1999.

84. Lundborg G, Zhao Q, Kanje M, Danielsen N, Kerns JM: Can sensory and motor collateral sprouting be induced from intact peripheral nerve by end-to-side anastomosis? J Hand Surg (Br) 19(3):277–82, 1994.

85. Mennen U: End-to-side nerve suture – a technique to repair peripheral nerve injury. S Afr Med J 89(11):1188–94, 1999.

86. Noah EM, Williams A, Fortes W, Terzis JK: A new animal model to investigate axonal sprouting after end-to-side neurorrhaphy. J Reconstr Microsurg 13(5):317–25, 1997.

87. Noah EM, Williams A, Jorgenson C, Skoulis TG, Terzis JK: End-to-side neurorrhaphy: a histologic and morphometric study of axonal sprouting into an end-to-side nerve graft. J Reconstr Microsurg 13(2):99–106, 1997.

88. Tham SK, Morrison WA: Motor collateral sprouting through an end-to-side nerve repair. J Hand Surg (Am) 23(5):844–51, 1998.

89. Viterbo F, Teixeira E, Hoshino K, Padovani CR: End-to-side neurorrhaphy with and without perineurium. Revista Paulista de Medicina 116(5):1808–14, 1998.

90. Mackinnon SE, Novak CB: Nerve transfers. New options for reconstruction following nerve injury. Hand Clin 15(4):643–66, ix, 1999.

91. Nath RK, Mackinnon SE: Nerve transfers in the upper extremity. Hand Clin 16(1):131–9, ix, 2000.

92. Herndon JH, Eaton RG, Littler JW: Management of painful neuromas in the hand. J Bone Joint Surg (Am) 58(3):369–73, 1976.

93. Herndon JH, Hess AV: Neuromas. In: Gelberman RG (ed.), Operative nerve repair and reconstruction. Philadelphia: JB Lippincott, 1991.

94. Tupper JW, Booth DM: Treatment of painful neuromas of sensory nerves in the hand: a comparison of traditional and newer methods. J Hand Surg (Am) 1(2):144–51, 1976.

95. Goldstein SA, Sturim HS: Intraosseous nerve transposition for treatment of painful neuromas. J Hand Surg (Am) 10(2):270–4, 1985.

96. Laborde KJ, Kalisman M, Tsai TM: Results of surgical treatment of painful neuromas of the hand. J Hand Surg (Am) 7(2):190–3, 1982.

97. Dellon AL, Mackinnon SE: Treatment of the painful neuroma by neuroma resection and muscle implantation. Plast Reconstr Surg 77(3):427–38, 1986.

98. Herbert TJ, Filan SL: Vein implantation for treatment of painful cutaneous neuromas. A preliminary report. J Hand Surg (Br) 23(2):220–4, 1998.
99. Dellon AL: The moving two-point discrimination test: clinical evaluation of the quickly adapting fiber/receptor system. J Hand Surg (Am) 3(5): 474–81, 1978.
100. Dellon AL, Jabaley ME: Reeducation of sensation in the hand following nerve suture. Clin Orthopaed Rel Res 163:75–9, 1982.
101. Moberg E: Objective methods for determining the functional value of sensibility in the hand. J Bone Joint Surg 40B(3):454–76, 1958.
102. Omer GE Jr: Methods of assessment of injury and recovery of peripheral nerves. Surg Clin N Am 61(2):303–19, 1981.
103. Rosen B, Lundborg G: A new tactile gnosis instrument in sensibility testing. J Hand Ther 11(4): 251–7, 1998.
104. Rosen B, Lundborg G: A model instrument for the documentation of outcome after nerve repair. J Hand Surg (Am) 25(3):535–43, 2000.
105. MacKinnon SE, Dellon AL: Surgery of the peripheral nerve. New York: Thieme, 1988.
106. Colditz J: Splinting for radial nerve palsy. J Hand Ther 1:18–23, 1987.

B.   BRACHIAL PLEXUS INJURIES

Claudia R Gschwind and Lisa Newell

DEFINITION AND PATHOLOGY

Injuries to the brachial plexus (spinal levels C5 to T1) occur after trauma, at birth, accidentally during surgery of the neck or shoulder, after radiotherapy, or they can be caused by tumours. In trauma, the mechanism of injury is downward traction of the arm and forcible widening of the shoulder neck angle[1] (Fig. 7.11). This leads to traction on the upper roots of the brachial plexus which provide shoulder and elbow function. A fall with an outstretched arm leads to a traction injury of the lower roots which provide hand function.

Clinical presentation is loss of motor function, loss of sensation and pain. The extent of this loss

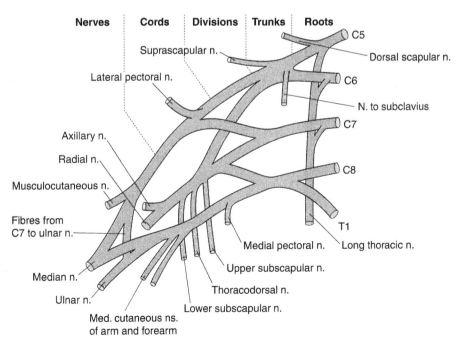

Figure 7.11   Anatomy of the brachial plexus.

depends on the severity and localisation of the injury within the plexus. Slow-velocity injuries usually cause a traction injury of the plexus. This can be simple neurapraxia or, in severe cases, disruption of the nerve (Sunderland classification I–V).[2] Rupture of nerves is, however, rare after slow-velocity injuries. High-velocity injuries after motor bike or water ski accidents not only lead to severe traction injuries or ruptures of trunks, cords and peripheral nerves but also can cause root avulsions.

INDICATIONS FOR SURGERY

High-velocity injuries presenting with a flail and insensate arm, or with complete loss of C5/C6 function, should be explored early in order to confirm root avulsions and to reconstruct the injured structures. The priorities of reconstruction are elbow flexion, shoulder stability, wrist extension, finger flexion and sensation in the hand. Depending on the number of roots avulsed, only limited reconstruction is possible.

Open injuries and sharp divisions of plexal structures are indications for immediate exploration and repair, as are injuries with severe vascular trauma. Low-velocity injuries (traction injuries through collisions on football fields, simple shoulder dislocations) usually lead to a lesser degree of internal neural damage. The axons may be disrupted but the endoneurial tube may be preserved. Useful nerve recovery by axonal regeneration is therefore possible; observation is indicated. If there is no clinical recovery after 3 months and the nerve conduction tests show no innervation of the muscle involved, exploration is undertaken.

SURGICAL CONTRAINDICATIONS

Restoration of C8 and T1 function (intrinsic function of the hand) has never been achieved in adults. If the clinical presentation suggests traction injury, rupture or avulsion of the C8/T1 roots or the lower trunk only, surgery is not indicated.[3]

SURGICAL TECHNIQUE

Through a longitudinal incision behind the border of the sternomastoid muscle, the supraclavicular plexus can be exposed after division of platysma and the omyhyoid muscle. If the infraclavicular plexus is to be explored, the incision is extended laterally, 2 cm below and parallel to the clavicle to the coracoid process, with an extension into the upper arm.

Two or three months after injury, dissection becomes difficult due to fibrosis of the neck muscles and the injured nerves. Tedious dissection is the main reason for the lengthy operating times. In early exploration, tissues planes are still preserved and dissection is therefore easier. For inspection of the infraclavicular plexus, the pectoralis minor is divided at its insertion on the coracoid. It is rarely necessary to osteotomise the clavicle for better exposure. All injured roots, trunks and cords are identified. Intraforaminal ruptures can be discovered by a gentle pull on the roots in early exploration. If there is macroscopic continuity but obvious traction injury of the neural structures, intraoperative electrical stimulation is used to assess axonal integrity. If there is no continuity by electrical stimulation, the injured segment of the nerve is excised back to healthy looking fascicular structures. Continuity is then restored with cable grafts of adequate length, usually harvested from the sural nerve. If one or several roots are avulsed, reconstruction of the plexus has to be carefully planned and the principles of priority of reconstruction apply.

Surgical planning takes into consideration that elbow flexion can reliably be restored by an intercostal nerve transfer to the musculocutaneous nerve if the patient is under 40 years of age and if the transfer is performed within 6 months after injury. This means – e.g. in the patient with all but one roots avulsed – we would plan shoulder fusion, intercostal nerve transfer for elbow flexion and distribute available axons of the extraforaminal ruptured nerves to the radial nerve and the median nerve. (Potential achievements: some shoulder abduction, elbow flexion and extension, wrist extension, some finger flexion and sensation.)

After intraplexal transfers and nerve grafts are performed the platysma is closed, and the pectoralis minor is reattached to the coracoid.

INTERCOSTAL NERVE TRANSFER

The principle of nerve transfer is to connect a distal nerve stump with the spinal cord and therefore with the central nervous system. This procedure is necessary, for example, after C5/C6 root avulsions (Fig. 7.12).

Through a transverse incision over the third intercostal space the third and fourth intercostal nerves are dissected out from the midaxillary line to the costochondral junction. They are then divided distally and, through a subcutaneous tunnel, pulled into a longitudinal incision in the upper arm, which exposes the musculocutaneous nerve at its entry into biceps. Under the microscope, two intercostal nerves are sutured to the musculocutaneous nerve as close to its entry into biceps as possible.

During surgery, the arm is abducted to 90 degrees and the head of the patient turned to the contralateral side. In over 75% of patients this procedure will restore elbow flexion at least against gravity, often to an M4 if the patient is under 40 years of age and the surgery is performed within 6 months of the injury. If the patient is older, or the nerve transfer performed at a later stage, results are less predictable. It takes between 6 and 10 months after intercostal nerve transfer for the first flicker in biceps to occur: this is usually connected to respiratory function, e.g. coughing or sneezing. Over the next 12–24 months, biceps strength increases and the patient will learn to use the transfer independently of respiratory function.[4]

OTHER NERVE TRANSFERS

The accessory nerve is often used as a transfer donor for restoration of shoulder function: e.g. to neurotise the suprascapular nerve. The hypoglossal, phrenic and nerves of the cervical plexus have also been used as donors. Some centres even divide the healthy contralateral C7 root and use long interpositional nerve grafts to restore function in a plexus injury with multiple root avulsions.

GENERAL COMMENTS

Brachial plexus injuries are often devastating physically, psychologically and socially. These injuries mainly affect young males involved in fast sports. Early exploration after high-velocity injuries has improved the functional and psychological management of these patients. Rehabilitation can be planned sooner. Even if all roots are avulsed, elbow flexion and shoulder stability can be restored in most cases. Even if elbow flexion is the only voluntary movement achieved, it is of great importance to the patient's body image and function. It turns a flail dangling arm to a limb with controllable elbow flexion, allowing for some use in ADL. Neuropathic pain still remains a problem after brachial plexus injuries, particularly for the first 2 years. It has been shown in many studies that surgery with reconstruction of plexal structures has a beneficial effect on the intensity of pain.[5]

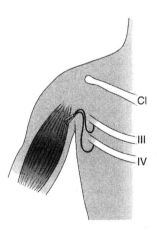

Figure 7.12 Principle of intercostal nerve transfer. (Redrawn with permission from Tonkin MA, Eckersley JRT, Gschwind CR: The surgical treatment of brachial plexus injuries. Aust NZ J Surg 66:29–33, 1996.)

Treatment of brachial plexus injury is challenging and usually means a long-term surgeon–patient relationship. It makes sense that the surgeon performing brachial plexus reconstruction is trained in hand and microsurgery and is familiar with upper limb function. It is, therefore, the same person who will also undertake the necessary secondary procedures (wrist fusion, muscle transfers).

HAND THERAPY ASPECTS OF BRACHIAL PLEXUS INJURIES

Preoperative management

The flail arm has to be supported to prevent subluxation of the glenohumeral joint and to stabilise the elbow:[6] this can be achieved with an arm sling and adequate patient education. If wrist extension is lost, a wrist extension splint will prevent stretching of the dorsal capsule and the extensor tendons. Due care needs to be taken with loss of sensibility and potential pressure areas. Stiffness of the fingers, particularly of the metacarpophalangeal joint, has to be prevented by passive exercises and, if needed, a night splint in a functional position. First-web contractures should likewise be prevented by stretching exercises and static splint. Range of motion in the shoulder and elbow joint is maintained with regular passive exercises. In the early days after injury, specific antioedema therapy may be indicated (e.g. effleurage massage and pressure bandaging).

Postoperative management

Return of nerve function is slow; therefore, the same principles apply as in preoperative management. After removal of stitches, scar management is helpful to prevent hypersensitivity and hypertrophic scar formation.

In the first 4–6 weeks, stretching of the nerve graft has to be avoided (head positioning). If the pectoralis minor muscle was detached, the arm is kept in a sling for 3 weeks before gradual shoulder mobilisation is begun. In these 3 weeks shoulder shrugging and gentle rolling exercises in the sling are permitted. Finger stiffness, particularly

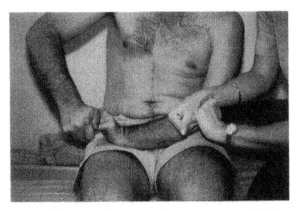

Figure 7.13 Instruction for maintenance of metacarpophalangeal joint flexibility.

metacarpophalangeal joint stiffness, must be prevented[7] (Fig. 7.13).

If it is decided intraoperatively that shoulder function is not achievable with nerve grafts or nerve transfers, the patient is scheduled for a shoulder fusion. This is usually performed after an intercostal nerve transfer for elbow flexion during the waiting period between transfer and the return of biceps activity. If a shoulder fusion is planned, stretching of the shoulder joint capsule is avoided. The shoulder is only brought through a functional range from 0 to 90 degrees of abduction and flexion. External rotation, however, should be passively maintained. After an intercostal nerve transfer, the arm is rested in a sling for 4 weeks with the usual precautions and maintenance of mobility of the other structures. Shoulder abduction is then started gently and abduction to 90 degrees is gradually obtained over a period of 6–8 weeks. Forceful and sudden abduction of the arm can lead to rupture of the nerve transfer.

If function is returning to a muscle, specific strengthening exercises are begun, progressing from antigravity to active assisted to resisted movement. After intercostal nerve transfer, biceps function is linked to respiratory action. Specific exercises are designed to improve strength in biceps. The patient is instructed in active assisted elbow flexion with deep inspiration. The flexion should be sustained for several seconds. Later

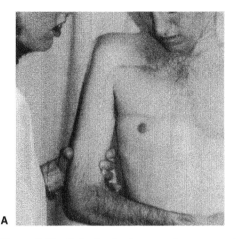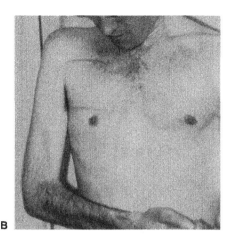

A   B

Figure 7.14 Patients after intercostal nerve transfer. A: Instructed active assisted elbow flexion with deep inspiration. B: Active assisted elbow flexion.

on, the patient is encouraged to flex his elbow without using respiratory function (Fig. 7.14). It has to be emphasised that during the waiting period for reinnervation of the hand and forearm musculature, all joints should be kept supple.

Neuropathic pain may respond to treatment with transcutaneous electrical nerve stimulation (TENS) (Chapter 7E) and in severe cases (rare) referral to a pain management clinic may be necessary.[8]

REFERENCES

1. Coene L: N.E.M. Mechanisms of brachial plexus lesions. Clin Neurol Neurosurg 95:24–9, 1993.
2. Sunderland S: Nerves and nerve injuries, 2nd edn. Edinburgh: Churchill Livingstone, 1978.
3. Narakas A: Brachial plexus surgery. Symposium of peripheral nerve injuries. Orthoped Clin N Am 12(2):303–23, 1981.
4. Nagano A, Tsuyama N, Ochiai N, Hara T, Takahashi M: Direct nerve crossing with the intercostal nerve to treat avulsion injuries of the brachial plexus. J Hand Surg 14A:980–5, 1989.
5. Bruxelle J, Travers V, Thiebaut JB: Occurrence and treatment of pain after brachial plexus injury. Clin Orthop 237:87–95, 1988.
6. Frampton VM: Management of brachial plexus lesions. J Hand Ther 1:115–20, 1988.
7. Frampton VM: Rehabilitation of the hand. In: Hunter J, Schneider L, Makin E, Callahan A (eds), Surgery and therapy, 3rd edn. Philadelphia: Mosby, 1990:630–9.
8. Frampton VM: Management of pain in brachial plexus lesions. J Hand Ther 9:339–43, 1996.

C. COMPRESSION SYNDROMES/ ENTRAPMENT NEUROPATHIES

W Bruce Conolly and Rosemary Prosser

INTRODUCTION

The peripheral nerves of the hand and upper limb, in their course from the neck (from the C5–T1

nerve roots) to the hand, are subject to compression in anatomical tunnels and spaces (Fig. 7.15).

Generally, there may be an increase in the contents of the tunnel, e.g. a space-occupying lesion such as a ganglion or other tumours, or a narrowing of the tunnel, e.g. post-traumatic fibrosis or anomalous or tight fascia/muscle. Any obstruction of venous return in the nerve causes congestion of the neurovascular plexuses, leading to fibrosis around and within the nerve. External pressures

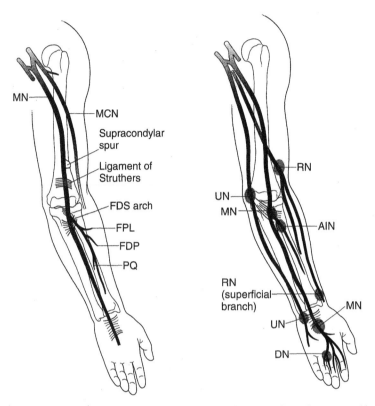

Figure 7.15 Sites of peripheral nerve entrapment at the arm, elbow, forearm and hand.

above 50 mmHg for 45 min have been reported to compromise conduction transmission.[1]

These conditions can occur not only after acute injury – e.g. distal radial fracture or 'occupational overuse syndrome' – but also after surgery, e.g. a carpal tunnel syndrome may develop after forced hand exercise to recover grip after fasciectomy. The therapist should recognise the compression syndrome and the need for conservative or even operative treatment and refer that patient back to the surgeon for review and assessment.

GENERAL PRINCIPLES

Clinical features

Pain, numbness, weakness and autonomic changes reflect the disturbed sensory, motor and autonomic functions of the nerve.

Differential diagnosis. Nerve signs and symptoms from non-compressive causes including peripheral nerve disease, diabetic neuropathy, spinal cord disease and motor neurone disease should be considered and excluded before diagnosis of a compression syndrome is made.

The classic compression syndromes include:

1. median nerve: carpal tunnel syndrome, pronator syndrome and anterior interosseous nerve syndrome
2. ulnar nerve: cubital tunnel syndrome and hypothenar hammer syndrome
3. radial nerve: posterior interosseous nerve syndrome and Wartenburg syndrome
4. digital nerve compression
5. thoracic outlet compression.

Conservative treatment

Conservative treatments for mild or intermittent compression syndrome include: splintage, rest from that occupation or activity known to be causing or aggravating the condition, anti-inflammatory medication and corticosteroid injection. Range of motion and tendon excursion should be maintained without aggravation of the compression syndrome.

Surgical treatment

Surgical decompression of the anatomical tunnel with or without neurolysis, or with nerve transposition, is indicated if conservative measures fail, i.e. the patient who has persisting sensory symptoms, motor weakness or muscle wasting. Results following decompression are more favourable if the decompression is done early; some authors[2] suggest this should be within 3 months.

MEDIAN NERVE

Carpal tunnel syndrome

Cause

Carpal tunnel syndrome (CTS) is the most common peripheral nerve entrapment. It is usually caused by an increase in the flexor tenosynovial mass, causing compression of the median nerve in the carpal tunnel (Fig. 7.16). It occurs most commonly in women of menopausal age. It also occurs in association with rheumatoid arthritis,

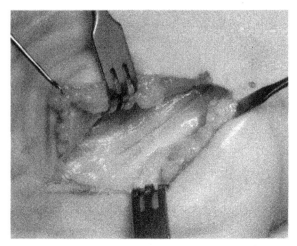

Figure 7.16 Open carpal tunnel release: intraoperative view of compression of the median nerve.

endrocrine conditions such as thyroid disease, obesity, diabetes and in pregnancy. CTS may also be familial.

Diagnosis

CTS is largely diagnosed on the clinical findings, but nerve conduction and electromyographic (EMG) studies should be carried out in cases being considered for surgery.

Clinical features

Clinical features include waking from sleep in the early hours of the morning with numbness and tingling in the median nerve distribution of the hand. There may be proximal radiation of the symptoms to the forearm or elbow. Associated weakness or clumsiness, paraesthesia aggravated by hand use and the feeling of the hand being swollen are often reported by the patient. Sustained wrist flexion for 1 min (Phalen's test) and tapping over the nerve in the carpal tunnel (Tinel's sign) may be positive. There may also be associated cervical nerve root irritation from cervical spondylosis (the 'double crush syndrome').

Conservative treatment

Therapy measures alone are most beneficial in those cases where there is a temporary increase in the flexor tenosynovial mass, e.g. pregnancy, and in some activity-related CTS.

Assessment

If the patient's subjective complaint indicates possible nerve compression, the therapist needs to assess all possible sites of nerve compression along the course of the nerve methodically. A positive Phalen's test and Tinel's sign at the wrist with no increase in symptoms with proximal testing is a good indication that the problem is an uncomplicated CTS.

Proximal testing may include sustained neck postures, e.g. side flexion, rotation and extension, palpation of the cervical spine in various neck

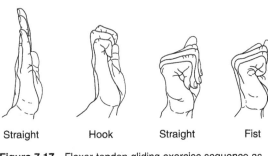

Straight   Hook   Straight   Fist

Figure 7.17 Flexor tendon gliding exercise sequence as recommended by Stewart and van Strein. (Reproduced with permission from Stewart K, van Strein G: Postoperative management of flexor tendon injuries. In: Hunter J, Mackin E, Callahan A (eds), Rehabilitation of the hand; surgery and therapy, 4th edn. St Louis: Mosby, 1995:443.)

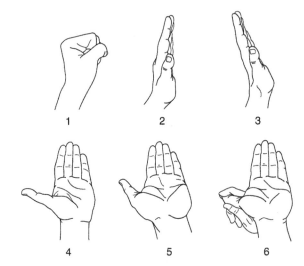

Figure 7.18 Median nerve gliding exercise sequence, as recommended by Byron. (Reproduced with permission from Byron.[12])

positions, combined movements and brachial plexus tension testing. Tests for thoracic outlet compression should also be done if compression at this level is suspected.

Monofilament testing[3] before and after provocative postures, i.e. wrist flexion for 3–5 min may aid in the diagnosis. Thenar muscle weakness and wasting may be evident in long-standing cases.

Treatment

Treatment includes rest from any aggravating activity, particularly repetitive activity. Wrist flexion postures should be avoided. Splinting of the wrist at night in neutral[4] or in a small degree of extension (10 degrees) may relieve night symptoms completely. Holding the wrist in neutral maximises the space in the carpal tunnel. If there is a particular aggravating activity or work task that cannot be avoided, then a working splint which supports the wrist close to the neutral position may be indicated.

Tendon gliding[5] (Fig. 7.17) and median nerve gliding exercises at the wrist level (Fig. 7.18) have been reported in the literature[6,7] to be beneficial in the conservative management regime.

Specific tips

Long-standing CTS or CTS that has proximal radiation of symptoms is unlikely to respond to conservative treatment. Even with surgical release of the flexor retinaculum, a complete recovery may not be realised.

CTS due to repetitive gripping may be due to well-developed lumbrical muscles gliding into the carpal tunnel area with full grip activity,[8,9] which increases the content and thus pressure in the carpal tunnel.[10] Prevention of full forceful grip and repetitive full grip activities should be considered if this is suspected.

If there is radiation of symptoms proximally, proximal structures must be assessed with particular attention to the other possible sites of compression at the elbow, e.g. the pronator or FDS arch, shoulder (pectoralis minor) or neck (thoracic outlet syndrome or cervical spine).

If there are cervical spine symptoms at the C5, 6, 7 level, the entire median nerve may become irritable. The proximal signs and symptoms need to be thoroughly evaluated and treated in conjunction with the CTS.

Surgical treatment

The carpal tunnel can be released (CTR) by the traditional open method or by endoscopic carpal tunnel release (ECTR) through a uniportal or biportal approach. The aim of surgery is to divide the flexor retinaculum and the related fascia of the distal forearm. Occasionally, flexor tenosynovectomy is indicated and, occasionally, an epineurotomy or endoneurolysis is indicated if there is an hourglass constriction of the median nerve.

Postoperative management

Generally, most patients require minimal postoperative therapy.

ECTR patients usually have their wrist bandaged after the procedure. The bandage may stay in place for up to 1 week. Use of the hand and full-range finger extension and flexion exercises are encouraged as soon as the discomfort of the operation allows, usually after 3–4 days.

Strong gripping with the wrist in flexion should be avoided until the flexor retinaculum is healed at approximately 6 weeks post-surgery. This position causes the flexor tendons to sublux volarly out of the carpal tunnel, which may result in irritation of the flexor retinaculum and symptomatic pillar pain.

Open carpal tunnel release (OCTR) patients are generally treated in the same manner: the recovery is usually slower than ECTR. Further hand therapy measures may be needed, depending on the findings at surgery. For example, an inflamed median nerve or a nerve severely compressed may require a plaster volar wrist resting splint for 7–10 days after operation. This is usually applied in the operating theatre at the surgeon's discretion.

These patients are instructed in full-range finger extension/flexion, tendon gliding exercises and gentle neural gliding exercises for the median nerve at the wrist level. Nerve gliding involving the whole brachial plexus[11,12] (Fig. 7.19) may be indicated in those patients with proximally radiating pain or more proximal symptoms in conjunction with CTS symptoms prior to CTR. Oedema control and scar management are carried out as necessary.

Those cases in which revision CTR is required need a different therapeutic approach. If scarring or fibrosis along the nerve is the major operative finding, then emphasis is placed on tendon gliding, nerve gliding and scar management.

Neuroma, particularly of the palmar cutaneous branch is also a common finding in revision

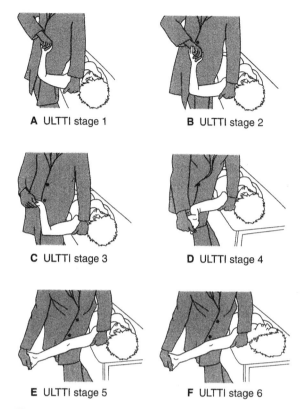

Figure 7.19 A–F: Brachial plexus gliding exercises: ULTT 1. Stages of brachial plexus, median nerve bias gliding. Butler refers to this as upper limb tension test number 1 (ULTT 1). (Reproduced with permission from Butler D: Mobilisation of the nervous system. Melbourne: Churchill Livingstone, 1991:149.)

surgery. Treatment needs to be directed towards decreasing pain and hypersensitivity. This can be largely managed with a desensitising programme, TENS, scar care and compression therapy in the form of a pressure garment/sleeve.

Complications

Complications of surgical decompression include iatrogenic injury to the palmar cutaneous nerve, the recurrent thenar branch or the median nerve itself or inadequate release of the flexor retinaculum. Other complications include haematoma, oedema, and wound infection.[13]

After surgery if the patient complains of weakness of grip and stiffness of the fingers in association with severe pain, reflex dystrophy – chronic regional pain syndrome (CRPS type 1) – should be suspected and investigated. Recurrent CTS can follow fibrosis of the median nerve or hyperplasia of the tenosynovium.

The pronator syndrome

Cause

This syndrome is rare but should be thought of if pain and paraesthesia in the median distribution (including the palm and thenar eminence) is associated with forearm pronation rather than at night as in the CTS.

The median nerve can be constricted by abnormal ligaments, e.g. the ligament of Struthers, the uncommon oblique ligament from the medial epicondyle to the supracondylar process above or at the elbow or in the upper forearm as the median nerve passes between the two heads of the pronator teres and under the fibrous arch of FDS.

Clinical features

There will be sensory loss in the distribution of the palmar branch as well as the major sensory branch of the median nerve; the motor deficit will include weakness of the long flexors of the thumb, index and middle fingers and FDS. There may be considerable reduction of grip strength.

Treatment

Most cases settle with conservative management but, if they do not, surgical release of the median nerve from above the elbow to the forearm is indicated. Recovery after such surgical decompression can be slow and incomplete.

Conservative management

Conservative management includes rest from aggravating activities or postures. Splintage with the wrist in neutral or slight extension and even supination may be necessary in severe cases. Forearm rotation can only be controlled in a splint if the elbow is included; therefore, elbow motion is secondarily limited to some degree in this situation.

The FDS is primarily activated with strong gripping. Activity modification involving avoiding pronation and strong or prolonged gripping activities may be necessary. Pronator teres (PT) and long flexor massage and stretches preceded by heat to reduce the resting tension of the pronator teres will aid in symptom relief.

Following surgical release, the same therapeutic principles are followed. Attention to muscle tendon glide and neural gliding in the form of appropriate stretches and flexor tendon gliding exercises, and neural gliding exercises involving the whole median nerve is emphasised.

Anterior interosseous syndrome

This may develop as a complication of a supracondylar fracture of the humerus in childhood or there may be compression under the fibrous arch at the origin of the pronator teres (PT). It can develop after closed forearm fractures, or can occur spontaneously.

Clinical features

The patient presents with a motor palsy – FPL, FDP of the index and sometimes middle finger and of pronator quadratus (PQ) – as in the pronator syndrome without sensory symptoms. PQ weakness can be tested by forearm pronation with a flexed elbow. This attempts to eliminate PT action. There may be forearm pain.

Treatment

As for the pronator syndrome. Muscle stimulation of the denervated muscle is controversial in the literature.[14] Daily stimulation for up to 20 min for each muscle is usually recommended if this treatment technique is to be used.

THE ULNAR NERVE

Cubital tunnel syndrome

Cause

The ulnar nerve may be entrapped:

- just above the elbow in the triceps muscle or by the arcade of Struthers

- in the cubital tunnel itself. It can occur after fractures, from direct injury or by fibrous bands or by cysts, bone spurs or arthritis
- in the upper forearm between the two heads of the flexor carpi ulnaris (FCU) muscle or Osborne's ligament.

Clinical features

Macnicol[2] reports significant increases in pressure on the ulnar nerve (171 mmHg) with maximum elbow flexion; this increases considerably (238 mmHg) if combined with 135 degrees of shoulder abduction. The cubital tunnel narrows up to 55% with elbow flexion, and the nerve is required to elongate 5 mm for every 45 degrees of elbow flexion.

The ulnar motor and sensory nerves to the hand are primarily affected. Nerve fibre size and length and sensitivity to pressure determine the degree of involvement. Mostly there is ulnar nerve distribution paraesthesia aggravated by elbow flexion, leading onto deteriorating handwriting and, for musicians, difficulty in playing a musical instrument. Later there may be clinical weakness of the interossei, particularly the first dorsal interosseous muscle. Hypothenar intrinsics are less involved than the interossei. There may be a positive Tinel tapping sign over the ulnar nerve in the cubital tunnel and clinical anterior subluxation of the ulnar nerve on full elbow flexion.

Conservative management

Activity modification and night-splinting of the elbow are the two most important factors in conservative management. Activities requiring repetitive or sustained elbow flexion should be avoided. If the patient reports symptoms at night this may be due to a flexed elbow sleeping posture. A night splint with the elbow held in a more extended position (approximately 30 degrees flexion) can often resolve night symptoms. Seror[15] reports good results when flexion beyond 60 degrees is prevented at night for a period of 6 months.

A volar splint of 1.6 mm thermoplastic material provides some minimal flexibility and clinically is tolerated better than the thicker more rigid

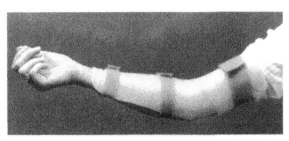

Figure 7.20 Elbow splint worn at night for relief of ulnar nerve compression symptoms. Wearing comfort can be improved by using the thinner thermoplastic material (1.6 mm) when fabricating the splint.

thermoplastics (Fig. 7.20). A neoprene sleeve with a thermoplastic strut may further improve comfort and tolerance. Care should be taken in the fabrication of these splints to avoid increasing external pressure over the cubital tunnel. Harper[16] advocates the drop-out splint as an alternative to the traditional long arm splint.

Sensibility monitoring can be useful in assessing the degree of sensibility symptoms and improvement gained from splinting.

More proximal joints and structures should also be evaluated. These include the cervical spine, thoracic outlet, pectoralis minor and brachial plexus.

Surgical treatment

This is indicated if there is continuing paraesthesia, and any degree of ulnar intrinsic weakness or wasting.

The types of surgical treatment include simple decompression, medial epicondylectomy, anterior transposition (subcutaneous or submuscular) and epineurotomy (Fig. 7.21). Generally, the surgery for patients less than 40 years old is more aggressive. In the older age group there is a risk of ischaemia after nerve transposition.

Postoperative care

At the time of surgery well-padded bandaging is applied to the elbow 20 degrees short of full extension. This gives good gentle compression to control swelling, aids the patient in maintaining an extended posture but still allows some movement of the elbow to glide the nerve. The well-padded bandage is usually maintained for 2 weeks.

A

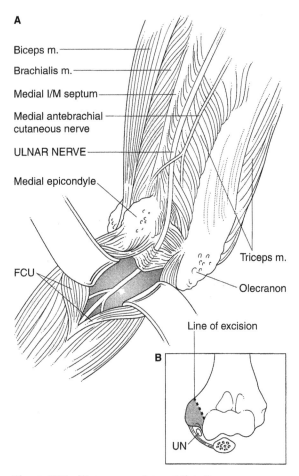

- Biceps m.
- Brachialis m.
- Medial I/M septum
- Medial antebrachial cutaneous nerve
- ULNAR NERVE
- Medial epicondyle
- FCU
- Triceps m.
- Olecranon
- Line of excision

B

UN

Figure 7.21 Ulnar nerve release at the elbow.

Within the first week the patient is instructed on active exercises for the shoulder, wrist, hand and the elbow. Gentle nerve gliding exercises are also commenced to prevent scarring and adhesions from tethering the nerve.

Good communication with the surgeon regarding the condition of the nerve and its blood supply is essential for the therapist to establish safe parameters for nerve gliding exercises.

When the sutures are removed, usually at 2 weeks postoperative, scar management involving massage and compression can be commenced. Care should be taken with compression garments and pads not to compress the nerve. In the early stages a foam pad and an elasticised circumferential bandage, e.g. Tubigrip, may be all

that is needed or tolerated. Monofilament testing can be helpful in monitoring recovery.

Complications

Complications include subluxation of the ulnar nerve from the cubital tunnel, persistence or recurrence of the ulnar nerve condition from scarring and/or ischaemia.

Ulnar nerve compression at the wrist (Guyon's canal): the ulnar tunnel syndrome

Cause

The cause may be traumatic, from repeated blunt trauma, as in the 'hypothenar hammer syndrome' or in cyclists from local pressure from the handle bar, from fractures of the hamate or from fractures of the fourth and fifth metacarpals. There may be a ganglion or space-occupying lesion in the canal, osteoarthritis of the pisotriquetral joint or thrombosis of the ulnar artery.

Clinical features

There may be pure sensory symptoms, or pure motor symptoms of the ulnar innervated intrinsics or a mixture of motor and sensory clinical features but, typically, the dorsal ulnar nerve sensation is spared. Allen's test for the presence of normal blood flow to the ulnar artery should always be evaluated.

Treatment

Surgical exploration and release is indicated if a mechanical cause is suspected.

Postoperative care

Nerve recovery may be monitored with sensibility testing two-point discrimination (2PD), moving 2PD and monofilament tests and muscle charting.

After removal of the sutures and postoperative bandaging at 2 weeks, scar care is commenced. Ulnar nerve gliding using the brachial plexus ulnar nerve bias gliding exercise can be used to facilitate the return of normal glide. This is particularly useful if the patient has a propensity to form dense scar tissue.

THE RADIAL NERVE

The radial tunnel (posterior interosseous nerve syndrome)

Cause

The radial nerve may be compressed (Fig. 7.22) as it passes:

- anterior to the lateral epicondyle between the brachialis and the brachioradialis
- deep to the ECRB (extensor carpi radialis brevis)
- deep to the arcade of Frohse and
- the fibrous arch in the proximal supinator muscle or
- between the two heads of the supinator itself.

There may be compression from an abnormal ligament, tight muscle, a fracture or dislocation or a space-occupying lesion.

Clinical features

Clinical features may include pain in the extensor/supinator muscle mass and along the line of the nerve aggravated by wrist flexion/extension and forearm rotation. There is weakness of wrist and finger (particularly middle finger) extension. Symptoms may be reproduced by resisted supination with a flexed elbow. This condition may be difficult to distinguish from or may be associated with tennis elbow or lateral epicondylitis. Nerve conduction studies are recommended.

Conservative treatment

A thorough and comprehensive assessment is necessary in order to isolate the problematic structures. The therapy programme follows the same guidelines for any nerve compression. Rest from aggravating activities, i.e. end range or prolonged wrist flexion and pronation. A splint maintaining the wrist in neutral or slight extension may be necessary for some activities in severe cases.

Stretching techniques for tight muscles, e.g. supinator and ECRB, should be done cautiously

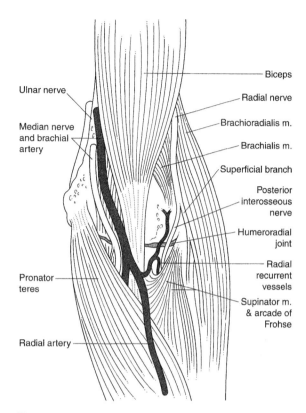

Figure 7.22 Anatomy of the radial nerve at the elbow.

so as not to exacerbate the compression. Active stretching techniques such as contract/relax combined with heat are less likely to irritate the nerve.

Modalities such as TENS and ultrasound may give temporary relief. In the authors' experience if, after 6–8 weeks, conservative measures have not helped, then further investigation or surgical release should be considered.

Surgical treatment

If the clinical features persist, the radial nerve is exposed between the brachialis and brachioradialis and dissected distally by dividing the fibrous origin of ECRB; the nerve is then dissected as it enters the supinator, care being taken to identify any possible cause of constriction such as fibrous bands in the arcade of Frohse, a ganglion or other tumours. Occasionally, a neurofibroma is found and needs to be resected and that area of nerve grafted.

Postoperative care

Postoperative therapy follows the same lines as any compression release: early active exercise, gentle nerve gliding exercises – in this case brachial plexus radial nerve bias gliding exercises – scar care and appropriate monitoring.

Wartenburg syndrome (cheiralgia paraesthetica): radial nerve compression at the wrist

Pathology

The radial nerve (the superficial radial nerve) at the wrist can be subject to compression or neuritis in association with de Quervain's condition or compression from a wrist watch, bracelets, sporting straps or a tight cast or splint. The neuritis can also follow injection to the area or follow scarring from surgery.

Clinical features

There is altered sensation in the first web space. This may be described as burning, pins and needles or pain. There may be a Tinel's sign at the point of compression in the distal forearm. Pain may also radiate proximally.

Conservative management

Conservative treatment is primarily aimed at relieving the pain and sensory discomfort. Gentle massage, TENS and comfortable compression are the primary techniques used. In the authors' opinion, nerve gliding should be done gently and cautiously, as the symptoms will be easily aggravated from strong stretching of the nerve.

Surgical treatment

Exploration and neurolysis is indicated after failed conservative measures.

Postoperative care

The superficial radial nerve is a sensory nerve. Treatment is aimed at reducing hyperaesthesia, by softening any scar around the nerve and gently increasing nerve glide.

Hyperaesthesia can be dealt with using a desensitisation programme (textures and mediums); a night compression bandage or pad may also be helpful in reducing nerve hypersensitivity/irritability. TENS can also be used to help decrease nerve irritability; placements along the nerve proximal to the surgery site are tried first. Scar care techniques can be combined with the desensitisation programme. Nerve gliding exercises focusing on radial nerve glide can be taught as part of the home programme.

OTHER ENTRAPMENTS AND SYNDROMES

Digital nerve entrapment

Pathology

The digital nerves can be compressed by a ganglion or bone spurs or post-traumatic fibrosis as they pass with the palmar digital artery from the hand into the finger in a tunnel between the superficial and deep intermetacarpal ligaments.

There may be repeated pressure on the nerve as can occur in a bowler or in a tennis player.

Clinical features

There may be burning pain or numbness or vasomotor changes in the digit.

Treatment

Local hand therapy measures and corticosteroid injections are usually helpful. Surgical release of the intermetacarpal ligament is indicated in unresolved cases.

Thoracic outlet syndrome (TOS)

The brachial plexus and the subclavian artery emerge from the cervical spine and the thorax into a triangular supraclavicular triangle bound by the first rib inferiorly, the anterior scalenus anteriorly, and posteriorly by the scalenus medius and superiorly by the clavicle. They then pass beneath the clavicle under the pectoralis minor and into the axilla. In this syndrome there is often an anatomical abnormality.

TOS has been described in the literature as cervical syndrome, scalenus anticus syndrome (Naffziger's syndrome), subcoracoid – pectoralis minor syndrome, costoclavicular syndrome and first thoracic rib syndrome.[17]

There are several risk factors: congenital – structural; post-traumatic – structural; and post-traumatic – postural.

Cause

The roots or trunks of the brachial plexus, especially the T1 root in the lower trunk and the subclavian artery, can be compressed by a cervical rib, an abnormal fibromuscular ligament arising from the C7 transverse process, after fracture of the clavicle or by tight fibrous bands in the scalene and pectoralis minor. Compression can be extrinsic by adjacent structure or intrinsic due to reactive perineural fibrosis from repetitive mechanical irritation by altered anatomy or posture.

Distal trauma such as a painful hand condition can cause nerve compression in the thoracic outlet. The guarding posture results in associated anatomical alterations in the thoracic outlet, e.g. elevation of the first rib, scalene muscle spasm. Above-shoulder activity decreases the size of the thoracic outlet and can further exacerbate symptoms.

Local trauma such as scalene tear or in a whiplash injury may lead to scar contracture and a delayed onset of thoracic outlet compression symptoms.

Clinical features

Pain in the shoulder and down the inner side of the arm that is worse after exercise and worse with activities with the arm above the head; however, pain may be diffuse in the whole arm. Sensory disturbance in the medial cord of the plexus or in the C8 T1 nerve root distribution in the hand (ulnar three digits), forearm and upper arm may be present. Intrinsic weakness and wasting due to T1 nerve root compression may be a presenting sign.

There may be associated vascular symptoms with a pale hand. Elevation of the limb above the shoulder may produce a diminished pulse. Adson's test may reveal a diminished radial pulse at the wrist level with or without ulnar-sided hand paraesthesiae with neck rotation to the

ipsilateral side and deep inspiration. Whitenack et al.[17] have described variations on this test which include shoulder abduction, elbow flexion and neck rotation to the contralateral side. The Roos test[18] is described as a 3 min elevated arm stress test. With the patient sitting, arms abducted 90 degrees and elbow flexed 90 degrees, the fingers are flexed and extended repeatedly while keeping the shoulder gently braced backwards. In a TOS, the patient will be unable to complete the test due to recurrence of symptoms (pain, numbness and perceived weakness). Rapid onset of symptoms indicates a more severe TOS.

Compression of the plexus in the neck at the site of irritation by direct pressure (Spurling manoeuvre) may cause local tenderness and reproduce symptoms. Tinel's sign may also be positive in the thoracic outlet region.

TOS may coexist with a brachioneuralgia or brachioplexopathy, in which there is primarily an irritation of the brachial plexus. The irritation may result from a number of pathologies, including cervical spine oesteoarthritis and disc lesions. A thorough neck examination, including spinal palpation and brachial plexus tension testing, is essential. All these patients need thorough investigations, including X-rays of the cervical spine, nerve conduction studies and, occasionally, angiography.

Conservative management

Conservative management falls broadly into six categories:

1. patient education
2. postural instruction
3. appropriate relative rest
4. stretching tight structures in a controlled manner
5. strengthening weak muscle in the shoulder girdle
6. neural mobilisation.

Patient education. Behavioural changes and patient compliance are vital to the successful treatment of these patients. The patient must have a good understanding of what causes the symptoms and what is required to improve them. The therapy programme can be very drawn out, requiring continuous patient compliance and long-term lifestyle changes.

Postural instruction. The classical good posture may aggravate these patients. A more slouched or flexed posture may decrease symptoms in the short term. Mechanically tight structures such as muscles and ligaments need to be stretched slowly over a long period of time. Return of 'good' posture may take some time and, in severe cases, may never be complete.

Appropriate rest. Rest should be relative for the irritable structure. Activity within pain limits should be encouraged. Several commercially available shoulder braces have been advocated in the literature.[19] The need for this type of brace and the suitability for each patient needs to be assessed on an individual basis.

Stretching tight structures. This category may include cervical spine mobilisation, muscle stretching, such as the scalene and pectoralis, anterior shoulder joint stretches and neural mobilisation, depending on the patient's presenting problems.

Strengthening. Usually, if the anterior structures are tight in the neck and shoulder, the corresponding posterior musculotendinous structures become lengthened and weak, particularly in inner range. The strengthening programme is aimed at gradually strengthening the posterior muscles as the antagonist muscles are gently lengthened. The aim is to produce a stable shoulder complex in an improved mechanical alignment.

Neural mobilisation. Neural mobilisation is included in mobilisation of tight structures. It bears particular reference here as too vigorous mobilisation or too rapid progression of neural mobilisation will retard the patient's progress, causing increased irritability, loss of patient confidence and compliance and thereby decreasing therapy effectiveness. Particular care should be taken to progress the programme slowly at a rate the patient and their tissues can cope with.

Treatment

Conservative treatment should always be tried first, but if there are objective neurological and vascular findings supported by investigations, surgical exploration and release of the compression is indicated.

REFERENCES

1. Adelaar RS, Foster WC, McDowel C: Treatment of cubital tunnel syndrome. J Hand Surg 9:90–5, 1984.
2. Macnicol M: Entrapment neuropathies. In: Lamb D (ed.), The paralysed hand. Edinburgh: Churchill Livingstone, 1987:169–87.
3. MacDermid J, Kramer J, Roth J: Decision making in detecting abnormal Semmes–Weinstein monofilament thresholds in carpal tunnel syndrome. J Hand Ther 7:158–62, 1994.
4. Burke DT, Burke MM, Stewart GW: Splinting for carpal tunnel syndrome; in search for the optimal angle. Arch Phys Med Rehab 75:1241–4, 1994.
5. Wehbe MA, Hunter JM: Flexor tendon gliding in the hand II: differential gliding. J Hand Surg 10A:575–9, 1985.
6. Sagerman S, Rooks M, Dry Ensor C: Carpal tunnel syndrome: an alternative method of conservative treatment. In: Leonard J, Willette-Green V (eds), Proceedings ASHT. J Hand Ther 6:54, 1993.
7. Rozmaryn L, Dovelle S, Rothman E, Gorman K, Olvey K, Bartko J: Nerve and tendon gliding exercises and the conservative management of carpal tunnel syndrome. J Hand Ther 11:171–9, 1998.
8. Siegel DB, Kuzma G, Eakins D: Anatomical investigation of the role of lumbricle muscles in carpal tunnel syndrome. J Hand Surg 20A:860–3, 1995.
9. Cobb TK, An KN, Cooney WP, Berger RA: Lumbricle muscle incursion into the carpal tunnel during finger flexion. J Hand Surg 19B:434–8, 1994.
10. Cobb TK, An KN, Cooney WP: Effect of lumbricle incursion within the carpal tunnel on carpal tunnel pressure: a cadaveric study. J Hand Surg 20A:186–92, 1995.
11. Butler D: Mobilisation of the nervous system. Melbourne: Churchill Livingstone, 1991:147–60.
12. Byron P: Upper extremity nerve gliding: programs used at the Philadelphia Hand Centre. In: Hunter J, Mackin E, Callahan A (eds), Rehabilitation of the hand: surgery and therapy, 4th edn. St Louis: Mosby, 1995:951–5.
13. McDonald RI et al: Complications of surgical release of carpal tunnel syndrome. J Hand Surg 3:70, 1978.
14. Low J, Reed A: Electrotherapy explained. Oxford: Butterworth Heinemann, 1994:39–116.
15. Seror P: Treatment of ulnar nerve palsy at the elbow with a night splint. J Bone Joint Surg (Br) 75B:322–7, 1993.
16. Harper B: The drop out splint: an alternative to the conservative management of ulnar nerve entrapment at the elbow. J Hand Ther 3:199–201, 1990.
17. Whitenack SH, Hunter JM, Jaeger SH, Read R: Thoracic outlet syndrome: a brachial plexopathy. In: Hunter JM,

Mackin EJ, Callahan AD (eds), Rehabilitation of the hand and upper limb, 4th edn. St Louis: Mosby, 1995:857–84.

18. Roos DB: Experience with first rib resection for thoracic outlet syndrome. Ann Surg 163:354–8, 1966.

19. Barbis J, Wallace K: Therapist's management of brachioplexopathy. In: Hunter J, Mackin E, Callahan A (eds), Rehabilitation of the hand; surgery and therapy, 4th edn. St Louis: Mosby, 1995:923–50.

D. TENDON TRANSFERS

W Bruce Conolly and Rosemary Prosser

INTRODUCTION

Disability in the hand and forearm resulting from loss of muscle function can be treated by transferring active muscles to substitute for those whose function has been lost. Such loss of function may be due to:

- Direct injury to the muscle or tendon, rupture from attrition, e.g. extensor pollicis longus (EPL) after Colles' fracture, or rheumatoid arthritis or
- Indirectly from nerve injury – e.g. brachial plexus, spinal cord or peripheral nerves – or following neurological disease, e.g. poliomyelitis, leprosy, motor neurone disease. The nerve injury may be irreversible or motor recovery may fail after nerve repair.

A paralysed hand can be improved by skilled surgery and therapy but it is not possible to return that hand to normal function.

Arthrodesis of the joint and tenodesis (this may be a static tendon transfer) are alternatives to dynamic tendon transfers. Dynamic tendon transfers transfer active muscle function: in this chapter they are referred to as tendon transfers.

INDICATIONS FOR TENDON TRANSFERS

1. The patient must have a particular need for a specific movement or function, be generally fit and be able to cooperate with the postoperative hand therapy programme.
2. Muscles must be available and expendable for transfer.
3. The joints need to be passively mobile so that the transferred motor is not overloaded.
4. Adequate skin and soft tissue cover, including adequate sensation, is also a prerequisite.

THE TIMING OF TENDON TRANSFERS

There are occasions when tendon transfers are advised early after nerve injury, e.g. a high lesion of the ulnar nerve. Reinnervation may take 18–24 months, and in the older patient reinnervation may be incomplete. Tendon transfer provides the patient with a hand that is functional in this time period.

In other cases, transfers are delayed until the full potential of nerve recovery is reached and the local tissue and the general condition of the patient is optimal for tendon transfer.

HEALING OF TENDON TRANSFERS

The transferred tendons are surgically sutured to a recipient tendon or bone. Immobilisation is required for 4 weeks for a tendon-to-tendon junction and 6–8 weeks for a tendon-to-bone junction. Sometimes a small joint arthrodesis is performed and immobilisation is required for 6–8 weeks. An arthrodesis in an insensate limb may require an immobilisation period twice as long as a normally sensitive limb.

In general, after 3–4 weeks of healing gentle careful movement can be carried out, at 4–5 weeks active exercise without resistance and at 6–7 weeks normal usage with light resistance only.[1]

POSTOPERATIVE COMPLICATIONS

Intraoperative surgical complications include poor healing from the surgical dissection, iatrogenic nerve damage, haematoma and infection, poor tendon junctions and inappropriate tension. Incorrect tension is one of the commonest causes of failure in tendon transfer.

Postoperative complications include joint stiffness, especially in the elderly, adhesions along the course of the tendon transfer and rupture of the tendon junction. Some patients are unable to learn to use a transfer due to their age, motivation or personality.

PREOPERATIVE ASSESSMENT: SURGICAL AND THERAPY

The patient's real functional needs must be established by:

1. a functional assessment
2. muscle strength evaluation
3. range of motion (ROM) charting, active and passive
4. assessment of 'trick' movements, hand balance and the use of the tenodesis effect
5. evaluation of the projected function of the tendon transfer in terms of use, ROM, strength, hand balance and the need for tenodesis movement
6. sensibility/sensory evaluation.

1. Functional assessment needs to be performed on an individual basis. Specific activities may need to be simulated. The use of splints to simulate the action of the proposed transfer may assist the therapist in assessing the impact of the tendon transfer on hand function, e.g. an opposition strap (see Chapter 7A).

2. Muscle charting will determine which muscles have been affected by the injury or nerve lesion and which muscles are available for transfer. Muscles to be transferred should be grade 5 strength because they will lose one grade of power after transfer and some further loss of strength occurs during the initial period of immobilisation. Reinnervated muscles are seldom strong enough to transfer. The transfer muscle should be matched in terms of strength and amplitude as much as is possible to that of the lost muscle.[2] Figure 7.23

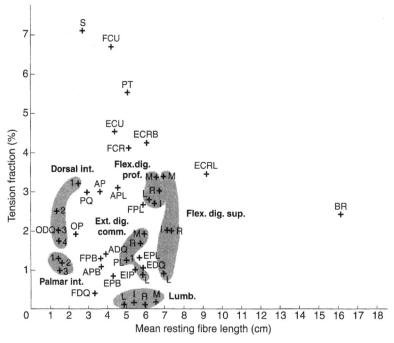

Figure 7.23 The relationship between fibre length and tension producing capability. Some muscle groups are highlighted for clarity. (Reproduced with permission from Brand PW et al.[3])

shows a graph depicting the tension fraction and mean resting fibre length of the wrist and hand muscles.[3] This can be helpful when evaluating transfer choices.

3. Range of motion charting will establish which joints and soft tissues are tight or contracted, e.g. the thumb web. These will need therapy treatment (see Chapter 2J) and, occasionally, surgical treatment prior to tendon transfer to restore ROM.

4. The balance of the hand and wrist and use of the tenodesis needs to be carefully assessed. If the patient is using the tenodesis to achieve grip and release, then it should be preserved at all costs. EPL and FPL (flexor pollicis longus) are often used as compensatory muscles to provide a more functional pinch when thenar muscle function is lost.

5. The proposed improvement in function and deficit in muscle action must be evaluated carefully. Splints to simulate the proposed action may be useful for the patient to evaluate his needs, e.g. Figure 7.24.

6. Re-education of a transfer is much slower if the sensation in the part being moved is not normal. Visual cues and joint proprioception will enhance re-education. The tendon transfer function will be enhanced if an insensitive part can be moved to a part with normal sensation, e.g. opposition of an insensitive thumb to the ulnar fingers of normal sensation. The patient's ability to cooperate with the postoperative programme, the time constraints and assistance both at home and in the workplace also need to be considered.

GENERAL COMMENTS ON SURGICAL TECHNIQUE

In general, incisions are made away from where the tendon sutures will be and away from the line of the transferred tendon. The tendons are tunnelled through subcutaneous tissue and not through scar, fascia or muscle.

The tension of the transfer is extremely important: most joins should be under some tension because most tendon to musculotendon joins stretch in the first 3 months. Meticulous surgical technique is necessary to avoid adhesions of the tendon junctions to the adjacent tissues.

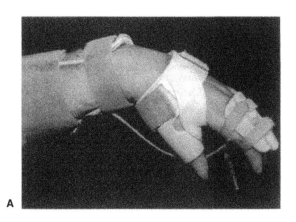

A

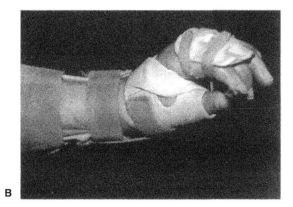

B

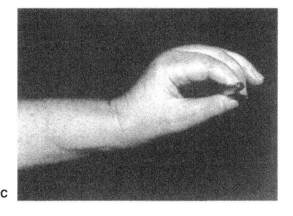

C

Figure 7.24 A tenodesis splint made and fitted for a patient with a brachial plexus palsy to simulate the possible function that would be gained following static tendon transfer. Possible extension (A) and flexion (B) is shown. In this case the static tendon transfers provided a tenodesis function for the thumb, index and middle fingers (C).

GENERAL COMMENTS ON TENDON TRANSFER

Tendon transfer procedures aim to improve coordinated motion by correcting instability and muscle imbalance. Correction is accomplished not by addition but by redistribution of the remaining muscle forces.

Design in tendon transfers should be simple, employ synergistic forces and accept a lower level of performance.

POSTOPERATIVE THERAPY

Aims of treatment

- Improve hand function
- Protection of the tendon transfer repair junction during healing
- Develop a functional range of motion using the transferred tendon
- Maintain or develop coordination of the transferred muscles
- Maintain tendon glide and limit unwanted adhesions
- Improve grip strength and general hand and arm strength
- Maintain mobility and restore strength to the unaffected joints and muscles.

Most tendon transfers in the past have been treated with 4 weeks of immobilisation, followed by a further 2–4 weeks of protected mobilisation in a splint.[1,3] This is the senior (surgical) author's preferred programme and is discussed in detail for radial, median and ulnar nerve tendon transfers.

An early passive motion postoperative programme utilising a splint with a dynamic component to protect the transfers (Fig. 7.25), similar to the Kleinert controlled passive motion flexor tendon programme, is being used in some centres. Good preoperative assessment of the patient's functional problem, motivation and circumstances, meticulous surgery and experienced hand therapy services are essential for this type of programme to be considered.

Immobilisation programme

- The tendon transfer repairs are protected with a cast or splint for 4 weeks (Table 7.2).
- Exercises for the unaffected joints/tendons can be commenced in the first postoperative week.
- Massage is commenced once the sutures have been removed if the operated area is accessible in the splint. Otherwise, it is commenced at 4 weeks when the splint is removed for exercises.

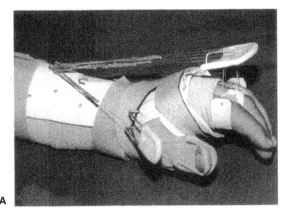 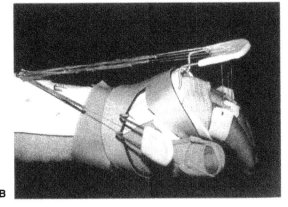

A   B

Figure 7.25 Controlled passive postoperative tendon transfer programmes require an experienced surgeon and therapist, and a well-motivated patient. The dynamic splint used following transfers for radial nerve palsy in a controlled passive programme has elastic traction, providing the extension force for the digits (A) and a flexion block to limit flexion (B) so that the transfer junctions are not stressed. A small digit-based splint is used to control thumb hyperextension. The dynamic splint is used for the first 6 weeks continuously, then intermittently over the next 2–4 weeks.

- Active transfer exercises are not commenced until 4 weeks post-surgery.
- The massage and exercise programme is used to mobilise the soft tissues, control scar adhesion and formation, restore joint range, and glide and re-educate the transferred musculotendinous unit.

The ultimate goal is to use the transferred tendons to achieve improved functional use of the hand.

The aim of the tendon transfer exercises is to change the cortical motor pattern from one motor function to another. For example, in a transfer to improve wrist extension using pronator teres, pronator teres cortical motor pattern needs to change from pronation to wrist extension. This is often termed muscle re-education or motor pattern relearning.

A tendon-to-tendon join needs continued protection when not under supervision until 6–8 weeks after surgery, or until the patient has gained active control, whichever is the longer. At 6 weeks, the splint can be removed during the day and light resistive activity is commenced.

At 8–10 weeks the splint can be discarded for light general daily activity. A graded resisted programme is started. Resisted exercise and activity should not be commenced until there is good active control of the transfer. An excessive sudden strain may rupture a tendon junction even after 3 months or it may stretch under long continued strain. For these reasons, 3–6 months of protection by splintage during sleep or whenever excessive strain may be exerted or during heavy activities is advised.

Specific tips

Some transfers require more re-education/ relearning than others. Transfer muscles that are not synergistic generally require more re-education, e.g. flexor digitorum superficialis (FDS) to finger extensors (extensor digitorum communis or EDC). Biofeedback or neuromuscular electrical stimulation may be useful adjuncts to the re-education phase.

Table 7.2 Postoperative programme

Postoperative time	Activity
Weeks 1–4	Immobilisation
Week 4	Commence active exercise, learning to use the transfer The splint is removed for exercises only
Week 6	Continue exercise training The splint may be removed for periods during the day Light activities are commenced
Weeks 8–10	Graded resisted exercise and activity are commenced The splint is discarded during the day; it is still worn for heavy activity and at night
Months 3–6	Full resisted activity is allowed including sport Protective splinting may be needed for some sports The splint is discontinued

Massage and heat are used as indicated to facilitate motion and glide of the tissue structures in the area of the reconstructive surgery.

Tendon transfer retraining is mentally very demanding. Even though only small movements are being done, the patient may feel exhausted from all the concentration and effort by the end of the day.

The exercise programme should not be painful. If the patient reports pain, the exercises should be reviewed. If the exercises are being done correctly, the therapist should be suspicious of postoperative complications, e.g. haematoma, impending rupture, nerve irritation. In this situation the patient requires immediate review by the surgeon.

Difficulty gaining transfer function may be due to rupture, adhesion or poor motor learning. Rupture may be diagnosed by palpation of the tendon transfer during attempted active motion. Moving the transfer from the shortened position to the lengthened position should produce some transfer motion at the peripheral joints. If joint motion is full and no transfer action occurs, rupture is suspected. Significant loss of motion overnight should also arouse suspicion.

Poor motor learning is usually characterised by inconsistent transfer action and poorly coordinated movement.

Adhesion of the transfer may be differentiated from rupture by decreased transfer length. Tendon transfer tension with contraction can be palpated; however, there is a reduced amplitude of motion.

TENDON TRANSFERS FOR RADIAL NERVE PALSY

A high radial nerve palsy, e.g. above the elbow, may involve all the extrinsic extensors and abductors of the hand and wrist. A low radial nerve palsy, below the elbow – e.g. posterior interosseous nerve palsy – spares the brachioradialis (BR) and extensor carpi radialis longus (ECRL).

The clinical problem may be as follows:

- Loss of wrist extension where replacement of extensor carpi radialis brevis (ECRB) is a priority.
- Loss of finger extension, which can be treated by tendon transfer or tenodesis.
- Loss of thumb extension, which can be treated by transfer to EPL. Some patients may also require arthrodesis of the metacarpophalangeal (MP) and/or interphalangeal (IP) joint in order to provide a stable thumb. The one transfer should not activate EDC and EPL.
- Loss of thumb metacarpal abduction–extension, some of which function is provided by the thenar muscles but can be supplemented by transfer to abductor pollicis longus (APL).

The following muscles are usually available for transfer:

1. Pronator teres (PT) is easily localised and re-educated.
2. Flexor carpi radialis (FCR) is a strong wrist flexor and easy to transfer. The impact on muscular balance of the wrist should be evaluated if FCR is to be used as a transfer. It can continue as a wrist flexor if it is attached to APL or EPL and these tendons are subluxed to the palmar aspect of the wrist.

Table 7.3 Tendor transfers for radial nerve palsy

Procedure	Transfer
Wrist extension	ECRB–PT. Combine this with a yoke to the base of the fourth metacarpal to balance the wrist extension
Finger extension	EDC–FDS of middle or ring fingers
Thumb extension	EPL–PL to re-routed EPL
Thumb abduction	APL–FCR

For abbreviations, see text.

3. Palmaris longus (PL) may be small and weak but may be useful for EPL transfer.
4. Flexor carpi ulnaris (FCU) is an ulnar wrist stabiliser as well as a flexor and removal may cause loss of flexion and ulnar deviation strength and balance. It has a limited amplitude and is not recommended for transfer.
5. FDS of the middle or ring fingers is strong and has good amplitude. Re-education from flexor to extensor may be challenging in some patients.
6. BR is often available. It has a good fibre resting length but clinically a small amplitude.

Table 7.3 shows the commonly performed tendon transfers for radial nerve palsy.

Surgical procedure (Fig. 7.26)

Wrist extension

The PT is mobilised in the upper forearm and stripped with its periosteal insertion from the radius. It is re-routed superficial to the BR, but deep to the superficial radial nerve. The PT is sutured to the ECRB just distal to the muscle tendon belly with the wrist in maximal extension, the forearm half pronated and the elbow flexed. A yoke is made to the base of the fourth metacarpal or the ECU insertion to balance wrist extension. The yoke is sutured to the PT–ECRB junction.

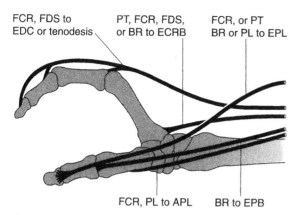

FCR, FDS to EDC or tenodesis

PT, FCR, FDS, or BR to ECRB

FCR, or PT BR or PL to EPL

FCR, PL to APL

BR to EPB

Figure 7.26 Basic muscle tendon transfers for radial nerve palsy:
- for wrist extension – PT to ECRB, alternates – FDS or FCR or BR
- for finger extension – FCR to EDC, alternates – FDS of middle or ring finger or tenodesis of EDC to ulna
- for thumb extension – PL to subluxed EPL, alternates – FCR or BR or PT
- for thumb abduction – BR to EPB, FCR or PL to subluxed APL
  Athrodesis of the thumb MP or IP joints may be useful.
For abbreviations, see the text.

Finger extension

The FDS of the middle or ring fingers is retrieved at the wrist level and transferred around the ulnar side of the forearm and sutured to the EDC slips of all four fingers, excluding the extensor indicus proprius (EIP) and extensor digiti quinti proprius (EDQ), proximal to the extensor retinaculum.

Thumb extension

The palmaris, if present, or the FCR, can be used and transferred to the EPL, which is released from Lister's tubercle: alternatively, the BR can be used. To gain some thumb abduction with extension, the APL and/or extensor pollicis brevis (EPB) tendons can be freed from their retinacular compartment and displaced palmarly. FCR can be used to motor this transfer at this level.

The hinge hand (The tenodesis hand)

If only one strong muscle remains, a useful hinge hand can be activated by a wrist extensor with tenodesis of the finger extensors and flexors and possibly the thumb. PT, BR or FCR can be used for a wrist extensor hinge hand.

Postoperative therapy

Splintage

The transfers are protected at the elbow, wrist and digit level for 6 weeks and a further 2 weeks at the wrist and digit level. The initial plaster splint/cast position requires the elbow to be held at 90 degrees, the forearm fully pronated, wrist in a moderate degree of extension, thumb in full palmar abduction and fingers extended. In some circumstances the IP joints can be left free while the MPs are held in full extension.

The sutures are removed at 2 weeks. At this time if a cast has been applied it is bivalved for removal of sutures (ROS) and then reapplied. It may be replaced by a thermoplastic splint, depending on its condition.

At 4 weeks postoperatively, the volar elbow section that becomes the dorsal forearm hood of the cast is removed. The long back slab gutter maintains the arm position. The dorsal forearm hood can be retained to be worn between exercise sessions to give greater stability if necessary.

The elbow section is removed completely at 6 weeks. The volar forearm splint is retained for a further 1–2 weeks, then used for travel and night-time for a further 2–6 weeks. Night splinting is required for 3–6 months.

Wound care and exercise

Massage. Massage is commenced at 2 weeks after suture removal if the incisions are accessible with the splint on. The splint is not removed at this time. If the incisions are not accessible, massage is commenced at 4 weeks when movement of the transfers is commenced.

IP joint motion. This activity is commenced within the first 2 weeks if the IPs are not splinted. Transfer motion is commenced at 4 weeks. Forearm pronation and wrist extension are started first. A few days later when these exercises are progressing satisfactorily, thumb palmar abduction and finger extension/EDC exercises are added.

The PT–ECR exercise. The patient is positioned with the elbows at approximately 90 degrees of flexion so that both forearms rest on the table with the wrists in some extension. Pronation of the unaffected arm is followed by pronation of the operated arm. Some wrist movement in the direction of extension should occur. This should be done second hourly. Gradually, the emphasis is moved from pronation to wrist extension. The elbow extension position should not be used until there is control of wrist extension with the elbow in flexion.

FDS–EDC exercise. The fingers are held with the IPs straight and MPs in some flexion and the wrist in extension; the IPs are flexed and the wrist is allowed to flex to a position of approximately 20 degrees of extension. This causes some tension in the FDS, which extends the MP joints. The patient is encouraged to actively extend the MP joints at the same time.

PL–thumb abduction exercise. With the wrist held in extension, the patient attempts wrist flexion (isometric flexion) to activate PL to produce some thumb abduction. Gradually, the emphasis is moved to active thumb abduction. The EPL transfer is dealt with in a similar manner.

Exercise progression. If IP joint exercises have not been commenced at 2 weeks they are started with transfer exercises at 4 weeks postoperatively: from 4–8 weeks, the exercises are upgraded; at 8 weeks, the patient starts to wean from the splint; from 8 to 12 or 14 weeks, a graded resisted exercise programme is pursued.

Specific tip

Maximal wrist extension and flexion may not be gained for 6 months. MP extension may also be slow.

The FDS to EDC transfer can be difficult to re-educate in some patients, particularly if simultaneous finger and wrist extension is required. The therapist aims to convert a flexor to an extensor. Biofeedback or neuromuscular electrical stimulation may be useful adjuncts in this situation.

TENDON TRANSFERS FOR MEDIAN NERVE PALSY

There may be:

1. A proximal high lesion above the elbow, where there is loss of FCR, PT, PL, flexor digitorum profundus (FDP) of the index and middle fingers, FDS, FPL, the thenar muscles and the radial lumbricals.

or

2. Lesion of the anterior interosseous nerve, which supplies FPL, and FDP to the index and middle fingers.

or

3. Injury at the wrist, where there is loss of thenar muscles and lumbricals to the index and middle finger. The loss of thumb opposition is the greatest functional loss.

In all these conditions, there is also loss of sensation to the dominant part of the hand, the thumb and index and middle fingers. This loss of sensation results in significant loss of overall function, particularly in co-coordinated fine manipulation in the hand, which cannot be compensated by any tendon transfer.

Transfers for median nerve lesions above the wrist

FPL can be motored by BR or ECRL. Loss of FDP to the index and middle fingers can be treated by side-to-side suture of the FDP tendons of the ring and little fingers. Poor thumb abduction and opposition, and pinch function, can be improved with an opponensplasty.

Opponensplasty

The following donor muscles are usually available:

1. FDS of the middle or ring finger. This is the best tendon for transfer. This muscle tendon unit has good strength, adequate length and a good excursion.
2. Extensor indicus (EI) or EDQ can be used but usually have a weaker action.

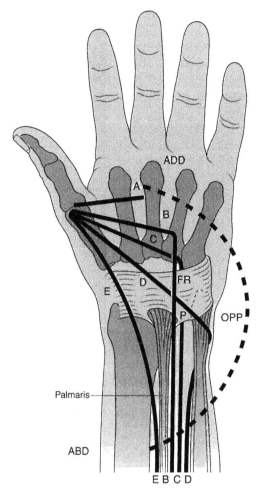

Figure 7.27 Main routes for thumb opposition tendon transfers, showing pulley sites relative to the movement required. The arc of possibility is indicated by the broken semicircle marked ADD (adduction), ABD (abduction) and OPP (opposition). The most frequently used types of transfer are: A Adductor replacement; the pulley is the second or third metacarpal. B The Thompson route; the pulley is the palmar fascia. This produces true opponens action. FDS is the common motor. C Guyon's canal; the pulley is the palmaris brevis or the palmar fascia. D Maximum abductor opponens pull; the pulley is at the pisiform on FCU. E Camitz route, the PL is fully dissected and becomes a weak abductor of the thumb without a pulley. Full adduction is (type A) through opposition (types B and C) to full abduction (type E).

3. FCR is a strong unit but has a shorter excursion and needs to be lengthened by a graft. An FCR transfer is influenced by wrist movement and tenodesis forces.

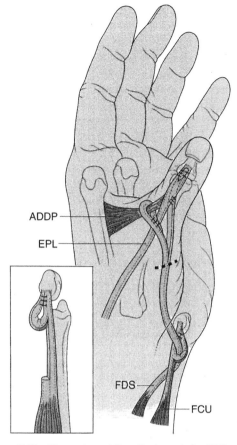

Figure 7.28 The route and the attachments for FDS opposition transfer are shown. The inset shows the pulley constructed at the wrist using half of FCU. See text for description.

4. APL can be detached from the metacarpal and re-routed around the palmaris as a pulley and re-attached.
5. ECRL can be re-routed around the ulnar border of the forearm through a pulley. The pulley is placed proximal at the pisiform for more abduction with opposition or more distal at the distal part of flexor retinaculum for more adduction with opposition (Fig. 7.27).
6. PL Camitz transfer.

Technique for the FDS opponensplasty

The FDS is taken from the radial side of the middle or ring fingers, retrieved at the wrist and transferred around a pulley at the distal part of FCU and tunnelled across the proximal palm. The two strips are inserted, one proximally to the adductor insertion – this slip crossing proximal to the MP joint – and the other distally, to the EPL just proximal to the IP joint (Fig. 7.28) – this distal slip controls any tendency to MP joint hyper-extension. The tension of this transfer is determined with the wrist at neutral and the thumb fully opposed, rotated and abducted.

Where there is a hypermobile proximal inter-phalangeal (PIP) joint of the donor digit, a PIP joint tenodesis should be carried out to prevent hyperextension of the PIP joint after taking the FDS tendon.

Camitz opponensplasty

The palmaris is elongated by taking continuous fibres of the palmar fascia to the base of the fingers to the tendon of abductor pollicis brevis (APB). No pulley is needed. The transfer is weak but produces some palmar abduction. This tech-nique is indicated in severe carpal tunnel syn-drome with thenar atrophy where this transfer can be carried out at the same time as the carpal tunnel release.

Postoperative therapy

Splintage

The initial postoperative plaster splint or cast should hold the wrist in approximately 30 degrees of flexion, the thumb fully abducted and rotated; the MP joint is flexed approximately 20–30 degrees and the IP joint able to fully extend. The fingers can be left free to move.

At 4 weeks the cast is bivalved. Half of the cast is retained for a further 2 weeks during the day and for up to 3 months at night. Alternatively, a thermoplastic dorsal splint can be made to replace the plaster splint/cast at week 1.

Wound care and exercise

If the hand is splinted (not cast) a controlled pas-sive postoperative exercise programme for the thumb can be used in the first 4 weeks. Passive flexion/opposition and active extension within

the splint can be started in the first postoperative week. If a cast is used, the thumb is immobilised up to the IP joint for 4 weeks.

Finger extension and flexion can be started within a few days following surgery. Thumb active IP extension and flexion can be started in the first week.

At 2 weeks post-surgery if a splint has been applied the sutures are removed and wound care commenced. If a cast is being used, this is done at week 4.

Active thumb opposition exercises are com-menced at week 4 post-surgery. The patient can monitor his own progress by palpating the trans-ferred tendon. This is performed by holding the wrist in a relaxed slightly flexed position.

For FDS transfer the donor digit, usually the ring finger, is flexed. This should produce some abduction of the thumb. The exercise is practised until a good range of motion is obtained. Once this technique is mastered, the patient should practise thumb abduction without finger movement. Func-tional pinch using all digits individually and as a gross function to oppose the thumb is the next progression, followed by functional pinch grip activities. From week 7 to 8, a graded resisted programme involving gross and pinch grip is instituted. Strong resisted work or sport is not permitted until week 12–16, depending on the activity and the strength of the transfer.

TENDON TRANSFERS FOR ULNAR NERVE PALSY

The motor lesion may be:

1. High, above the elbow, with loss of FCU and FDP of the ring and little fingers and all ulnar innervated intrinsics or
2. Low, where the loss is primarily in the hand. All the intrinsics are lost, except those of the thenar eminence on the radial side of FPL and the lumbrical to the index and middle fingers.

Transfers for low ulnar nerve palsy

• Loss of finger intrinsics is usually the primary problem; this can be improved by a dynamic or static transfer procedure. Dynamic tendon transfers can be direct into the intrinsic lateral bands or use the lasso technique. Static procedures include capsuloplasty or intrinsic tenodesis to hold the MP joints in flexion.

- The ulnar nerve controls the thumb MP joint in slight flexion and the IP joint in extension. Often the median innervated thenar muscles provide enough support and control of the MP joint, and in this situation surgery is not indicated. MP joint arthrodesis can be considered if the joint is functionally unstable.

- Adductor pollicis can be replaced by using EI if pinch is weak and a functional problem. Alternatives for thumb adduction are BR lengthened with a tendon graft or FDS of the middle or ring fingers passed across the palm to the adductor insertion using the distal end of the palmar fascia as a pulley.

- If loss of index abduction is a functional problem, EI or a slip of APL or FDS can be transferred to the interosseous insertion on the radial side of the proximal phalanx. If BR is used it is transferred through the space between the third and fourth metacarpals across the back of the wrist.

Intrinsic transfers

Static intrinsic transfers

1. Capsuloplasty involves excision of an ellipse transversely from the palmar plate of each MP joint and the defect closed by strong suture to produce MP joint flexion. This procedure can be complemented by palmar dermatodesis.

2. Intrinsic tenodesis utilises a free graft attached to the flexor retinaculum at the wrist or to the ulnar bone and sutured to grasp the lateral band of the radial side of each of the fingers holding the MP joints in flexion at 90 degrees.

Dynamic intrinsic transfers. The two donor tendons most commonly used are the FDS and ECRB.

FDS dynamic transfer. One FDS, e.g. from the ring finger, can be divided into four slips or the FDS of each of the fingers can be taken individually

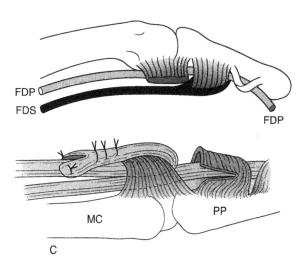

Figure 7.29 The Zancolli lasso operation for ulnar nerve palsy. An incision is made in the A2 pulley distal to the MP joint. The superficialis tendon is divided through the hole in the A2 pulley. The proximal stump is pulled through the incision into the A2 pulley and is attached to itself in the form of a loop or lasso with side-to-side sutures. Enough tension is applied to produce mild MP joint flexion so that the interphalangeal joints can be extended by the extensor tenodesis when activated by palmar wrist flexion.

and divided into half: one-half is used to flex the MP joints along the lumbrical canal; the remaining half can be tenodesed to prevent PIP hyperextension (Fig. 7.29).

The Zancolli lasso procedure.[4] The divided slip of FDS is passed under the A2 pulley and turned back over and sutured to itself.

Enough tension is applied to produce mild MP joint flexion so that the interphalangeal joints can be extended by the extensor tenodesis when activated by wrist palmar flexion. Such a technique does not increase the power of grip; it may reduce it slightly, because of the extra extensor tension on PIP flexion.

The Brand EEMTT (extensor–extensor mini tailed transfer). This is a dynamic tendon transfer popularised by Brand.[5] The ECRB is taken from the base of the third metacarpal, retrieved above the extensor retinaculum and elongated by four tendon grafts (using the plantaris). Each tail is transferred between the metacarpals volar to the intermetacarpal ligament and sutured to the

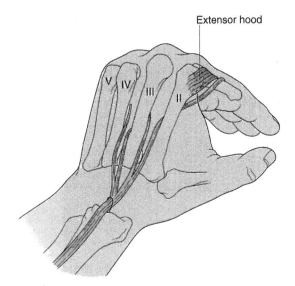

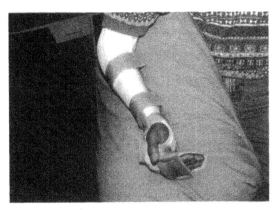

Figure 7.31 The static splint used following ulnar nerve transfer at 3–4 weeks post-transfer. The elbow is held in flexion, the wrist in approximately 30 degrees extension, the MPs in maximal comfortable flexion and the IPs in full extension.

Figure 7.30 The ECRB to intrinsic transfer using four tendon grafts attached to the distal end of ECRB. See text for description.

lateral intrinsic expansion of each finger on the radial side (Fig. 7.30).

The transfer should be sutured with the wrist extended, the MCP joints fully flexed and the fingers fully extended at the IP joints with the elbow at 90 degrees of flexion.

Postoperative therapy – EEMTT

Splintage

The postoperative cast or splint position is elbow flexion, wrist extension, full MP flexion and IP extension. The thumb is left free to allow some lateral pinch against the radial edge of the splint.

At 3–4 weeks, the plaster cast is bivalved; the volar half is kept as a resting splint for a period of 3 months. Alternatively, a volar thermoplastic splint can be made and fitted for this purpose (Fig. 7.31). At 6 weeks, the splint can be cut down to free the elbow. At 8 weeks, weaning from the splint in the day can be commenced. The splint will be required at night for at least 4 months, and often up to 6 months.

Wound care and exercise

Thumb exercise in terms of extension and flexion, abduction and opposition is encouraged in the first week.

At 2 weeks, the sutures are removed and wound care is commenced.

From week 3–4 intrinsic exercises are practised. With the wrist and IPs extended, passive small-range MP extension and flexion is practised. With the forearm and fingertips resting on the table, the wrist is extended, producing an intrinsic plus movement (MP flexion and IP extension). Within a week the exercise is progressed to MP joint flexion on verbal instruction, without any accompanying wrist extension (ECRB motion).

By week 5–6, there is enough control to allow wrist extension from neutral and MP flexion with the hand in various positions, e.g. with the hand in the palmar or lateral position or with the hand in the dependent position. At week 7–8, light co-coordinated functional movement using the transfer is the primary aim. Full resisted activity is not recommended until week 12 post-surgery.

Specific tip

It is important to protect these transfers from overstretching in the first 4–6 months. The patient is instructed to avoid strenuous activity, heavy lifting or forces that passively extend the MP joints for at least 6 months. A protective MP blocking splint may be worn in at-risk situations, e.g. during gym weightlifting programmes for at least 6 months.

EPL TRANSFER

EPL rupture after Colles' fracture is a well-documented complication following distal radial fractures. It commonly occurs 8–10 weeks following the fracture. The rupture is the result of the EPL tendon being worn away as it rubs across the roughened fracture site at Lister's tubercle. Primary repair is not the treatment of choice, as diagnosis is often delayed; thus there is a tendon gap and the tendon ends may be in poor condition. Tendon transfer offers restoration of EPL motion[6] with good results.[7] EIP is the tendon of choice for this transfer. It is in the anatomic area, reasonably matched for length and excursion and does not produce a functional deficit. EDQ can be used as an alternative to EIP.

Surgical procedure

EIP is dissected from the hood. The tendon is withdrawn just proximal to the extensor retinaculum, and routed subcutaneously across the dorsum deep to the superficial nerve and venous plane, to the thumb. It can then be interwoven into the MP joint mechanism or attached to the distal stump of the EPL. A temporary suture is used to assess the tension. With the wrist flexed, the thumb hyperextends at the MP and trapezimetacarpal (TMC) joints. With the wrist extended, the thumb should passively flex to reach the little finger.

Postoperative therapy

Splinting

The postoperative splint is usually volar and holds the wrist in 30 degrees of extension and the thumb in extension and some abduction at the trapezial

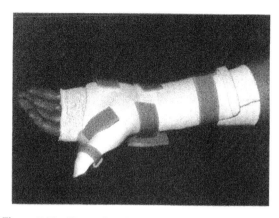

Figure 7.32 The static splint used after EI to EPL transfer. It is important to hold the thumb in maximal comfortable IP hyperextension if hyperextension is to be restored after the tendon transfer. It is our experience that the amount of hyperextension of the IP of the thumb is quite variable between individuals and should be splinted in accordance with each individual patient.

metacarpal (TMC) joint, extension at the MP joint and hyperextension at the IP joint (Fig. 7.32). The degree of IP hyperextension will depend on the patient's individual hypermobility at this joint. The splint is worn for 6 weeks and then for a further 2–3 weeks for travel and at night.

Wound care and exercise

Wound care in the form of massage and lux soaks is commenced as soon as the sutures are removed at 2 weeks.

Active thumb extension is commenced at 3–4 weeks post-surgery. Gross active thumb extension is tried first; if this cannot be achieved, index finger and thumb extension together is used. The patient quickly learns to differentiate thumb extension. This transfer is one that often requires minimal or no re-education. Perhaps this is due to the synergistic action and close proximity of EI to EPL.

Isolated extension of the IP and MP joints are commenced approximately 1 week after gross active extension. Particular attention to end-range IP hyperextension is necessary to regain this range, which is functionally very important for pinch grip activities.

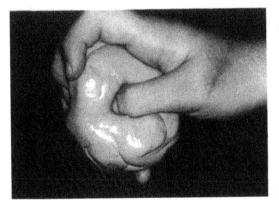
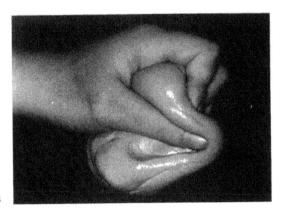

A   B

Figure 7.33 A: At 6–8 weeks resisted thumb extension exercises can be commenced. B: Very light grade putty exercises can be upgraded over the next 6 weeks.

At 6 weeks, light resisted exercise and activity (Fig. 7.33), particularly involving the pinch grip, is commenced. Full resisted activity is not recommended until 12 weeks post-surgery.

Specific tip

It is our experience that if the IP joint is not held in hyperextension, functional hyperextension used with a pinch grip may be difficult to restore.

REFERENCES

1. Warren G: Tendon transfers. In: Conolly WB (ed.), Atlas of hand surgery. New York: Churchill Livingstone, 1991:215–21.
2. Brand P, Hollister A: Clinical mechanics of the hand, 3rd edn., St Louis: Mosby, 1999:100–84.
3. Brand PW, Beach RB, Thompson DE: Relative tension and potential excursion of muscles in the forearm and hand. J Hand Surg 6A(3):209–19, 1981.
4. Zancolli E: Structural and dynamic bases of hand surgery, 2nd edn, Philadelphia: Lippincott, 1979:169–98.
5. Brand P: Tendon transfers for correction of paralysis of intrinsic muscles of the hand. In: Hunter J, Schneider L, Mackin E (eds), Tendon surgery in the hand. St Louis: Mosby, 1987:439–49.
6. Schneider L, Rosenstein R: Restoration of extensor pollicis longus function by tendon transfer. Plast Reconstr Surg 71:533–7, 1983.
7. Millender L, Nalebuff E, Albin R, Ream J, Gordon M: Dorsal tenosynovectomy and tendon transfer in the rheumatoid hand. J Bone Joint Surg 56A:601–9, 1974.

E. PAINFUL CONDITIONS – THE HAND

Victoria Frampton

INTRODUCTION

Pain is a complex perceptual experience. There is a uniform sensation threshold in all people. However, the pain perception threshold may vary'. Pain may be described as 'an unpleasant sensory and emotional experience associated with actual or potential tissue damage, or described in terms of such damage'.[1]

An understanding of the mechanisms involved in the perception of pain helps to clarify when there is actual damage or just an emotional experience. This understanding helps focus and direct our treatment methods in the rehabilitation of hand injuries.

PAIN MECHANISMS AND PAIN PATHWAYS

Classification

Pain can be divided into two types:[2]

1. First pain:
   - sharp
   - well-localised
   - carried quickly to consciousness
   - ceases as soon as the stimulus is removed (e.g. a pinprick).
2. Second pain or true pain:
   - dull
   - throbbing or aching
   - not localised
   - spreads well beyond the original site of injury.

Pain transmission

From the periphery to consciousness:

- nociceptors (pain receptors) connect with small unmyelinated, slow conducting afferent C fibres
- nociceptors connect with small myelinated, faster conducting afferent A delta (Ad) fibres
- fast 'first pain' may be carried by Ad fibres
- slow 'second pain' may be carried by C fibres, e.g. a blow to the hand results in a sharp intense, localised pain (fast first pain) immediately followed by dull, throbbing ache, not localised (slow second pain).

Detection of injury, transmission of pain and perception is more complex but provides a basis for understanding how normal afferent pathways can be modulated to relieve pain.

Gate control theory

This innovative theory[3] provides an explanation to the therapeutic value of many modalities used for pain relief:

- Slow-conducting C fibre afferents carrying painful stimuli.
- Faster-conducting Ad fibres carrying painful stimuli.

- Fast-conducting large Aβ afferent fibres carrying stimuli of light touch.
- Presynaptic inhibition. Stimulation of Aβ fibres blocks continuing transmission of C and Ad fibres, preventing the passage of the painful stimulus reaching consciousness.

Aβ fibres are susceptible to vibration, rubbing and electrical currents. They provide the pathway for pain modulation.

PAIN FOLLOWING NERVE INJURY

Physiological and pathological changes take place peripherally and centrally following nerve damage.[4] Examples of nerve injuries where pain may be present:

- neuroma – nerve division; axonotmesis, neurotmesis
- brachial plexus – avulsion injuries
- 'neuritis' – pain experienced following minor trauma, regenerating nerve or partial division
- chronic regional pain syndrome type I (CRPS).

Pathophysiological changes following nerve damage:

- Spontaneous electrical discharges at nerve endings.
- Following nerve division, the proximal nerve stump is the site for sprouting nerve fibres that form a knot or neuroma. Electrical firing spreads from the neuroma site and proximally along the length of the nerve.
- Nerve sprouts are sensitive to light mechanical stimuli. They are spontaneously active. Tapping over the neural sprouts produces a referred paraesthesiae to the part of the skin originally supplied by the nerve but which does not as yet have a pathway to that site.[5]
- C fibre increased sensitivity. Symptoms of sympathetic disturbance are generated from abnormal responses of C fibre sprouts.[6] The sympathetic system is normal, but C fibre abnormal response produces increased sympathetic activity.[7] It may be this process which forms the basis of symptoms seen in CRPS.
- An abnormal increase in firing of dorsal horn cells.[8]

• Avulsion pain experienced following deafferentation injuries, e.g. avulsion of the brachial plexus, phantom limb or digit pain following amputation and spinal cord injuries, result in characteristic-type pain. The absence of any afferent stimulation may be the cause of the abnormal increased firing of dorsal horn cells.[8] Loss of normal central inhibition results in unsuppressed firing of cells in the dorsal horn.

• Abnormal central patterns of pain established.[9] Abnormal peripheral discharges may be responsible for the concurrent changes that are occurring at spinal level and higher centres. New abnormal pain patterns become established, producing further abnormal peripheral nerve discharges. The autonomous circle of peripheral and central effects of nerve damage needs to be broken in order to relieve chronic pain following nerve injury.[10] A surprising number of patients experience pain following nerve injury. A comprehensive approach is required to treat these patients effectively.[11]

Pain in avulsion injuries has been described at length.[9,12–14]

PAIN FOLLOWING TRAUMA OR SURGERY

Pain is a common symptom following trauma. The hand therapist must recognise characteristics of painful conditions following surgery which signal potential hazards: e.g. pressure of external tight suturing, internal haematoma and inflammation indicating infection. Identification of a tight plaster following fracture of the forearm or hand is vital to avoid further complications.

Pain of this nature may be identified as 'acute pain' (Table 7.4). Clinical signs associated with this acute pain may be swelling, redness and heat.

CHARACTERISTICS OF PAIN

Pain management for the therapist falls into three categories:

• acute pain
• chronic pain
• intractable pain.

Table 7.4 Pain behaviour and characteristics

Pain	Behaviour	Characteristics
Acute	• Immediate onset • Spontaneous • Response to external stimuli and analgesia • Localised • Intermittent	• Sharp • Stabbing • Burning
Chronic	• Insiduous onset • Delayed • Constant • Variable to ADL	• Burning • Crushing • Aching
Intractable	• Paroxysms of pain • Constant • Unaffected by analgesia or external stimuli	• Electric shock • Shoots/cramp • Burning

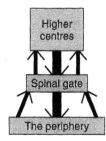

Figure 7.34 The autonomous pain pathway cycle.

It is important to recognise the different types of pain and the mechanisms which produce them in order to select and apply modalities most appropriately. Table 7.4 summarises pain behaviour and characteristics and how they might be identified. The passage of pain is a dynamic autonomous cycle (Fig. 7.34). An alteration at any part of the cycle will influence the perception of pain.

PAIN – ASSESSMENT, TREATMENT AND MANAGEMENT

Assessment

An objective and subjective assessment of pain is essential to establish the pathology of the pain, the treatment methods and to provide a baseline

Visual analog scale

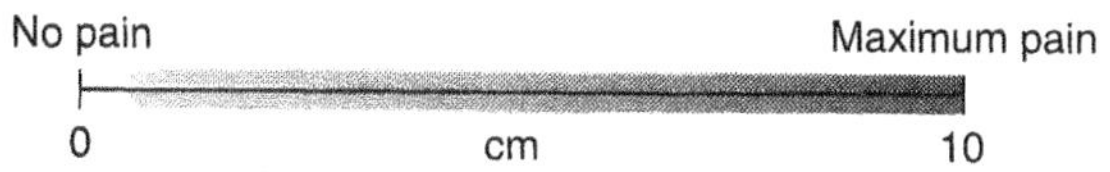

No pain   Maximum pain

0   cm   10

A

Behavioural analysis

• Nature of pain	• State – increasing
• Onset	– decreasing
• Distribution	– static
• Irritability	• Sleep disturbance
• Aggravating factors	• Medication
easing	

B

Figure 7.35 A, B: Quantitative behavioural analysis of pain.

from which to monitor success of treatment. There are many methods of pain assessment. Two practical methods for the hand therapist are:

A quantitative analysis. Using a 10 cm horizontal line, pain can be quantified between 0 and 10 on a visual analogue scale (VAS). This can be recorded before and after treatment and gives a somewhat subjective but reproducible visual record that can demonstrate improvement in the relief of pain.

Behavioural analysis of pain. A record of pain characteristics and behaviour provides a baseline of information that can be compared with subsequent measures following treatment. It is also a means by which the pathology of pain might be identified (Table 7.4). A record of pain irritability, e.g. onset of pain following 2 min active use of the hand, sets a target to improve on with treatment (Fig. 7.35).[15]

Treatment and management

The natural response to pain is one of spasm and guarding. An animal's response to pain is mirrored in the human:

- first response – often no pain at all
- second response – agitation, aggression and guarding
- third response – quiet, solitary, antisocial behaviour.

The therapist is often faced with the patient in the second or third stage. Treatment must be

Table 7.5 Pain-relieving modalities

Electrical modalities
- TENS
- Interferential
- Ultrasound
- Megapulse
- Laser
- Ice
- Biofeedback

Physical modalities
- Mobilisation 'Maitland'
- Soft tissue mobilisation
- Scar management

Re-education modalities
- Splinting (resting/dynamic)
- Desensitisation programmes
- Sensory re-education programmes
- Stress-loading programmes
- Exercise programmes

comprehensive and focus not only on the injury but also on restoring the limb to full function and as part of the normal body image.

Pain may accompany injury and disease but is not always a contraindication to mobilisation. Rehabilitation is a balance between rest to allow healing and mobilisation to restore function. For example, following laceration at the wrist, immobilisation is required following nerve repair; earlier mobilisation is required for the tendon repairs.

A wide variety of pain-relieving modalities are available to the hand therapist (Table 7.5). Successful treatment lies with a comprehensive assessment, leading to an accurate diagnosis and cause of pain. This approach focuses and directs treatment methods towards:

- a neurogenic problem – TENS/interferential
- a soft tissue or joint disorder – soft tissue techniques/ultrasound, laser, etc.
- an inflammatory problem – anti-inflammatory drugs/splinting.

Pain management should not be prescriptive or exclusive, but should be directed towards pain pathology and a comprehensive rehabilitation programme.

MANAGEMENT OF CHRONIC PAIN FOLLOWING NERVE INJURY

Peripheral nerve

Following nerve damage, the spontaneously firing, electrically active nerve may be damped down or stopped by application of vibration or electrical stimulation.[4] Transcutaneous electrical nerve stimulation (TENS) is a recognised and established form of effective pain relief.[10]

Brachial plexus avulsion injury

The deafferentation of the spinal cord and consequent unsuppressed firing of the dorsal horn cells may be altered by external stimuli. TENS applied on dermatomes supplied from roots unaffected (T2–C4) can restore an artificial input and may reduce firing in the dorsal horn cells.

Partial nerve injury

Causalgic symptoms have been well described following partial nerve injury.[7,9,11] Symptoms of hyperaesthesia or 'hyperpathia' may be seen in minor injuries such as compression injuries or following minor trauma. Symptoms of pain to light touch (hyperpathia) and sympathetic dysfunction may result from abnormal behaviour of C-fibre activity, producing symptoms of sympathetic dysfunction. These symptoms may be seen in nerve compression syndromes. The symptoms may persist after decompression, e.g. carpal tunnel or, if more widespread, may lead to CRPS. Transcutaneous electrical nerve stimulation can help to reduce symptoms of hyperaesthesia, but more often is most effectively used in combination with guanethidine blocks.

TENS is also thought to stimulate endogenous opiate peptides (morphine-like substances naturally produced within the body). This may be another mechanism by which TENS can relieve pain in nerve injury. TENS is a tool to help relieve pain, but must form part of the whole treatment programme for patients suffering from chronic pain.[10] Central changes established in chronic pain cases need prolonged stimulation and rehabilitation to reverse or modify the abnormal patterns. Programmes of normal functional activities must be used in conjunction with TENS. A summary of how TENS may work to relieve pain and reverse abnormal pain mechanisms can be seen in Table 7.6.

TENS

Machine parameters

Of the full spectrum of electrical current frequencies available for therapeutic uses, TENS uses a low-frequency current.[13] TENS machines are powered by a 1.5 V battery.

The amplitude is adjustable from 0 to 50 μA (μA into an electrode impedance of 1 kΩ).

The waveform is an asymmetrical biphasic balanced square wave with a 0 net DC component (Fig. 7.36) that prevents build-up of long-term positive–negative ion concentrations under electrodes or within the tissues.[16] The pulse width is fixed at 200 μs. Some machines provide variable pulse widths ranging from 50 to 300 μs.

The pulse frequency or rate is variable on most machines: 1–150 Hz. A variety of different pulse frequencies are available on some machines:

- continuous pulse
- burst pulse

Table 7.6 TENS – Pain relief mechanisms

Gate control	Presynaptic inhibition	Blocking transmission of C-fibre afferents
Direct inhibition	Mechanical inhibition on electrically active firing nerve	TENS proximal to firing neuroma or nerve compression subdues electrical firing
Restore artificial afferent input	Reduce unsuppressed firing of dorsal horn cells that have lost normal afferent inhibition	TENS provides alternative inhibitory stimulation
Endogenous opiate peptides	Naturally produced 'morphine-like' substances	TENS stimulates endorphins and may lead to pain relief

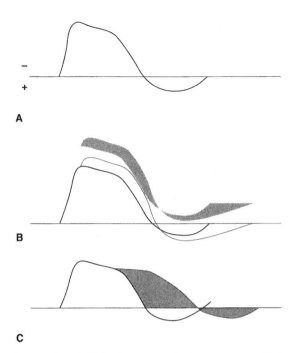

Figure 7.36 A: Biphasic asymmetrical square wave with 0 net DC components. B: Balanced net DC component on increased amplitude. C: Increase in pulse width equals increase in energy.

- frequency modulated pulse: constant stimulus with variable frequency.[13]

Variable frequency and burst-type stimulation machines are advocated in some cases of chronic pain. Benefits of TENS may fall with time.[17]

Adaption of the nervous system to regular repetitive stimuli may account for this.[18,19]

Electrodes and lead wires. Electrical stimulus is delivered via electrical cables through malleable conductive electrodes placed on the skin through into the underlying tissues. Variable-sized electrodes are available.

Electrode placement. The principles of electrode placement are founded on an understanding of the pain mechanisms involved with a particular condition (Table 7.7).

TENS APPLICATION IN NERVE INJURY

For a stimulus to be effective it must reach a certain intensity at a certain minimum speed and be

Table 7.7 Electrodes placement

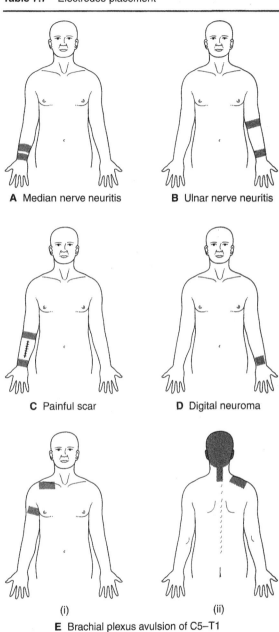

A Median nerve neuritis   **B** Ulnar nerve neuritis

C Painful scar   **D** Digital neuroma

(i)   (ii)
E Brachial plexus avulsion of C5–T1

of a certain duration. The relationship of amplitude and pulse width determines the adequate stimulus. Short pulse widths require high amplitudes to produce adequate stimuli; wider pulse widths require lower amplitudes to produce adequate stimuli. Aβ afferent nerve fibres are recruited by impulses of low amplitude, high frequency and short duration. Ad afferent nerve fibres can be recruited by impulses of higher amplitude, lower frequencies and longer pulse widths.

Research has shown prescriptive parameters cannot be given, as results of different trials are not consistent.[20,21] Patients should be encouraged to try a variety of different frequencies and mode stimulation to find their optimum parameters for pain relief.[13,22] A guideline is given as a direction below.

Neuritis, neuroma and nerve compression

Median nerve irritation following carpal tunnel decompression

Symptoms of hyperaesthesia and painful responses to light touch can be exacerbated following carpal tunnel decompression of the median nerve.

Electrode placement. Small pads (4 cm × 4 cm) in parallel on the anterior aspect of the forearm over the median nerve course 2 cm apart distal pad as close to the painful hyperaesthetic area, but *not* on the hyperaesthetic skin. Low pulse width and a frequency of around 50 Hz is an indication to start stimulation.

Digital and nerve neuroma

Following damage or division of a digital nerve, painful neuromas can result in painful hyperaesthesia and can seriously limit rehabilitation of associated injuries to the finger.

Electrode placement. One small pad (4 cm × 4 cm) over the anterior aspect just proximal to the distal wrist crease anterior surface of the wrist (for median nerve supplied digital nerve). Distal pad small butterfly or cut-down small pad wrapped around the lateral border of the finger just proximal to the hyperaesthetic area on the finger. Machine stimulation similar to median nerve compression above.

Ulnar nerve neuritis

Compression of the ulnar nerve at the elbow can give rise to widespread pain and painful

hyperaesthesia with painful symptoms throughout the medial aspect of the forearm and hand.

Electrode placement. Large pads (4 cm × 8 cm) placed horizontally. Proximal pad – proximal to the ulnar nerve above the elbow. Distal pad – horizontally in parallel pad just above the wrist crease of the medial aspect of the forearm. Electrode parameters similar to the above two examples.

Painful scar

Electrode placement. Small or large, depending on the size of scar; above and below the scar, not touching the hyperaesthetic or painful area and parameters, as above.

Avulsion pain

Brachial plexus avulsion injuries

In these injuries there is no longer any viable pathway to conduct from the anaesthetic limb into the spinal cord. It is important to use pathways to the spinal cord that remain intact and are adjacent or close to those roots that have been avulsed. For example, in a total brachial plexus avulsion injury of C5–T1 the dermatomes of T2 and C4 must be used. Careful assessment of skin sensation is essential prior to applying electrodes.

Electrode placement. Large pads (4 cm × 8 cm): the proximal pad superior to the clavicle or over upper fibres of trapezius as close to the anaesthetic skin as possible. Alternatively, over the cervical spine. Distal pad – on the medial side of the arm distal to the axilla. A variety of different positions can be tried, depending on the roots that have been avulsed.[13]

Electrical stimulation. Wide pulse width and high frequency (80 Hz). (This is a starting point and emphasis needs to be made on the importance of trying alternative parameters.) The wide pulse width and high-intensity current is only possible due to denervation. Muscle contraction would be stimulated in a normally innervated arm with these parameters.

Systematic application of electrodes over successive sessions will lead to a more successful outcome.[23] Patients turn to such frequencies and patterns of stimulation for reasons of comfort that may be unconnected with specific pain control mechanisms.[10,22] Patients should try a variety of different frequencies and modes of stimulation to find those that are most appropriate for the relief of their pain. If TENS is successful initially, but falls in time, then burst-mode alternative pulse frequencies may overcome this adaption and accommodation of the nervous system.

Duration of treatment

For chronic pain patients, particularly in deafferentated cases, prolonged stimulation is required consistently to produce an effect: the recommended 8 hours a day is a good starting point.

Important points to consider

- The choice of electrode placement should compliment functional use of the limb. When applying TENS, the first choice should be to allow freedom of the hand for functional use; however, if relief is not imminent, then a more distal position on to a finger may be indicated.
- Careful monitoring is essential for successful results of TENS. A regular record of electrode placement, pain VAS, pain behaviour, electrode parameters and duration of treatment should take place on each application.[13]
- Systematic and sequential placement of electrodes and electrical parameters is essential for good results. Do not change more than one variable in each treatment: e.g. do not alter placement and electrical parameter on the same visit.
- Accurate assessment of the patient and appropriate selection of suitable candidates for TENS.
- Pain may only be reduced at first and not obliterated.
- The patient's expectations must be rationalised prior to treatment.
- The objectives must be clearly set prior to treatment.

- It is essential to motivate the chronic pain patient and incorporate TENS pain relief with a full rehabilitation programme.

Sources of poor results

Patient. Inappropriate patient selection.
Technique

- Poor electrode placement
- Inadequate securing of electrodes to the body
- Insufficient treatment time
- Random change of placement and parameters

TENS equipment

- Flat batteries or poor connection
- If carbon electrodes – worn pads
- Overuse of disposable electrodes
- Flimsy cables associated with some cheap machines
- Alternative parameters not explored.

Review. Poor monitoring and documentation available for comparative evaluation.

CHRONIC REGIONAL PAIN SYNDROME TYPE I (REFLEX SYMPATHETIC DYSTROPHY)

The pathophysiology associated with chronic regional pain syndrome (CRPS) is similar to isolated nerve irritation, but more widespread. For this reason and for its complexity it deserves separate attention. CRPS can spontaneously occur following minor trauma, following minor surgery such as carpal tunnel decompression, and following fractures, such as Colles' fractures. Without intervention, CRPS progresses from the acute stage of the red-hot swollen hand to one of a shiny, atrophic, osteoporotic hand with complete dysfunction and alienation of the hand from the body. Lee-Langford[24] classified CRPS into different clinical types:

Minor causalgia. Damage to minor peripheral nerve. Symptoms affecting small part of hand.

Minor trauma. No specific nerve injury, but spontaneous symptoms following minor injury, e.g. crushed finger, fracture dislocation or sprain or penetrating wound.

Shoulder hand syndrome. CRPS-like symptoms in the hand following a stiff and painful shoulder. Spontaneous or insidious onset or following trauma.

Major traumatic dystrophy. Symptoms produced following major trauma, such as a crushed hand or Colles' fracture.

Major causalgia. Symptoms produced from partial nerve injury of a major nerve. The symptoms of causalgia from partial nerve injury of major nerves are well-recognised and can be related to those with minor causalgia.

Predisposing factors

- Poor or disturbed circulation, e.g. Raynaud's disease.
- Hot/cold clammy hands preoperatively can predispose to postoperative problems following minor surgery.

Management, early diagnosis and early intervention

Researchers and writers vary on their approach to management of CRPS. Some researchers advocate early intervention with active mobilisation, whereas others prefer pain control and not aggressive mobilisation in the first stage. As CRPS can present in the different clinical classifications, recipe book remedies for successful treatment should be flexible, problem-orientated and reflect the severity of the case. In some cases, early mobilisation may be indicated and each case should be taken individually. The priorities must be to prevent alienation of the hand at an early stage and to maintain the hand as part of the full body image.

Stages of CRPS

Stage 1

- Burning pain of 3 months' duration
- Hand is soft, swollen, hot and often sweaty
- Pain is intense and increasing
- Hyperpathia (abnormal, painful response to light touch)
- Osteoporosis not present before 3 weeks, but may be evident after the fifth week.[5]

Stage 2

- Pain increasing
- Change in swelling from soft to hard
- Redness and heat reduced
- Less sweating
- Demineralisation may increase, continuing for the next 9 months.

Stage 3

- Constant pain reduced; pain on movement
- Shiny, wasted fingers with pencil pointing of the fingertips
- Atrophic, shiny appearance and osteoporosis are the focus of symptoms and signs at this stage
- Complete dysfunction and alienation of the hand.

Treatment of CRPS

Medical management must be accompanied by active therapy.

Early stage management

- Guanethidine blocks, where abnormal sympathetic symptoms predominate, are the first line of treatment.[11] Blocks should be initiated as soon as CRPS is suspected. Passively moving the affected part during the procedure is encouraged. Blocks are most successful when followed immediately by therapy. It is important to coordinate therapy services with the application of guanethidine blocks. Normal patterns of movement must be established as soon as pain is relieved. The patient must observe and fully participate in these movements.
- Blocks may be repeated, given every 2 days if necessary. Three blocks in 1 week is usually adequate, but more may be necessary.
- Evaluation is essential to record the response and encourage progression of active movement and function.
- Sympathectomy may be indicated if relief from repeated blocks is unsustained.
- Carbamazepine and other antispasmodic drugs may be useful in symptoms of shooting or spasmodic pain.

- Therapy management must be coordinated between pain relief and mobilisation. Attention must be made to avoid any unnecessary increased vascularity with active movement that may add to a highly vascular hand, particularly in the first stage.
  - Aggressive, effective, consistent elevation.
  - Electrical modalities, diapulse, interferential and TENS.
  - Vibration.
  - TENS is the treatment of choice, as it allows functional use of the arm and delivers the pre-scribed prolonged input that is required in this chronic pain condition.

Successful treatment will depend on realistic goals and management of pain in the context of a complete rehabilitation programme. Close monitoring is essential. The use of TENS is very valuable.

Electrode placement. Electrodes must be placed close to the painful area, but not touching, if hyperaesthesia is a major symptom. If pain is on one aspect of the hand, the pad should be placed in parallel over that aspect. If pain is glove-like, then pads placed circumferentially around the forearm proximal to the pain is the placement of choice (large pads).

Exercise. An exercise programme should be selected so that it is effective and simple. Five simple exercises that mobilise joints and elasticity of soft tissue are preferable to 20 more elaborate exercises. Bilateral activities should be encouraged and a few effective exercises should be taught.[25,26]

Continuous passive motion. Continuous pas-sive motion has proved very effective.[27] This may be applied at any stage and may be worn contin-uously or as the pain permits.

Splinting. The use of splints in the early stages is controversial: it requires careful supervision and application. Flexion gloves are a useful adjunct to treatment, but application should be for short, closely supervised periods and should not increase pain. Corrective splints are useful in the late stages of the condition. In the early stage, resting splints may encourage disuse and alienation.

Middle stage management

At this stage, all treatment techniques apply as for early stage. However, splinting may be more useful at this stage, particularly if contractures are present. There is still a need to ensure that the splint does not act as a reminder of the loss of function of the hand or cause an increase in pain.

Late stage management

There is often little to offer the patient at this stage. However, there are occasions when intrepid surgeons are prepared to operate on these hands. In most therapists' experience, surgery often exacerbates CRPS problems. However, in the very chronic late stage, capsulotomies of meta-carpophalangeal joints can be considered with close monitoring, and early mobilisation can be successful in some cases.

CONCLUSIONS

The therapist forms the focus of coordinated care for the nerve-injured patient. Continuity and trust is essential for a long-term good prognosis for these chronically disabled patients. Successful treatment relies upon accurate diagnosis, realistic and attainable goals and a full partnership with the patient and their carers.

REFERENCES

1. Merskey H: Pain terms: A list with definitions and notes on usage. (Recommended by the International Association for the Study of Pain chaired by Merskey.) Pain 6:249–52.
2. Bowsher D: Acute and chronic pain and assessment. In: Wells P, Frampton V, Bowsher D (eds), Pain management in physiotherapy, 2nd edn. London: Butterworth Heinemann, 1993:11–17.
3. Melzack R, Wall PD: Pain mechanism: a new theory. Science: 150:971–8, 1965.
4. Wall PD, Gutnik M: Properties of afferent nerve impulses originating from a neuroma. Nature 248:740, 1974.
5. (a) Tinel J: Le signe due "fourmillement" dans les lesion des nerss peripherique. Press Med 47:388, 1915.
   (b) Moldaver J: Tinel's sign. Its characteristics and significance. J Bone Joint Surg 60a:412, 1978.

6. Loh L, Nathan PW: Painful peripheral states and sympathetic blocks. J Neurol Neurosurg Psych 41:664–71, 1978.

7. Wallin G, Torebjork E, Hallin R: Preliminary observations on the pathophysiology of hyperalgesia in the causalgic pain syndrome. In: Zotterman Y (ed.), Sensory function of the skin in primates. Oxford: Pergamon Press, 1976:489–502.

8. Loeser JD, Ward AA: Some effects of deafferentation on neurons of the cat spinal cord. Arch Neurol 17:629–36, 1967.

9. Wyn Parry CB: Pain in rehabilitation of the hand. London: Butterworths, 1981:126–46.

10. Frampton V: Transcutaneous electrical nerve stimulation and chronic pain. In: Wells P, Frampton V, Bowsher D (eds), Pain management in physiotherapy, 2nd edn. 1994:89–91.

11. (a) Withrington RH, Wyn Parry CB: The management of painful peripheral nerve disorders. J Hand Surg 9B(1):24–8, 1984.
(b) Wyn Parry CB, Withrington RH: The management of painful peripheral nerve disorders. In: Wall PD, Melzack R, eds, Textbook of pain, 1st edn. Edinburgh: Churchill Livingstone, 1984:395–441.

12. Frampton V: Therapist's management of brachial plexus injuries. In: Hunter J, Schneider L, Mackin E, Callahan A (eds), Rehabilitation of the hand: surgery and therapy. St Louis: Mosby, 1990:630–9.

13. Frampton V: Transcutaneous electrical nerve stimulation (TENS). In: Kitchen S, Bazin S (eds), Clayton's electrotherapy, 10th edn. 1994:287–305.

14. Frampton V: Brachial plexus lesions. In: Salter M, Cheshire L (eds), Hand therapy principles and practice. Oxford: Butterworth-Heinemann, 2000:181–95.

15. Bond MR, Pilowsky I: Subjective assessment of pain and its relationship to the administration of analgesics in patients with advanced cancer. J Psychosomat Res 10:203, 1966.

16. Mannheimer JS, Lampe GN: Clinical transcutaneous electrical nerve stimulation. Philadelphia: Davis, 1984.

17. Loeser JD, Black RG, Chirstman A: Relief of pain by transcutaneous stimulation. J Neurosurg 42:308–34, 1975.

18. Thompson JW: The role of transcutaneous electrical nerve stimulation (TENS) for the control of pain. In: Doyle D (ed.), International symposium on pain control 1986. London: Royal Society of Medical Services, 1987:27–47.

19. Pomeranz B, Niznick G: Codetron, a new electrotherapy device overcomes the habituation problems of conventional TENS devices. Am J Electromed First Quarter: 22–6, 1987.

20. Tulgar M, McGlore F, Bowsher Z, Milos JB: Comparative effectiveness of different stimulation modes in relieving pain, Part 2, A double blind controlled long term clinical trial. Pain 47:157–62, 1991.

21. Johnson MI, Ashton CH, Thompson JW: The consistency of pulse frequency and pulse patterns of transcutaneous electrical nerve stimulation (TENS) used by chronic pain patients. Pain 44:231–4, 1991.

22. Johnson MI, Ashton CH, Thompson JW: An in-depth study of long-term users of transcutaneous electrical nerve stimulation (TENS). Implications for clinical use of TENS. Pain 44:221–9, 1991.

23. Woolf SL, Gersh HR, Rao VR: Examination of electrode placements and stimulating parameters in treating chronic pain with conventional transcutaneous electrical nerve stimulation (TENS). Pain 11:37–47, 1981.

24. Lee-Langford L: Reflex sympathetic dystrophy. In: Hunter J, Schneider L, Mackin E, Callahan A (eds), Rehabilitation of the hand, 3rd edn. St Louis: Mosby, 1990:763–86.

25. Webbe MA, Hunter JM: Flexor tendon gliding in the hand, Part II, Differential gliding. J Hand Surg 10A: 575, 1995.

26. Van Strien G: Post-operative management of flexor tendon injuries. In: Hunter J, Schneider L, Mackin E, Callahan A (eds), Rehabilitation of the hand, 3rd edn. St Louis: Mosby, 1990:401.

27. Woods Z, Withrington RH: Continuous passive motion as a treatment modality in reflex sympathetic dystrophy. Proceedings from the British Society for Surgery of the Hand, Autumn meeting, 1992.

F. OTHER NEUROLOGICAL CONDITIONS: CEREBRAL PALSY

Claudia R Gschwind and Lisa Newell

DEFINITION AND PATHOLOGY

Cerebral palsy is not a specific disease of the brain but a congenital disorder caused by pre-, peri- or postnatal insults affecting various parts of the central nervous system, resulting in motor disorder, cognitive, sensory and developmental dysfunction and/or convulsive disorders. Clinically, cerebral palsy may present with severe intellectual impairment with motor dysfunction, speech disorder, deafness and blindness, or in less severe cases with normal intelligence and only minimal spasticity in one limb. It is of clinical importance for the hand surgeon to distinguish between predominantly pyramidal spastic disorders and extrapyramidal dystonic manifestations. The latter motion disorders are characterised by variable and unpredictable change of tone. Often, we find a mixed pattern of motor disorder. Emotional stress and positioning of the limb can increase tone; stretch reflexes are present, sometimes even clonus. During sleep the affected muscles (with no myostatic contracture) are completely relaxed.

GENERAL CONSIDERATIONS

About 20% of patients with cerebral palsy and upper limb involvement will benefit from upper limb surgery. The surgical goal is dependent on the severity of the disorder. In severe cases it can simply be to facilitate patient care and hygiene. In mild cases hand function is helped by releases of joint contractures, weakening of spastic muscle groups by tenotomy or muscle slides or augmenting weak muscle groups by tendon transfers. Joint fusions may be considered.[1,2]

Children with cerebral palsy are managed by a team of physicians and therapists. They manage the overall care of the patient and, if appropriate, refer to the hand surgeon when life-threatening (e.g. convulsive) or more pressing medical problems (spinal problems, renal problems) are stabilised. The ideal age for surgery in these children is between 4 and 7 years of age, before spastic muscles have undergone myostatic changes and involved joints have become stiff.

The most common pattern of presentation in upper limb spasticity is that of internal rotation and adduction of the shoulder, flexion contracture of the elbow, pronation deformity of the forearm, wrist and finger flexion with thumb flexion and adduction (Fig. 7.37). It is important to assess these children on several occasions, together with their therapists and parents, to learn how they use the affected arm. Some children may simply neglect the limb, whereas others may use it as an assist arm when stabilising objects. Some children have simple function with grasp and release under poor control. In milder cases, independent grasp and release are present and under good volitional control. Repeated examinations allow recognition and documentation of joint deformities, range of motion, hand sensibility, functional level, cooperation and the general neurological condition.[3]

PREOPERATIVE THERAPY

Patients with cerebral palsy normally have regular sessions with neurotherapists, who work on improving posture and tone to reduce the effects of spasticity. They also perform passive and active range of motion (ROM) exercises, and joint and soft tissue stretches and work on maximising function in activities of daily living (ADL). Rigid lightweight plastic splints can help stabilise joints and maintain position. Serial plasters can be useful to overcome soft tissue and joint contractures. Recurrence of deformity is, however, common when splinting is ceased. Splints can be used in preoperative assessment: e.g. the ability to extend the fingers with the wrist in extension can be observed. Soft fabric splints allow more mobility but provide less stability. Elastic enveloping stockings have recently been introduced by some therapists to modify muscle stretch reflexes and to control muscle firing patterns by even, circumferential pressure. These stockings have to be worn for a prolonged period of time and they interfere with sensory feedback. All splints are cumbersome and are unpopular with the patients in hot weather.

SURGICAL INDICATIONS

Shoulder and forearm

Shoulder joint releases are only indicated in severe adduction and internal flexion contractures when normal hygienic requirements and functional hand placement are made difficult. Elbow contractures of more than 70 degrees will also impede useful positioning of the hand in space and should, therefore, be released.

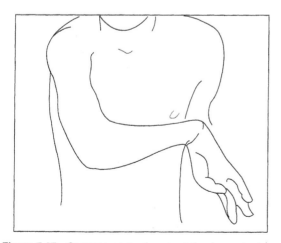

Figure 7.37 Common postural presentation in cerebral palsy.

Pronation deformities of the forearm are treated according to their main deforming force.[4] If active supination beyond neutral is present, no specific procedure is indicated.

If active supination is possible but does not go beyond neutral, a pronator quadratus release is performed. At the same time, most patients require a flexor aponeurotic release for wrist deformity. This latter procedure also decreases pronatory forces and facilitates supination.

If there is no active supination, and passive supination of the forearm is easy, an active transfer, i.e. pronator teres rerouting procedure, is indicated. If there is no active supination and passive rotation is tight, a release of pronator quadratus and the flexor pronator mass (or flexor aponeurotic release), including pronator teres, is performed. These releases may unmask weak but active supination.

Wrist and hand

The wrist flexion deformities are assessed in a similar fashion.[2] If finger extension is possible with the wrist in neutral or slight flexion (to 20 degrees), a flexor aponeurotic release can be considered. This release may improve wrist extension with combined extension of the fingers to initiate grasping. If the wrist is held in marked ulnar deviation and in some flexion, a flexor carpi ulnaris (FCU) tenotomy is advisable. If extension is beyond neutral but in marked ulnar deviation, an extensor carpi ulnaris (ECU) to extensor carpi radialis brevis (ECRB) transfer may be preferable in order to rebalance wrist extension. If the fingers can only be extended when the wrist is flexed beyond 20 degrees, a release of the flexor pronator side, i.e. a flexor aponeurotic release, is indicated. If, however, the child has no active wrist extension, an active transfer is needed. An FCU transfer to ECRB will provide wrist extension. This transfer for wrist extension should, however, only be considered in the presence of active wrist flexion, i.e. an active flexor carpi radialis (FCR), and must be combined with release of the finger flexors. Otherwise, a wrist extension deformity and further finger flexion will occur.

In very severe flexion deformities, only an aggressive release of the flexor pronator musculature and a transfer for wrist extension can overcome the deformity. In some cases, lengthening of the flexor pronator mass alone is not enough, and the skeleton has to be shortened by a proximal row carpectomy. An alternative in severe cases is wrist fusion with a flexor pronator slide; however, this is irreversible and the tenodesis effect of wrist extension is lost. Thumb adduction and flexion contractures should also be assessed to find where the main deforming force lies.[5] If it is an intrinsic adduction flexion caused by spasticity in the thumb adductor, the first dorsal interosseous and the flexor pollicis brevis (FPB) muscles should be released. In this group of intrinsic spasticity of the thumb, the interphalangeal (IP) joint is extended.

If the main deforming force is extrinsic, i.e. spasticity of the flexor pollicis longus (FPL), the metacarpophalangeal (MP) joint and IP joint are flexed, and FPL should be released. The third group of patients show combined extrinsic and intrinsic spasticity, and the abductor pollicis longus (APL), extensor pollicis brevis (EPB) and extensor pollicis longus (EPL) tendon may be weak or stretched out. Abduction can be improved by tendon transfers. Brachioradialis, flexor digitorum superficialis (FDS), FCR, FCU or extensor carpi radialis longus (ECRL) can be used to augment EPL, abductor pollicis brevis (APB) or APL function. In some cases, with good EPL function, an EPL to EPB transfer is sufficient.

It is important to also address joint instabilities, e.g. hyperextension instability of the MP joint. This is achieved by sesamoid arthrodesis or, in severe cases, by MP joint fusion.[6] Failure to recognise hyperextension instability of the MP joint may lead to recurring adduction deformity.

If MP adduction deformity cannot be controlled by tendon transfers, a carpometacarpal (CMC) joint fusion is indicated.

Swan-neck deformities of the fingers may be due to extrinsic tightness. After correction of wrist flexion deformity, this tightness may be corrected because extensor activity is rebalanced. If surgery of the wrist does not improve the swan-neck deformity, lengthening of the extrinsic extensors

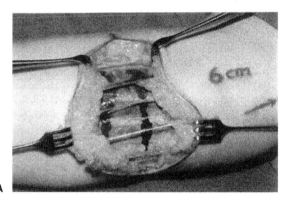
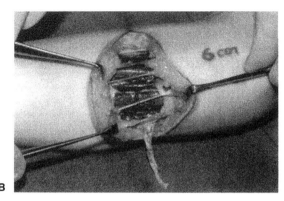

Figure 7.38 A, B: Flexor aponeurotic release. A fascial strip and the septa are divided.

over the proximal phalanx, or translocation of the radial lateral band, may be necessary.

SURGICAL PROCEDURES

Elbow release

Release of flexion contracture of the elbow is performed through a lazy Z incision on the anterior aspect of the elbow. Z lengthening of the biceps tendon is usually not sufficient to correct the deformity. Incision of the brachialis aponeurosis and, occasionally, release of the anterior capsule is necessary. If this still does not provide sufficient release, the brachioradialis muscle is released from the supracondylar ridge.

Flexor aponeurotic release

Through a transverse incision 6 cm distal to the medial epicondyle, a 2-cm strip of the flexor pronator aponeurosis is excised, and the underlying septa divided. In children who have no myostatic contracture, this is sufficient to lengthen the flexor pronator musculature (Fig. 7.38).

Flexor pronator slide

This procedure is performed if several centimetres of lengthening is necessary or, in adults with spasticity, detachment of the whole flexor pronator mass from the medial epicondyle is performed.

Pronator quadratus release

Through a longitudinal incision over the radial distal forearm, the pronator quadratus is detached from its radial insertion. It then retracts back to the interosseous membrane.

PRONATOR TERES REROUTING

Through a longitudinal incision in the volar upper forearm, the tendon of pronator teres is lengthened with a step cut. The portion inserting into the radius is rerouted around the bone and the tendon is then repaired. Contraction of pronator teres then produces supination (Fig. 7.39).

FCU transfer

FCU is divided just proximal to the pisiform bone as in a simple FCU tenotomy. It is then rerouted around the ulnar border of the forearm and woven into the ECRB tendon. This transfer also produces some degree of forearm supination due to the course of the tendon transfer. It is vital to assess FCR activity before proceeding to this transfer.

Flexor pollicis longus tenotomy

This is an intramusculature tenotomy that allows the divided FPL tendon to slide 1–2 cm distally, while still being attached to muscle fibres.

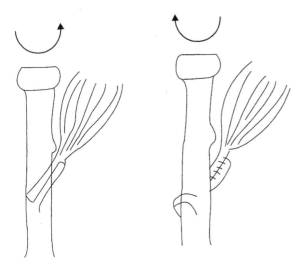

Figure 7.39 Pronator teres is rerouted and becomes a supinator. (Redrawn with permission from Gschwind and Tonkin.[4])

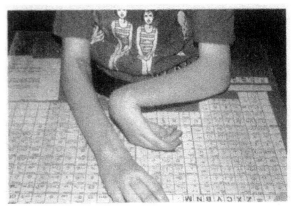

Figure 7.40 Patient with severe bilateral pronation/flexion contracture after proximal row carpectomy, flexor aponeurotic release, FCU and ECRB transfer on her right side.

Thumb surgery

Surgical procedures for the spastic thumb are normally performed through a longitudinal incision on the dorsum of the thumb extending to, and over, the first dorsal compartment. Adductor release from the third metacarpal is performed through palmar incision following the thenar crease. The position of the thumb is assessed intra-operatively, and if tendon augmentation is needed the best line of pull for metacarpal abduction is identified. An active transfer is then used to maintain abduction (i.e. brachioradialis to APL, FCU to APL). Surgery of the MP joint can also be performed through the same longitudinal incision in the thumb. After removal of the superficial cartilage, the radial sesamoid is fixed into a small prepared recess in the metacarpal neck and held with non-absorbable transosseous sutures. This capsulodesis is tightened at about 10–20 degrees of flexion, thereby preventing hyperextension at this joint. A temporary K-wire holds the joint in about 30 degrees of flexion for 6 weeks.

Lateral band transfer

Through a mid-lateral radial incision of the digits the lateral band is transposed to the palmar aspect of the proximal interphalangeal (PIP) joint. The band is held behind a sling formed by the radial slip of FDS and the volar plate. Tension can be adjusted to extend the distal interphalangeal (DIP) joint. Care must be taken not to tighten the translocation too much or a PIP flexion contracture may ensue.

POSTOPERATIVE MANAGEMENT

Procedures for elbow contracture normally precede surgery for wrist and finger deformities. Plaster immobilisation in 10–20 degrees of elbow flexion is maintained for 5 weeks.[7]

Surgery for pronation deformity and wrist and finger contractures are usually combined. The arm is immobilised with the elbow in 60 degrees of flexion, the forearm is supinated and the wrist in 40–50 degrees of extension. The MP joints are kept in about 30 degrees of flexion, with the IP joints extended. After 5 weeks, the plaster is removed and specific exercises with a hand therapist are commenced. These exercises are aimed at restoring active motion with an emphasis on function, beginning with active assisted exercises and progressing to gentle resistance, depending on the ability of the patient. In between sessions with the therapist, the parents or carers are instructed to do a simple exercise programme (e.g. fist formation, grasp and release, forearm supination). A thermoplastic splint is usually worn at night, and intermittently during the day, for 2 months. Exercise programmes consist of 4–6 sessions per day. It is important to maintain active pronation and wrist and finger flexion.

Surgery for the thumb is best performed after correction of wrist deformity. It is also easier to hold the thumb alone in the correct position. After 5 weeks (6 weeks when K-wire fixation for sesamoid arthrodesis or joint fusion was necessary) the exercise programme, with 4–6 sessions per day, is begun. The exercises are designed to facilitate grasp and release with the thumb out of the palm. A thermoplastic splint at night and intermittently during the day is used to maintain position.

Three months postoperatively it is decided if further splinting is necessary (Fig. 7.40). Most children have learned to perform some playful tasks, which encourages use of the hand and arm in the desired fashion.

REFERENCES

1. Zancolli EA, Goldner LJ, Swanson AB: Surgery of the spastic hand in cerebral palsy: Report of the Committee on Spastic Hand Evaluation. J Hand Surg 8:766–72, 1983.
2. Zancolli EA, Zancoilli E: Surgical rehabilitation of the spastic upper limb in cerebral palsy. In: Lamb DW (ed.), the paralysed hand. Edinburgh: Churchill Livingstone, 1987:153–68.
3. Koman LA, Gelberman RH, Toby ED, Poehling GG: Cerebral palsy: management of the upper extremity. Clin Orthop 253:62–74, 1990.
4. Gschwind C, Tonkin M: Surgery for cerebral palsy. Part 1. Classification and operative procedures for pronation deformity. J Hand Surg 391–5, 1992.
5. Manske PR: Redirection of extensor pollicis longus in the treatment of spastic thumb-in-palm deformity. J Hand Surg 10A:553–60, 1985.
6. Tonkin MA, Beard AJ, Kemp SJ, Eakins DF: Sesamoid arthrodesis for hyperextension of the thumb metacarpophalangeal joint. J Hand Surg 20A:334–8, 1995.
7. Tonkin MA: The upper limb in cerebral palsy. Mini-symposium: cerebral palsy. Curr Orthopaed 9:149–55, 1995.

G.   OTHER NEUROLOGICAL CONDITIONS: HAND SPASTICITY – CONSERVATIVE MANAGEMENT

Judith Wilton

Hand dysfunction across the broad range of diagnoses from cerebral palsy, stroke, post-traumatic head injuries and dementia is generally a consequence of altered motor function. Factors which contribute to deformity, contracture and dysfunction are:

- altered levels of consciousness
- decreased sensibility and awareness of the affected limb
- spasticity or paralysis, leading to abnormal posture and resting positions of the limbs
- lack of purposeful intent to move and use the limb.

In planning therapeutic intervention, it must be remembered that the hand cannot be considered in isolation from the rest of the body, and that these clients are faced with significant challenges in movement for the rest of their lives. Methods to treat the deformity, with indications and contraindications for splinting and casting in long-term management of dysfunction, are considered in this section of the chapter.

HAND DEFORMITY

Identification of the altered muscle function and its associated contribution to deformity are determined during active opening and closing of the hand. Key issues are:

- spasticity or paralysis of wrist muscles
- the impact of wrist position on the length, and active motion of, extrinsic finger muscles

- the presence of spasticity in the intrinsic muscles and influence on position of the metacarpophalangeal (MCP) and proximal interphalangeal (PIP) joints of the fingers
- contracture of the thumb web space combined with spasticity in adductor pollicis and/or flexor pollicis brevis muscles.

An extensive description of deformities found in the hand of clients with neurological dysfunction along with recommended splinting intervention may be found in Wilton.[1]

INTERVENTION

Empirical research into therapeutic techniques has focused on the contribution of splinting and casting in remediation of hand dysfunction. Whereas direct comparisons cannot be made due to the differences in research design, sample diagnoses and intervention procedures investigated, the trends do support the continued use of casting and splinting modalities. Review articles by Neuhaus et al[2] and Reid[3] focus on the different practices and published studies. However, the bottom line for every therapist working with clients with hand dysfunction secondary to neurological conditions is achievement of the client's objectives rather than a prescription of therapy based upon published studies and statistics.

INDICATIONS AND RECOMMENDATIONS FOR SPLINTING AND CASTING OF THE HAND

Modification of spasticity

The exact neurophysiological effects of splinting and casting on spasticity are undefined. It is proposed that inhibition results from altered sensory input from cutaneous and muscle receptors during the period of splint or cast application. Immobilisation, applying gentle continuous stretching of the spastic muscle at submaximal passive range of motion (ROM), is seen to reduce spasticity by altering the threshold response to stretch of the muscle spindle and Golgi tendon organs in the antagonist and agonist muscles. The effects of neutral warmth and circumferential contact are also thought to contribute to modification of spasticity seen following casting.

Splints designed to address spasticity are worn when spasticity is most severe (Fig. 7.41). There are no gains to be made by wearing splints at night if there is minimal evidence of spasticity during sleep.

Prevention or modification of contracture

The biomechanical effects of splinting and casting relate to changes in the length and extensibility of muscle and connective tissue.

Application of low-load prolonged stress to the contracted tissues at the end of their available range allows histological changes to occur in the tissues in response to the position imposed. Where daily passive range of movement, posturing or splints do not adequately maintain range, casting may be indicated (Fig. 7.42).

Tardieu and Tardieu[4] suggest the increase in passive ROM seen on removal of casts in hemiplegic and cerebral palsy clients results from the lengthening of connective tissue elements along with addition of sarcomeres to the muscle fibre.[5,6] Loss of ROM seen after not wearing a cast or splint is due to reaccommodating of the muscle to the shorter length by the loss of sarcomeres. Therefore, the requirement is to increase and then *maintain* the ROM.

Aggravation in muscle contracture in cerebral palsy clients also results from lack of muscle adaptation as the bone becomes longer. Tardieu and Tardieu[4] suggest conservative intervention has no effect in this instance, with surgery necessary to modify the passive ROM.

Improvement in function of the limb

Reduction of spasticity and/or contracture, and modification of deformity to facilitate biomechanically efficient patterns of motor action, offer the potential to improve voluntary function. The essential prerequisite is that the client must demonstrate purposeful intent to use the hand.

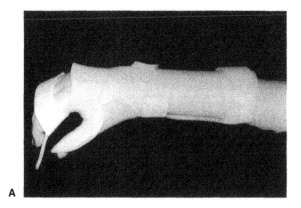

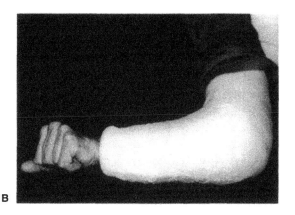

Figure 7.41   A, B: Spasticity reduction splint.

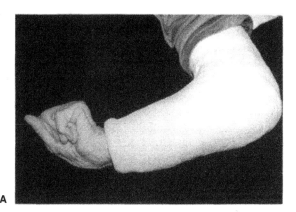

Figure 7.42   A, B: Elbow cast.

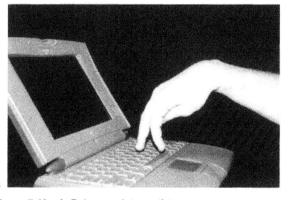

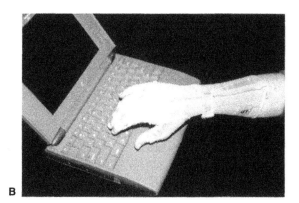

Figure 7.43   A, B: Lycra wrist gauntlet.

Appropriate positioning and control of the wrist and the thumb are the keys to function of the hand.

Where a variety of postures are required in task performance, rigid immobilisation is not conducive to function. Correction of the wrist deformity should not compromise finger extension sufficient for reach to grasp an object. Custom-made dynamic lycra wrist splints (Fig. 7.43) provide exciting new developments in facilitating functional performance. Thumb abduction is best achieved by more rigid thermoplastic splinting.

Long-term management

Post-discharge from rehabilitation facilities, it is not uncommon to see regression in patients with spasticity. Benefits gained from rigorous therapy programmes may have a longer duration if appropriate positioning is provided through bivalved casts or splints worn for specified periods during the day.

Spasticity and contracture that leads to the hand being tightly fisted can result in maceration of the skin, injury from the finger nails digging into the palm of the hand, and skin and nail infections from an inability to open the hand so that it may be cleaned. Intervention is required early when signs of the persistence of this posture are evident to prevent deterioration. Individually fabricated palmar rolls to extend the fingers or commercial lamb's wool spacers are recommended.

CONTRAINDICATIONS AND PRECAUTIONS TO CASTING AND SPLINTING

Precautions to the use of splinting as a therapeutic intervention pertain to the integrity and sensibility of the skin, and the viability of the peripheral vascular system.

Casting is contraindicated when continued monitoring is not possible and in the presence of conditions such as significant oedema, impaired circulation or the presence of heterotropic ossification. The responsibility of the therapist for safe and effective application of splints and casts applies in inverse proportion to the responsibility assumed by the client.

REFERENCES

1. Wilton JC: Splinting and casting in the presence of neurological dysfunction. In: Wilton JC, Hand splinting: principles of design and fabrication. London: WB Saunders, 1997:168–97.
2. Neuhaus BE, Ascher ER, Coulton BA et al: A survey of rationales for and against hand splinting in hemiplegia. Am J Occup Ther 35:83–90, 1981.
3. Reid DT: A survey of Canadian occupational therapists' use of hand splints for children with neurological dysfunction. Can J Occup Ther 59:16–27, 1992.
4. Tardieu Y, Tardieu C: Cerebral palsy. Mechanical evaluation and conservative correction of limb joint contracture. Clin Orthopaed Rel Res 219:63–9, 1987.
5. Tabary JC, Tabary C, Tardieu C, Tardieu G, Goldspink G: Physiological and structural changes in the cat's soleus muscle due to immobilisation at different lengths by plaster casts. J Physiol 224:231–44, 1972.
6. Williams PE, Goldspink G: Changes in sarcomere length and physiological properties in immobilised muscle. J Anat 127:459–68, 1978.

8

Sporting injuries

A. INJURY TO THE HAND AND WRIST IN SPORT

W Bruce Conolly, Mark Perko and Rosemary Prosser

GENERAL PRINCIPLES

Hand therapists and surgeons are being called upon to treat sport- and exercise-related injuries more and more. About one-third of all such injuries occur in the hand and wrist. Fortunately, the majority are minor, and treatment is straightforward. However, some major injuries are not recognised until it is too late for effective treatment.

Many of these injuries are sports-specific and an understanding of the mechanism of injury, the requirement of the sport and the needs of the athlete or enthusiast is important to the diagnosis and treatment.

History taking with special reference to the mechanism of injury must never be omitted. The anatomical structures in the hand are intricate, complex and confined. This makes careful and precise observation and palpation mandatory for clinical diagnosis.

Failure to X-ray and failure to re-X-ray (e.g. fractured scaphoid) will often lead to misdiagnosis.

Hand and wrist injuries are common, because of the involvement of the hand and wrist in a wide range of sporting and functional activities.

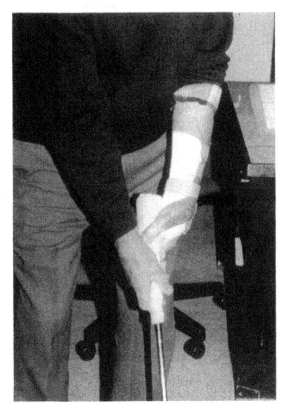

Figure 8.1 Modification of equipment: the grip on this man's golf club was made larger with a grip-enhancing material to increase grip adhesion. It was also necessary to support the left osteoarthritic wrist with a wrist support to maintain the wrist in maximal extension.

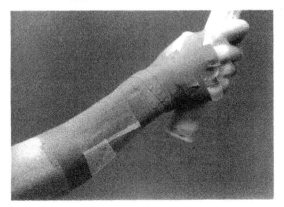

Figure 8.2 Taping is often preferred by the athlete in competition: it is not bulky and provided it is applied correctly can give appropriate support. Tape should be reapplied during competition breaks, as it tends to loosen and stretch out slightly with vigorous motion and perspiration. Taping for a tennis player with ulnar carpal instability is shown here.

CLASSIFICATIONS

Sporting injuries may be classified as relatively minor – e.g. abrasions, contusions and sprains, fracture of the neck of the fifth metacarpal – or major e.g. fractures involving the proximal interphalangeal (PIP) joint, scaphoid fracture, scapholunate ligament rupture.

Hand injuries may also be classified according to the tissue of injury: ligaments, joints, bones, tendon, neurovascular structures, skin and soft tissue.

Injuries may also be classified as open or closed from direct or indirect force – traction, compression, avulsion, twisting, angulation – or repetitive stress injuries.

Rehabilitation usually involves some type of support splinting and an exercise programme. Modification of the sporting equipment (Fig. 8.1)

and/or technique may also be necessary in order for the athlete to return to the sport: this should be done in conjunction with the coach. Splinting or taping (Fig. 8.2) may also be necessary to enable an early return to sport following the injury.

Many people become involved following hand injuries in an athlete. The injured person himself is often young and will have two careers – a sporting career and a business or professional career. The involvement of the team coach, therapist, the team doctor and family members will also affect treatment.

LIGAMENT INJURIES IN THE HAND AND WRIST

Ligament injuries[1] are the most common of all sporting injuries in the hand and wrist. They have minimal signs but maximal disability and are often badly treated. The common ligament injuries in the athlete include:

- lateral ligament injury of a digit, e.g. ulnar collateral ligament (UCL) of the metacarpophalangeal (MP) joint of the thumb (skier's thumb)
- hyperextension injury of a digit, e.g. of the PIP joint, leading to rupture of the palmar plate or lateral ligaments

- scapholunate ligament injury at the wrist caused by a fall on the outstretched hand.

Ligament injuries may be classified as:

1. sprain
2. rupture
3. dislocation
4. fracture dislocation.

Sprain injuries to ligaments and joint capsules

Here there is no instability. The management should be supportive strapping and early range of movement within the limit of discomfort. An X-ray should always be taken to exclude a hidden fracture. One must be sure that it is a sprain, i.e. incomplete tearing of fibres, and not a rupture.

Ligament rupture

Ligament rupture occurs in the thumb at the UCL, in the fingers at the palmar plate or lateral ligament of the PIP joint. Complete ligament ruptures are best treated by surgical repair.

Skier's thumb

Anatomy and pathology

When a skier falls, the pole forces the thumb into abduction and extension, stressing the UCL of the MP joint of the thumb. There may be rupture of the UCL at its mid-substance or at either end and there may be a fracture or fracture dislocation of the metacarpophalangeal joint. This injury can also occur in ice hockey and in other games.

Diagnosis

There will be tenderness over the site of ligament rupture, with significant bruising and swelling. The joint will probably be unstable: always compare with the other thumb MP joint. There is often less pain with a complete rupture than with a sprain or an incomplete rupture.

The ligament may be displaced and become lodged between the ruptured end of the ligament and its attachment to the base of the proximal phalanx (Stener lesion).[2]

Management

The first-aid management should include ice packs and strapping for gentle compression and support to avoid further damage.

If one suspects a complete rupture, surgical repair is indicated. Following this, immobilise the repaired ligament for 4–6 weeks in a splint. Begin early interphalangeal joint exercises in the first postoperative week. Gentle thumb MP extension/flexion exercises can be commenced at 4 weeks. Strengthening exercises for the thumb and grip are not commenced until 6 weeks postoperatively. Incomplete ruptures may be treated conservatively with a thumb spica for 5–6 weeks.

Healing and complications

Incomplete diagnosis and incomplete management may lead to permanent instability of this ligament system, with weak grasp and later osteoarthritis.

Specific tip

If IP flexion is not at least half-range by 2 weeks, passive flexion exercises need to be commenced and/or an IP flexion strap worn for 30 min twice a day or more (Fig. 8.3).

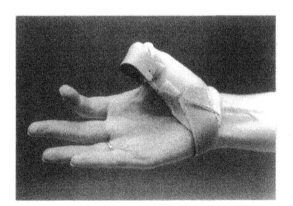

Figure 8.3 A skier's thumb UCL injury requires a splint for protection so that the ligament does not stretch out while it is healing. A flexion strap is worn intermittently for 30 min twice a day or longer if flexion is not 50% of the contralateral side by 2 weeks post-injury.

PIP joint dislocation

Dislocation can occur at any joint level. At the PIP joint level it can be particularly disabling for both grasp and release. Reduction may seem easy but the joint may redislocate just as easily due to instability.

PIP joint dislocations are common in ball sports, particularly football. The force of the football hitting the fingertip hyperextends the PIP joint, causing an avulsion of the distal attachment of the volar plate at the base of the middle phalanx. This may cause an avulsion fracture.

Reduction under a local anaesthetic digital block with traction and a volar directed force over the dorsally displaced middle phalanx will usually suffice.

Therapy for simple dislocations

If a dislocation has been reduced and is stable and there is no associated fracture, simple buddy strapping and early range of motion (ROM) exercises will suffice.

If the joint is only stable in flexion at the PIP joint, an extension block splint in 30 degrees of flexion will be required for 4–6 weeks.

If the injury is more severe and the joint unstable, then direct repair of the fracture or the ligament system may be necessary.

Therapy for severe dislocations

Where the dislocation is associated with a soft tissue and skin wound, often with exposure of the flexor tendons, the wound should be thoroughly cleaned prior to reducing the dislocation to avoid and minimise the chance of infection. Always X-ray after reduction of dislocation to check the accuracy of the reduction and the absence of fracture.

Post-reduction therapy for severe dislocations

Following reduction, the joint should be protected in a dorsal blocking splint in approximately 30 degrees of flexion for 4–6 weeks. Distal interphalangeal (DIP) joint exercises should be commenced within a few days. If the joint is stable, PIP joint exercises in the splint can also be started in the first week. End-range extension should be avoided for approximately 3 weeks. If there is some concern regarding stability and surgical treatment has been ruled out, PIP exercises should not be commenced for 4 weeks.

The patient may develop a flexion contracture due to the soft tissue injury involved in the dislocation. This can be remedied by night-time extension splintage, which is usually commenced 4–6 weeks following reduction. Minor flexion contractures can be treated with a neoprene sleeve, which provides a gentle extension force while still allowing flexion (Fig. 8.4); this type of sleeve may also be appropriate when returning to sport.

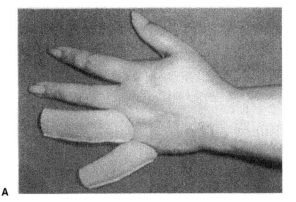

A

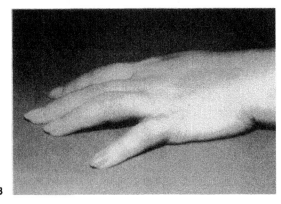

B

Figure 8.4 A neoprene sleeve (A) provides both support for the joint and a gentle extension force to alleviate minor PIP flexion contractures for the PIP joint following ligamentous injury (B) at this level.

Specific tips

DIP joint exercises are important. DIP flexion glides the flexor tendon, intrinsics, long extensors and oblique retinacular ligament, all of which can become gummed down in the healing tissue at the PIP joint level.

Scapholunate ligament injuries

The scaphoid is the key to normal carpal kinematics and wrist stability. When the ligaments connecting it to the lunate and the volar radius are ruptured by a dorsal extension, ulnar deviation and supination injury, the scaphoid separates from the lunate and rotates vertically, causing carpal collapse. If untreated, this can lead to disabling instability and oesteoarthritis.[3]

The clinical features include diffuse wrist pain and tenderness over the scapholunate ligament dorsally. The wrist is swollen and movement restricted. There may be a wrist haemarthrosis. Displacement of the scaphoid will lead to collapse of the midcarpal joint. The scaphoid shift test (Watson test) will be positive. This is positive if there is dorsal pain over the scapholunate interval and increased mobility of the scaphoid; sometimes there is a click as the scaphoid jumps over the rim of the radius. X-ray may show a gap between the scaphoid and lunate.

Acute scapholunate ligament injuries should be treated primarily by surgical open reduction and ligament repair. Postoperative therapy is described in Chapter 3F.

FRACTURES IN THE HAND AND WRIST

Fractures[4] are common in contact sports. The type of fracture should be diagnosed and checked for displacement, rotation, alignment and joint involvement.

Fractures of the thumb

Intra-articular fractures need to be distinguished from extra-articular fractures as they require more comprehensive treatment, particularly reduction.

Fractures of the base of the metacarpal

Extra-articular fractures of the first metacarpal can be managed by a thumb spica cast for 3 or 4 weeks.

Intra-articular fractures of the thumb include Bennett's fracture. This fracture is often caused by clenched fist injury due to the axial compression load across the first carpometacarpal (CMC) joint. This is really a fracture dislocation which requires reduction of both fracture and the dislocated first metacarpal at the CMC joint.

In the past, K-wire fixation after reduction was advised but open reduction internal fixation (ORIF) with a screw (Fig. 8.5) gives better fixation and is the preferred method (if the avulsed fragment of bone involves more than one-third of the joint surface). An unrecognised and untreated Bennett's fracture dislocation can lead to osteoarthritis of the CMC joint.

Fractures of the metacarpal neck and shaft

A fracture analogous to the Bennett's fracture can occur at the base of the fifth metacarpal and require similar treatment.

Most metacarpal shaft fractures are stable. Rotational alignment should always be checked by assessing digit alignment with the fingers flexed; the malalignment may not be obvious with the finger extended.

Metacarpal neck fractures, e.g. boxer's fracture of the fifth metacarpal neck

Substantial angulation (up to 40–50 degrees) can be accepted because of the great mobility of the CMC and the MP joint of the little finger.

Angulation is not acceptable in neck fractures of the index and middle fingers.

Phalangeal fractures

Phalangeal fractures are more difficult to treat. If they are undisplaced and stable, buddy strapping will suffice. Follow-up check X-ray to detect

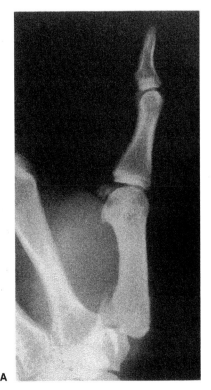 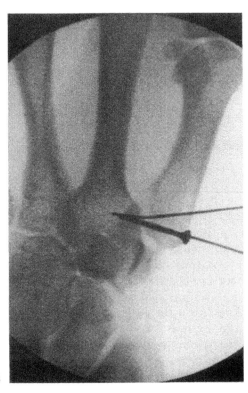

A   **B**

Figure 8.5 Bennett's fracture (A) treated by open reduction and internal fixation (ORIF) with a screw (B).

subsequent displacement of the fracture may be necessary in some cases, e.g. spiral fractures.

A displaced or unstable fracture requires reduction and internal fixation. This allows most athletes to return to their sport earlier than with conservative treatment and with fewer complications.

Therapy for hand fractures

All fractures of the metacarpals and phalanges requiring splinting need to be splinted in the position of safe immobilisation (POSI). The injured digit plus the adjacent one or two digits should be splinted; other digits can be left free. Early return to sport can be facilitated by protection of the fracture with a lightweight thermoplastic splint (1.6 or 2.4 mm). The splint needs to comply with the sports code requirements for the athlete's particular sport. Generally, splints need to be padded externally and taped so that the splint cannot injure other players.

Metacarpal fractures. The IP joints can be left free to move in the case of a metacarpal fracture. The patient should be instructed in ROM exercises for all joints which do not have full range. Emphasis should be placed on MP flexion and EDC (extensor digitorum communis) glide for metacarpal fractures. Gradually, as the patient begins to use the hand, the splint can be exchanged for buddy straps, which should be worn for a further 2–3 weeks.

Phalangeal fractures. Many of these fractures require splintage in the POSI position. ROM exercises should be commenced as soon as the fracture is stable, preferably in the first week. Emphasis should be placed on maintaining full extension while gaining flexion. PIP extension splintage intermittently during the day or at night may be required (see Chapter 2B).

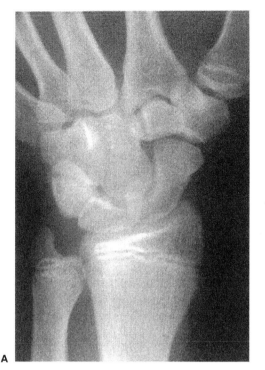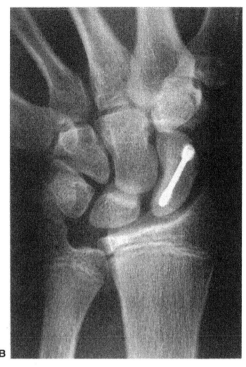

A   B

Figure 8.6 X-ray of fracture of the scaphoid (A) requiring open reduction and internal fixation (ORIF) (B).

Fractures of the wrist and carpal instability

Fractures of a scaphoid

These fractures represent the most common and potentially most severe of all carpal bone injuries. Any patient who presents with a painful swollen wrist following a fall on the outstretched hand should be suspected of having a scaphoid fracture or a scapholunate ligament injury.

It is characterised by tenderness and some swelling in the anatomical snuff box. A full series of X-rays with anteroposterior (AP), lateral and oblique views and with radial and ulnar deviation of both wrists are required for comparison.

If there is a suspicion of fracture, a scaphoid cast should be applied for 7–10 days and then the X-ray repeated. If there is doubt, a bone scan should be arranged. Scaphoid fractures present a challenge in management and require vigilance. Even seemingly innocuous fractures can become displaced and fail to unite. Follow-up X-rays

(at 10 days) during the period of casting are necessary. Fractures that are displaced from the outset and the proximal pole fractures, even if undisplaced, are associated with a high incidence of long-term complications and are usually managed best by internal fixation (Fig. 8.6).

The indications for surgical reduction and internal fixation include fractures displaced greater than 1 mm, malrotated fractures, scaphoid fractures associated with carpal instability such as scapholunate dissociation and trans-scaphoid perilunate dislocations of the carpus, and some oblique and proximal pole fractures. ORIF in most cases leads to an earlier (6–8 weeks) return of function and ability to work. This in itself in some cases may be an indication for ORIF.

Fractures of the hamate

These fractures often occur in golfers in a non-dominant hand after striking the club on hard ground. The clinical features include point tenderness over the hamate hook. X-ray may not show this fracture except on carpal tunnel views. A computed tomography (CT) scan may be required. Many of these fractures fail to unite. Excision may be the best long-term treatment.

Fractures of the triquetrium

Dorsal avulsion fracture of the triquetrium is the next commonest carpal injury. There is tenderness over the dorsal aspect of the triquetrium. An X-ray will show the ligamentous avulsion fracture.

Treatment is conservative and involves 3 weeks of immobilisation, followed by an exercise programme to regain mobility and strength. Strong forearm rotation or wrist radial deviation should be avoided for at least 6 weeks.

Fractures of the distal radius

Displaced comminuted fractures will require reduction and, in young patients because of the likelihood of residual collapse following initial reduction, supplementary stabilisation with K-wires or an external fixator may be necessary. Postoperative therapy should follow the same lines as described for distal radial fractures (Chapter 3D).

Fractures of the radial styloid

These fractures may be associated with scapholunate ligament injury even though the fracture is not displaced. If there is a scapholunate ligament injury, management will be more complicated.

Simple radial styloid fractures can be managed in a cast. Scapholunate ligament rupture requires surgical repair.

TENDON INJURIES IN THE HAND IN SPORT

There may be ruptures of the extensor tendons (DIP joint – baseball finger, PIP joint – buttonhole deformity, or the interphalangeal joint of the thumb). There may be rupture of the FDP (flexor digitorum profundus) tendon of the finger (rugby finger).

In general, extensor tendon ruptures which are closed injuries can be treated conservatively with splintage (see Chapter 2E). Closed ruptures of the flexor apparatus are best treated surgically as soon as possible; otherwise, the proximal tendon stump will retract and make reattachment too difficult. For postoperative care, see Chapter 2D.

If diagnosis of FDP rupture is delayed and not made until 3–5 days after injury, it may be inadvisable to attempt surgery but to treat the patient conservatively and concentrate on restoring full movement of the MP and PIP joints. Flexor tendon reconstruction at a later date or DIP joint stabilisation may provide a better functional outcome.

Tenosynovitis can occur from repetitive actions, as in the FCR (flexor carpi radialis) or FCU (flexor carpi ulnaris) tendons of the wrist, or in the first extensor compartment with involvement of the APL (abductor pollicis longus) or EPB (extensor pollicis brevis) tendons (de Quervain's condition) or the ECR (extensor carpi radialis) tendons, the ECU (extensor carpi ulnaris) tendons or the 'intersection syndrome' (see Chapters 2D and 2E).

NEUROVASCULAR INJURIES

Neurovascular injuries include 'bowler's thumb' (neuroma in continuity of the ulnar digital nerve of the thumb from the constant pressure of a bowl), racket ball syndrome, ulnar nerve syndromes and compartment syndromes.

Bowler's thumb

Hand therapy

Hand therapy measures include modification of the grip for bowling and perhaps a change in the ball.

Adaptive devices to protect the nerve from pressure may also be successful. These can be fitted either to the ball or the thumb. Neoprene and silicone elastomere or putty are helpful in the fabrication of these custom-made adaptive devices. If the neuroma proves troublesome in other daily activities, techniques such as the use of TENS (transcutaneous electrical nerve stimulation) and/or desensitisation may be helpful (see Chapter 7E).

Surgery

In resistant cases, an ulnar digital neurolysis can relieve the problem.

Racket ball syndrome – carpal tunnel syndrome

In racket ball and in other sporting activities – such as rowing, wind surfing and cycling – where prolonged gripping is required, there can be an enlargement of the flexor tenosynovium within the carpal tunnel with secondary compression of the median nerve.

Conservative treatments often suffice, but in resistant cases carpal tunnel decompression may be indicated. In athletes, endoscopic release avoids the interthenar scar and enables an earlier return to sport.

Hand therapy

Conservative management includes stretching the long flexors before and after the sporting activity. Ice, elevation and compression should be applied immediately after the sporting activity if swelling is noted. A splint made of soft material such as neoprene with thermoplastic ribs may be useful depending on the activity causing the carpal tunnel compression. Sporting technique may need modification. In the case of long-distance cycling, alterations in the handle bars, e.g. forearm bars, will decrease the pressure on the carpal tunnel.

Ulnar nerve syndromes

The ulnar nerve can also be trapped at the wrist by a ganglion or by ulnar artery occlusion, in which case the treatment should be directed at the cause.

Ulnar artery thrombosis can occur from a repetitive impact, as in cycling, because of the constant vibration of the bicycle handle, and in sports such as volleyball, handball or karate, where repetitive impact occurs.

Ulnar artery thrombosis presents with local tenderness and swelling, at the hypothenar eminence, ischaemia, often with a painful white ring and little finger. Microemboli may be present.

A bruit may or may not be audible. Prompt referral should be arranged for reconstructive vascular surgery.

Compartment syndromes

There may be increased pressure in the fascial compartment of the forearm, wrist or hand. Severe forearm pain coming on after prolonged vigorous activity may be associated with clinical tension in the forearm compartment. This is seen often in rowers, kayakers or motorcycle racers. If the condition does not respond to local therapy and rest, surgical decompression may be required.

Hand therapy

Conservative management involves completely resting the injured muscles if pain is acute in a POSI resting splint for the hand and/or wrist. Splinting should not be prolonged, e.g. 1–14 days. Local electrophysical agents such as ultrasound, interferential, laser and cryotherapy may prove to be helpful. Massage and appropriate stretching is important. Once the episode has settled, the upper limb should be assessed with particular attention to the length, strength and balance of the musculature. Both concentric and eccentric strength should be evaluated. Following this, an appropriate exercise programme involving both stretching and strengthening exercises is constituted. The rowing/kayaking athlete, coach and therapist may need to discuss the particular stroke technique. Size and shape of the oar/paddle handle and blade may also need scrutiny.

SKIN AND SOFT TISSUE INJURIES

These include abrasions, contusions, calluses and blisters.

Blisters

Blisters occur on the foot and hand. They are best prevented by a common-sense approach to factors known to precipitate them, e.g. proper-fitting socks, footwear and gloves.

The aim of treatment of a blister is to promote healing and prevent infection. Treat by cleaning the blister and skin with antiseptic; aspirate tense blisters with a fine-gauge needle and inject a small dose of tincture of benzoin. If the blister is broken, trim the overlying skin and protect the floor of the blister with a tincture of benzoin and apply protective tape.

Calluses

Treat by light abrasion with a pumice stone. If the callus is large, treat by softening in a warm antiseptic bath and then paring with a fine scalpel.

'Boxer's knuckle'

This condition may include a mild bursa or synovitis or partial or complete rupture of the dorsal capsule of the MP joint of a finger.

Conservative measures are required for all but the ruptured hood, which may need surgical repair. Conservative measures include the fabrication of protective devices that can at least be worn in training sessions. Massage and local electrotherapy modalities are worth exploring but are not always useful. A change in training schedule is necessary in order to give the joint time to heal.

PAEDIATRIC INJURIES

Children and adolescents require specific consideration of their injuries because they are skeletally immature and have open growth plates.

About one-third of all skeletal fractures in children involve the growth plate. Growth plate injuries may be complicated by disturbances in growth, leading to deformity. There may be involvement of the joint surface.

In adolescents, epiphyseal plate injuries are more likely; in the younger child and the skeletally mature person, a ligament or tendon injury is more likely.

Where the growth plate injury is in association with an intra-articular fracture, anatomical reduction, either closed or open, is indicated. With any growth plate injury, the patient should be followed up on a regular basis to recognise and monitor any potential growth disturbance.

One of the more common paediatric hand injuries is a fracture separation of the distal phalangeal epiphysis, which may present as a pseudo mallet finger. X-rays are essential. Anatomical reduction is indicated.

REFERENCES

1. Posner MA: Ligament injuries in the wrist and hand. Hand Clin 4 November, 1992.
2. Stener B: Displacement of the ruptured ulnar collateral ligament of the metacarpophalangeal joint of the thumb. J Bone Joint Surg 44B:869, 1962.
3. Herbert T: The fractured scaphoid. St Louis: Quality Medical Publishing, 1990:173–94.
4. Barton NJ: Fractures of the hand. J Bone Joint Surg 664:159–67, 1984.

B. INJURY OF THE ELBOW AND SHOULDER IN SPORT

Mark Perko

For a comprehensive treatment of the elbow and the shoulder, the reader is referred to Chapters 5 and 6, respectively.

Participation in sports can place considerable demands on both the shoulder and the elbow. Injuries can occur from overuse or direct trauma. Overuse injuries can be reduced by appropriate training and conditioning. Acute injuries will always occur, but attention to participant safety, game codes and the playing environment will reduce these risks. The goal of treatment is to restore function as quickly as possible, but treatment decisions will be influenced by the player, family, friends, coaches and financial interests. Overall, the safety of the player should be paramount and other demands should be weighed carefully against appropriate treatment.

CONTACT SPORTS

Acute injuries to the shoulder and elbow are common. Dislocations and fractures are usually violent injuries due to the strength and speed of the participants. A thorough clinical assessment with adequate radiographs and follow-up reviews are mandatory. Neurological or vascular injuries, although uncommon, can be overlooked; if detected later, recovery can be prolonged. Rotator cuff tears can complicate both dislocations and neurological injuries and are especially difficult to detect in the presence of neurological weakness or a painful shoulder. In most cases, the pain from a dislocation should subside within 1–2 weeks. Persisting pain or failure to regain function should alert the treating clinician to the possibility of other injuries.

The treatment of anteroinferior shoulder dislocations will vary between the acute and chronic. Although arthroscopic repair in acute dislocations is often advocated and achieves better results than conservative therapies, to date its success rate does not match that of a delayed open repair. Timing is also a consideration. Injuries early in the season are more often treated conservatively, with a trial return due to prolonged recovery following surgery. Recurrence in the conservatively treated group, although high, is not necessarily imminent.

Elbow dislocations are usually stable after reduction and splintage should be avoided. Motion should be encouraged, to avoid a flexion contracture. Orthotic protection is only necessary in cases where the elbow is unstable after reduction. Oral indomethacin can be used to reduce the incidence of heterotopic bone and should be commenced early with more serious injuries. Any associated fractures should be treated along usual principles.

Hyperextension injuries to the elbow are often seen in the tackling player and can produce prolonged symptoms without any apparent injury.

Recurrent olecranon bursitis can also be difficult to manage. Appropriate protection and drainage are usually sufficient, but excision is sometimes necessary.

THROWING SPORTS

Throwing is a complex movement, requiring sequential and coordinated muscle contraction. It follows a sequence of wind-up, cocking, acceleration, release or deceleration and follow through. The shoulder joint achieves high angular velocities and ligamentous restraints and neuromuscular control must resist these forces. The potential for injury is high and can be due to improper mechanics, poor dynamic stability or fatigue.

The elbow is also exposed to large valgus stresses in the acceleration phase of throwing, which can lead to valgus overload and injury to the medial collateral ligament. Adolescents are more likely to sustain a separation of the medial epicondyle. Fragmentation of the epiphyses of the capitellum and radial head may occur with excessive pitching.

TENNIS

Injuries in tennis are common and the majority are classified as overuse. The stresses on the shoulder and elbow are not dissimilar to throwing. Rotator cuff tendinopathy and lateral and medial epicondylitis are common complaints. Treatment will usually include a period of rest followed by appropriate conditioning.

SWIMMING

Swimming is a popular recreational pastime, but problems usually only occur in competitive swimmers. Shoulder pain is a common complaint in those engaged in a regular training programme. Poor stroke technique is the most likely cause. It can be actual incorrect technique or simply deterioration in technique due to fatigue. Remedies may include changes in technique, decreased training intensity in the pool or use of additional weight programmes for strength and endurance.

GYMNASTICS

Injuries are commonly due to overuse, resulting in tendonopathies. Falls from apparatus or during tumbling can result in more serious injuries. The upper limb is weight bearing in many routines, and adequate strength and endurance are necessary. Appropriate conditioning and strength training, especially in male gymnasts, will help to alleviate many problems. Acute elbow injuries such as dislocations or supracondylar fractures are not uncommon. In adolescents, avulsion of the medial epicondyle or osteochondritis of the capitellum can occur.

CONCLUSIONS

The elbow and shoulder will continue to be prone to injury with the ever-increasing demands placed by sporting pursuits. As understanding of the biomechanics of these two joints improves, so will training techniques and treatments.

FURTHER READING

Andrews JR, Wilk KE (eds): The athletes' shoulder. Edinburgh: Churchill Livingstone, 1994.

Morrey B (ed.): The elbow and its disorders, 2nd edn. Philadelphia: WB Saunders, 1993.

Rockwood CA, Matsen FA (eds): The shoulder. Philadelphia: WB Saunders, 1990.

9

Occupational overuse injuries of the upper limb

Amelia Lucas

INTRODUCTION

Work-related overuse syndromes affecting the upper limb are not a new phenomena. Ramazzini[1] documented upper limb pain in Scrilies in the 18th century. One hundred and sixty years ago, the British Civil Service reported symptoms of pain and fatigue in the arms of their writers and attributed this to the introduction of the steel rule.[2] Writer's cramp was covered by the British Workman's Compensation Act in 1906 and within 3 years almost 60% of the workforce were reporting symptoms of muscle weakness, pain or cramp: they blamed the new technology.[3] 'The Australian epidemic peaked in the mid-80s.[4]

WHAT IS OCCUPATIONAL OVERUSE SYNDROME?

There are many varied opinions as to the definition of this syndrome, its aetiology, pathophysiology, or indeed whether such a condition exists. Diverse opinions have been offered by psychologists, rheumatologists, orthopaedic and hand surgeons, neurologists and physicians.

Box 9.1 illustrates this diversity.

Lam[5] concluded that '… the concept of repetitive strain injury (RSI) is not occupationally caused in its current context, but is compensation caused.'

Boyling[6] defined this syndrome as

a concentric term for those conditions characterised by discomfort or persistent pain in their muscles, tendons and other soft-tissues. This can be a clearly defined condition or an ill-defined symptom complex.

Box 9.1 Synonyms for regional upper limb pain syndrome

- Occupational cramp/occupational neurosis
- Writer's cramp/telegraphist's cramp
- Occupational over-use syndrome
- Cumulative trauma disorder (CTD)
- Rapid movement disease
- Repetitive strain injury (RSI)
- Occupational cervicobrachial syndrome
- Regional fibrostic syndrome
- Work-related upper limb disorder
- Golden wrist/kangaroo paw
- RSI (rampant social iatrogenesis)
- RSI (retrospective salary increase)

Butler[7] states that

RSI is the common name given to the symptom complex of upper limb and trunk pain ... there the aggravating factor appears to be repetitious activity. One underestimated factor ... is abnormal physiology and mechanics of the nervous system during movement.

He cites clinical studies by Elvey et al[8] and later Quinten et al[9] supporting neural involvement.

Albert[10] considers that:

in over-use injury, tendinitis becomes a principal problem ... and is due to the gradual biologic process of tissue breakdown ... muscle becomes fatigued, but preset force levels are still required to complete a specific activity ... the tendon is selectively overloaded as a compensatory mechanism and eventually becomes inflamed.

A generally accepted 'definition' of this syndrome has been difficult to achieve, since each medical specialty approaches examination and diagnosis within the limitations of their own field of expertise. However, most agree that it is a syndrome affecting the musculoskeletal system and associated with excessive repetitive or eccentric stresses, rather than a disease process.

Since physiotherapy skills *are* primarily related to disorders of the musculoskeletal system, they are in an ideal position to contribute to a more global understanding of this syndrome, which requires a knowledge of:

- posture and movement analysis
- arthrokinematics
- biomechanics and pathomechanics (articular and neural)
- muscle testing – length, strength and endurance

- joint-testing – including passive tests
- palpatory skills
- neural mobility testing.

The following definition is based on applying the above statements to a very large patient population referred with a diagnosis of 'RSI' over many years:

Overuse syndrome is an isolated lesion or a combination of soft tissue and articular disorders associated with prolonged static postures or excessive movement demands. The location distribution and progression of symptoms can be explained in terms of the biomechanically integrated function of the neuromuscular–articular system.

The demands placed on the upper limb and trunk in various occupations are analogous to those imposed on the lower limb during many sports and athletic pursuits. These 'industrial athletes'[11] are susceptible to the same neuromuscular–articular disorders as their 'athletic counterparts'. Unfortunately, 'industrial athletes' do not always have the benefit of adequate training, conditioning, monitoring and immediate post-injury care.

AETIOLOGY

Figure 9.1 proposes a concept for the development of the overuse syndrome.

CLINICAL MANIFESTATIONS

Butler[7] agrees that an anatomical basis for symptoms and signs of overuse syndrome is possible and that 'such a basis includes recognition of the potential for different parts of the system to contribute simultaneously and of the contribution of non-neural structures'. He also agrees with Lucas that a consistent pattern of signs and symptoms does exist but has failed to be recognised.

Subjective components

History

A typical history has many of the following features:

- gradual, insidious onset of symptoms
- a change in normal working activities, e.g. extra overtime, increased output

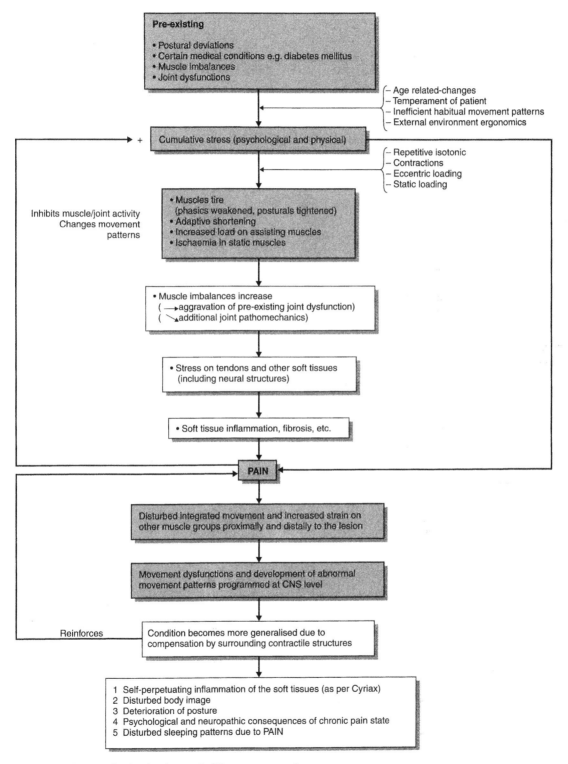

Figure 9.1   Concept for the development of the overuse syndrome.

- returning to work after a period of absence or illness
- change in the physical work environment, e.g. operating fault in equipment, new keyboard, different work station
- an increase in psychological stress due to personal relationships, or conflict with staff and management at work.

Symptoms

Initially, patients often report a feeling of tiredness, heaviness or vague aching in either the wrist forearm or cervical spine/shoulder girdle region. This occurs during the course of the working day or after work. These early symptoms usually settle overnight or after a weekend of rest. Patients perceive this as a mild strain, although they cannot recall a specific injury: therefore, it is often unreported.

Symptoms usually progress, with discomfort and pain spreading either more proximally from the wrist/forearm or more distally in the case of the cervical/shoulder region being the initial site.

Pain is often accompanied by soft tissue oedema in isolated or multiple muscles or tendons. Pain also interferes with performing normal activities of daily living and interrupts sleeping. Symptoms may no longer settle with rest outside normal working hours.

The persistence, severity or generalisation of symptoms together with advice from co-workers and fellow sufferers often prompts the patient to seek advice and treatment. However, some sufferers remain at work until pain and dysfunction become disabling. This may be due to fear of losing their job or other socioeconomic reasons.

Objective components

Posture

The patient often presents with postural deviations in the upper body and upper limb, which usually manifest as a forward head alignment, increased thoracic kyphosis, shoulder girdle protraction (with depression or elevation), internal rotation at the glenohumeral joint and slight flexion at the elbow. These postural deviations become more pronounced, as more structures become involved, and are probably a combination of muscle imbalances, adverse neural tension and compensatory antalgic positions.

Figure 9.2 is that of an overuse syndrome sufferer and is typical of the majority of patients.

The forward head alignment results in upper cervical extension and neurovascular entrapment (particularly at O/C1). This is often the cause of headaches. Eccentric stress on the posterior cervical muscles, attempting to control the weight of the head, causes ongoing pain. This is compounded by the weight of the protracted shoulder girdle and upper limb stressing the trapezius and rhomboid muscles. Shortening in the pectoralis minor and scalenii muscles can irritate neural structures and cause adverse neural tension.

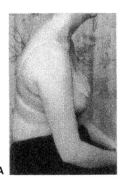 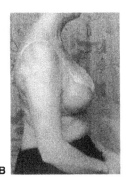 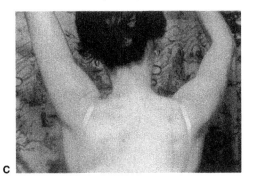

Figure 9.2 A: This patient's posture is typical of the overuse syndrome. Note the forward head alignment, depressed sternum, increased thoracic kyphosis and protracted and depressed shoulder girdle. B: This is the patient's attempt at correcting her posture. Muscle imbalances are severe enough to prohibit a biomechanically efficient alignment. C: Muscle imbalances prevent full range active elevation of the gleno-humeral joint.

Muscular–articular–neural disorders

Associated with this syndrome are:

Wrist and hand. Comprises tendinitis, tenosynovitis, e.g. de Quervain's, wrist or digital ganglions; stenosing – tenosynovitis of the flexor tendons, pathologies of the triangular fibrocartilage; ulnocarpal laxities and hypermobility of the distal radioulnar joint usually associated with repetitive pronation/supination, especially in the closed-chain situation where the hand is fixed reversing the normal radioulnar mechanics; hypermobility of the first carpometacarpal joint or between the trapezium/trapezoid scaphoid articulation (often associated with forceful or repetitive radial deviation/thumb extension activities); median nerve compression in the carpal tunnel (carpal tunnel syndrome); or ulnar nerve compression in the canal of Guyon.

Elbow/forearm. Comprises myositis in the flexors, extensors, pronators or supinators; lateral epicondylitis; proximal radiohumeral joint dysfunctions usually resulting from repetitive or forceful use of the biceps; entrapment of the median nerve at the cubital fossa (pronator syndrome); or the ulnar nerve in the cubital tunnel (cubital tunnel syndrome).

Cervical spine/shoulder region. Comprises biceps and rotator cuff tendinitis, subacromial bursitis, suprascapular nerve entrapment, neurovascular symptoms associated with entrapment of the brachial plexus and vascular structures in this region. This often results from repetitive or sustained activities above the shoulder level.

Clinical experience suggests that a vast majority of overuse patients display commonly recurring pain patterns, patterns of the muscle imbalances, distribution of articular dysfunctions and location and nature of soft tissue involvement. These common patterns occur too frequently to be considered coincidental.[11] They are discussed in the following section.

ASSESSMENT

A keystone to the understanding of assessment and other aspects of upper limb overuse syndrome, particularly its progression, is the concept of the upper limb components forming part of one complex – a biomechanically linked – functional segment,[12] which also includes the cranium, mandible, cervical and upper thoracic spine.

These components are anatomically different but inextricably integrated by virtue of proximity, neural and muscle influences, evolutionary and/or embryological development. Their functional interdependence demands that disruption in one component results in compensation by another. Soft tissue and joint involvement is often predictable and consistent with the biomechanics and movement dynamics of the work demands.

All aspects of the neuromuscular–articular components of this complex should be assessed:

- postural deviations and altered movement patterns
- cervical and upper thoracic joints, first rib, joints of the shoulder/girdle and upper limb both for hypomobility and hypermobility.

Common presentations are:

- hypomobility at C7 and T2 and O/C1 and C2/3, radiohumeral joint
- hypermobility at C5/6/7; distal radioulnar joint, ulnocarpal joint and joints on radial side of the wrist.

Muscles are examined for length, strength and endurance. Common presentations are:

- shortening in scalenii, pectorals, rotator cuff group, biceps, wrist and finger extensors or flexors, thumb adductors and flexors
- weakness in scapular stabilisers, triceps, wrist and finger extensors. Comparisons should be made with the unaffected side (Fig. 9.3).

Neural mobility tests

Neural mobility becomes progressively more compromised as the syndrome progresses and mobility between neural tissues and their interface is affected.

Upper limb tension tests and slump tests are described by Butler,[7] who also suggests a

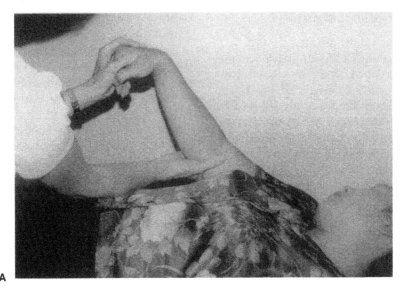

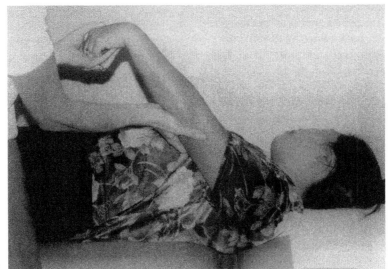

Figure 9.3 A, B: The shortening in the wrist and finger extensors on the affected side compared to the unaffected side. Note the difference in the amount of available wrist flexion.

sympathetic involvement in the pain associated with the syndrome.

INVESTIGATIONS

Radiology, pathology and electrical studies are generally not helpful in the diagnosis or assessment, except as a method of excluding factors such as arthropathies, disc pathologies or other bone or soft tissue disorders. Electromyography (EMG) studies are helpful in detecting and monitoring nerve compression or entrapment.

DIFFERENTIAL DIAGNOSIS

Differential diagnosis can be considered as having two components:

- differentiating overuse syndrome from other disorders

- differentiating *between* components of the neuromuscular–articular system to identify the structures affected by the syndrome.

Differentiating this syndrome from other disorders may be made on the basis of the history. A typical history would include insidious onset, typical pattern of progression of symptoms and repetitive nature of the work.

Differentiation *between* structures is simple in the early stages when only an isolated structure is involved, e.g. tendinitis in wrist/finger extensors. However, it becomes a great challenge when multiple structures – muscles, tendons and joints – are affected. Since these form the interface for neural tissue, this also ultimately becomes implicated.

Differentiation and lesion localisation would then involve the interpretation of specific tests to identify contractile from non-contractile structures, intra-articular as opposed to extra-articular structures, and any neural involvement.

TREATMENT PRINCIPLES

Treatment is directed at the affected soft tissues and joints and may involve:

- soft tissue massage techniques
- joint mobilisations, manipulation or stabilisation
- muscle stretching, strengthening and task-specific conditioning
- neural mobilisation
- home exercises
- auto-stretches, mobilisations
- retraining posture and movement patterns
- electrotherapeutic modalities.

The ultimate goals are to relieve pain and restore normal function to all components, improve their integration and maintain that status to minimise recurrences.

In the initial stages, when very few structures are involved, this goal can be achieved in a short period of time, e.g. a couple of weeks. However, as the condition progresses, and becomes multifactional and chronic, complete resolution of pain and return to normal function may take many months to achieve. In a percentage of these

patients it cannot be fully achieved and they require chronic pain management strategies.

Surgery can compound the problem unless specific, organic reversible pathology is diagnosed beforehand.

CASE STUDY

Subject: Mrs R
Age: 37
Dominant hand: right
Occupation: machine operator (3 years)

History

The patient presented 27 March 1997, complaining of pain around the lateral aspect of her right elbow, some 6 weeks prior to presentation. The onset of soreness developed when she was using her knife to cut through very hard plastic. She was performing this job constantly for some 6 hours. Normally her job has more variety, although it does involve regular and frequent use of knives. Mrs R continued to work, thinking that the soreness was a mild sprain and would resolve. However, symptoms persisted and she reported them some 2 weeks after onset.

The company doctor diagnosed RSI and prescribed Voltaren gel. He also suggested that she change her movement patterns and use the knife differently with more force from the shoulder to offload stress on the forearm. She remained at work and instituted the advice given. However, she subsequently developed soreness in the anterior upper arm region, anterior aspect of her right shoulder, and symptoms at the elbow increased.

Mrs R then consulted her own doctor, who prescribed Anaprox (naproxen) and referred her for physiotherapy and ordered selected duties.

General health

Mrs R is an obese woman with poor posture who also suffers from asthma that requires regular medication. Mrs R presented with a 6-week history of right lat epicondyle pain after performing a job requiring the use of a knife to cut hard plastic for 6 hours per day. She subsequently developed soreness in the right anterior upper arm and shoulder.

Pain location and behaviour

- Pain was reported as constant.
- Aggravating factors were those activities requiring elbow flexion, lifting or supination of the forearm.

Neurological signs and symptoms

Mrs R reported occasional vague 'numbness' in the hand, which seemed unrelated to specific postures or activities. There were no positive neurological or vascular signs.

Neuromuscular–articular examination

The following is a summary of the main findings on the neuromuscular–articular examination.

Active movements

The following movements were restricted in inner range and painful:

- right cervical rotation
- right shoulder elevation and abduction
- elbow flexion and extension.

Passive movements

The range in the shoulder was full but painful. Right cervical rotation, elbow flexion and extension remained restricted and painful.

Muscle tests: resisted tests

The following areas were *painful* and slightly weak (compared to the unaffected side):

- wrist and finger extensors
- supinator
- biceps
- brachialis
- pectorals major and minor
- scapular stabilisers were weak but *not* painful.

Muscle length tests

The wrist and finger extensors, supinator, biceps and pectoralis minor had shortened when compared to the unaffected side.

Endurance

Repetitive isotonic contractions caused early fatigue and pain when applied to the above muscles.

Specific joint testing

There was reduced mobility at C7/T1/2 on the right and the right radiohumeral joint. These joints were also acutely tender on palpation.

Neural mobility tests

Upper limb tension tests were difficult to perform and interpret due to the pain and shortening in the affected muscles and were reserved to a later stage in the course of treatment when the soft tissue soreness and muscle extensibility had improved.

Head and neck flexion and slump tests did not reproduce the patient's symptoms.

Diagnosis

On the basis of the history and the distribution of muscle and joint involvement, the patient does have an overuse syndrome, affecting the structures most involved with the specific task she had performed at the time.

The extensors, supinator, biceps and brachialis and pectorals together with the C7→T2 and radiohumeral joints are the main components affected.

Goals of treatment

- To reduce soft tissue inflammation
- To improve muscle extensibility, strength and endurance
- To mobilise restricted joints
- Retrain posture and review her movement patterns at work, the tools she uses and her method of gripping those tools
- Monitor her progress at work and identify any further risk factors.

Comments

This case study illustrates:

- the typical history of an overuse patient
- the integration between muscles and joints that results in a number of structures becoming affected
- on biomechanical analysis, the structures affected are consistent with the causative occupational activities described by the patient, and also consistent with the present movements aggravating pain.

A multidisciplinary approach is the key to success. This not only involves interaction between those treating the patient – GP, specialist and physiotherapist – but also cooperation with workplace personnel – occupational therapist, occupational health nurse, ergonomist and management.

Preventative strategies at the workplace are paramount in minimising the incidence and recurrence of the syndrome. They include pre-employment screening; adequate job training; attention to ergonomics at work stations; provision for job rotation; adequate rest breaks; fitness activities, e.g. institution of pause-gymnastics; workplace education programmes; and encouraging early reporting of symptoms.

ERGONOMICS

Any external or environmental factors which may compromise or constrain any anatomical part, normal body alignment or efficient and economical physiological movements require some form of adaptation and compensation by the neuromuscular–articular components of the upper quarter either locally, or in a more generalised way. These factors include equipment and tool design, furniture design and location, restrictive clothing and poor lighting or temperature control.

Accumulation of the resultant environmental stressors may eventually cause soft tissue or articular failure and a combination of any one or a combination of the pathologies previously mentioned.

Ergonomics and environmental work-site factors (Fig. 9.4) are as critical to the prevention and

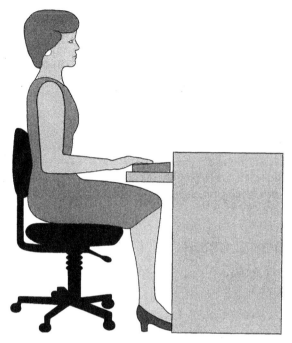

Figure 9.4   Correct keyboard posture.

management of upper limb overuse syndrome as correct footwear, terrain and equipment are to athletes.

PATHOPHYSIOLOGY

The pathophysiology of many of the separate entities previously mentioned are already well-documented. The issue of physiological changes in muscles affected by overuse is still unresolved. Dennett and Fry[13] took muscle biopsies from the affected dorsal interosseous muscle in 29 women with chronic, painful overuse syndrome and 8 volunteer controls. Structural differences in the overuse syndrome group included increased type 1 fibres with type grouping; decreased type 2 fibres; type 2 fibre hypertrophy; increased internal nuclear count mitochondrial changes; and various ultrastructural abnormalities. The changes were also related to clinical severity. They concluded that these changes point to an organic cause but were uncertain these changes resulted directly from the disorder or other primary factors produced by the syndrome.

Evans[14] concluded that 'delayed-onset muscle soreness is most likely caused by structural damage in skeletal muscle after eccentric exercise and may take as long as 12 weeks to repair.' 'Industrial athletes' do not have this option.

Eccentric muscle loading in the upper limb is underrated and needs more study. Entrapment neuropathies in the upper limb result from compression against unyielding fibrous or muscle aponeurotic bands.[15] A precipitating factor is repetitive movement, especially in exaggerated joint positions. Ischaemia and ultra neural fibrosis can result.

CONCLUSION

Occupational overuse syndromes of the upper limb is a broad, descriptive term for a cluster of musculo–articular–neural disorders. The pathologies of many of these have been described but remain controversial. They are well known in sports medicine. There are many parallels between the sporting athlete and the industrial athlete regarding physical demands, and also many disparities in training, management and prevention of this syndrome.

The progression of this syndrome is less well understood. However, the concept of the upper limb as part of a biomechanically linked functional segment, which includes the cervical spine and upper thoracic region to T4, that needs to be appropriately balanced in terms of muscle, soft tissue and joint function, may offer an explanation.

REFERENCES

1. Ramazzini B: De morbis artificum. Diatriba padua 1713 [translated by Wright WC] Chicago: University of Chicago Press, 1940.
2. Bell C: Partial paralysis of the muscles of the extremities. In: The nervous system of the human body. Washington: Duff Green, 1833.
3. Great Britain and Ireland Post Office: Departmental Committee on Telegraphist's Cramp Report. London: HMSO, 1911.
4. Reilly P: Repetitive strain injury: from Australia to the UK. J Psychosom Res 39(6):783–8, 1995.
5. Lam SJS: Repetitive strain injury (RSI) or cumulative trauma disorder (CTD) as legal and clinical entities. Med Sci Law 35(4):279–86, 1995.
6. Boyling J: Upper limb disorders in the workplace. OC PPP In Touch 61, 1991.
7. Butler D: Mobilisation of the nervous system. Edinburgh: Churchill Livingstone, 1994.
8. Elvery RL, Quinter JL, Thomas AN: A clinical study of RSI. Austral Fam Phys 15:1314–19, 1986.
9. Quinter J, Elvery RL, Thomas AN: Regional pain syndrome. Med J Austr 146:230–1, 1987.
10. Albert M: Eccentric muscle training in sports & orthopedics, 2nd edn. Edinburgh: Churchill Livingstone, 1995.
11. Lucas A: Assessment and treatment of industrial overuse syndrome (upper-limb). A clinical manual for physiotherapists, 2nd edn (out of print).
12. Lucas A, Atkinson B: Dimensions and principles of orthopaedic manipulative therapy. Course notes for Masters students in Health Science. Charles Sturt University, 1995.
13. Dennett X, Fry HJH: Over-use syndrome: a muscle biopsy study. Lancet April 23: 905–8, 1988.
14. Evans W: Exercise-induced skeletal muscle damage. Phys Sports Med 15(1), 1987.
15. Dixon L: The nerve composition syndromes of the upper-limb. Patient Management March 1987.
16. Cyriax J: Textbook of orthopaedic medicine, Vol. 1. Diagnosis of soft-tissue lesions, 6th edn. London: Baillière Tindall, 1977.

Appendix 1: American Shoulder and Elbow Score

ELBOW ASSESSMENT FORM (DRAFT)
AMERICAN SHOULDER AND ELBOW SURGEONS

NAME:		DATE:
AGE:	HAND DOMINANCE: R L AMBI	GENDER: M F
DIAGNOSIS:		INITIAL ASSESS: Y N
PROCEDURE/DATE:		FOLLOW-UP: M Y

PATIENT SELF-EVALUATION

DO YOU EXPERIENCE PAIN IN YOUR ELBOW? (Circle correct answer)	YES	NO

MARK WHERE YOUR PAIN IS

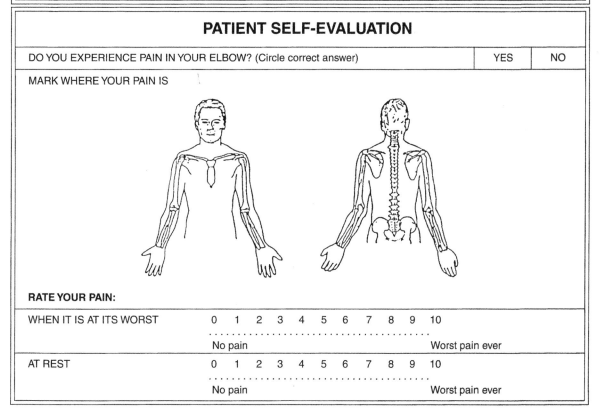

RATE YOUR PAIN:

WHEN IT IS AT ITS WORST	0 1 2 3 4 5 6 7 8 9 10
	No pain Worst pain ever
AT REST	0 1 2 3 4 5 6 7 8 9 10
	No pain Worst pain ever

LIFTING A HEAVY OBJECT	0 1 2 3 4 5 6 7 8 9 10	
	No pain	Worst pain ever
WHEN DOING A TASK WITH REPEATED ELBOW MOVEMENTS		
	0 1 2 3 4 5 6 7 8 9 10	
	No pain	Worst pain ever
AT NIGHT	0 1 2 3 4 5 6 7 8 9 10	
	No pain	Worst pain ever
ARE YOU SATISFIED WITH YOUR ELBOW SURGERY? (if applicable)		
	0 1 2 3 4 5 6 7 8 9 10	
	Not at all satisfied	Very satisfied

CIRCLE THE NUMBER THAT INDICATES YOUR ABILITY TO DO THE FOLLOWING ACTIVITIES: 0 = **Unable** to do; 1 = **Very** difficult to do; 2 = **Somewhat** difficult; 3 = **Not** difficult

ACTIVITY		RIGHT ARM	LEFT ARM
1. DO UP TOP BUTTON ON SHIRT		0 1 2 3	0 1 2 3
2. MANAGE TOILETTING		0 1 2 3	0 1 2 3
3. COMB HAIR		0 1 2 3	0 1 2 3
4. TIE SHOES		0 1 2 3	0 1 2 3
5. EAT WITH UTENSIL		0 1 2 3	0 1 2 3
6. DO USUAL WORK - DESCRIBE:		YES NO	YES NO
7. DO USUAL SPORT - DESCRIBE:		YES NO	YES NO

PHYSICIAN ASSESSMENT

RANGE OF MOTION (degrees)	RIGHT	LEFT
FLEXION		
EXTENSION		
FLEXION/EXTENSION ARC		
PRONATION		
SUPINATION		
PRONATION/SUPINATION ARC		

# STABILITY
0 = severe instability; 3 = moderate instability; 5 = no instability

INSTABILITY	RIGHT	LEFT
VALGUS, VARUS, or POSTEROLATERAL ROTATORY (specify)	0 1 2 3 4 5	0 1 2 3 4 5

STRENGTH
(RECORD MRC GRADE)

0 = no contraction; 1 = flicker; 2 = movement with gravity eliminated;
3 = movement against gravity; 4 = movement with some resistance;
5 = normal power

	RIGHT	LEFT
TESTING AFFECTED BY PAIN?	Y N	Y N
FLEXION	0 1 2 3 4 5	0 1 2 3 4 5
EXTENSION	0 1 2 3 4 5	0 1 2 3 4 5
PRONATION	0 1 2 3 4 5	0 1 2 3 4 5
SUPINATION	0 1 2 3 4 5	0 1 2 3 4 5

# SIGNS
0 = none; 1 = mild; 2 = moderate; 3 = severe

SIGN		RIGHT	LEFT
ULNOHUMERAL TENDERNESS		0 1 2 3	0 1 2 3
RADIOCAPITELLAR TENDERNESS		0 1 2 3	0 1 2 3
MEDIAL FLEXOR ORIGIN TENDERNESS		0 1 2 3	0 1 2 3
LATERAL EXTENSOR ORIGIN TENDERNESS		0 1 2 3	0 1 2 3
MEDIAL COLLATERAL LIGAMENT TENDERNESS		0 1 2 3	0 1 2 3
POSTERIOR INTEROSSEOUS NERVE TENDERNESS		0 1 2 3	0 1 2 3
IMPINGEMENT PAIN IN FLEXION		0 1 2 3	0 1 2 3
IMPINGEMENT PAIN IN EXTENSION		0 1 2 3	0 1 2 3
OTHER TENDERNESS – specify:		Y N	Y N
CREPITUS – location:		Y N	Y N
SCARS – location:		Y N	Y N
ATROPHY – location:		Y N	Y N
DEFORMITY – describe:		Y N	Y N
ULNAR NERVE TINELS		Y N	Y N
OTHER JOINTS LIMITING ACTIVITY: SHOULDER/WRIST		Y N	Y N

OTHER PHYSICAL FINDINGS:

EXAMINER'S NAME:

_____   _____ DATE

ASES ELBOW FUNCTION INDEX (DRAFT)

		RIGHT	LEFT
PAIN (25)	{(50-VAS) ÷ 2}		
MOTION (30)	**FLEXION-EXTENSION ARC** >120: 20 120–90: 15 90–60: 10 30–60: 5 <30: 0		
	PRO-SUPINATION ARC >120: 10 120–90: 7 90–60: 5 30–60: 2 <30: 0		
STABILITY (5)			
FUNCTION (30)	Total Score × 2		
STRENGTH (10)	Total Score ÷ 2		
TOTAL SCORE (100)			

Index

Note: page numbers in *italics* refer to
figures and tables

Printed and bound by CPI Group (UK) Ltd, Croydon, CR0 4YY

03/10/2024

01040345-0011